F

IS FOR FITNESS

REAL EXERCISE, REAL RESULTS

ASHLEY KALYM & ABBIE CUMMINGS

First published in 2019
Kindle Direct Publishing

Photographs Matt Marsh
Text Design Ashley Kalym
Cover Design Ashley Kalym
ISBN 9781795813921

CONTENTS

1. *Introduction*

We're here to tell you that you've been doing it wrong. Endless miles of running, hours and hours on the bike, and countless aerobics classes haven't worked. The reason's simple: you've been doing the wrong exercises!

We know how difficult it is to know what exercises are the right ones to do. The media, celebrities, and fitness personalities are everywhere these days, and you can't go a day without a new Instagram star telling you how to lose weight, tone up, or get in shape.

So what makes our method any different? Why should you trust us more than any of these other sources?

First, we are going to give you common sense, scientific reasons as to why you should be doing certain exercises and avoiding others. The exercises we propose in this book have stood the test of time, and have been and are used by some of the greatest athletes, coaches, and trainers worldwide.

Second, we are not going to lie to you, or sugar coat things, or otherwise pull the wool over your eyes. We will tell you exactly what to do, and why, in order to get the body you want.

Third, both of us have many years of training many different types of people, and we have seen what works and what doesn't first hand. Lots of cardio training *DOESN'T WORK!* Resistance training ***DOES!***

1.1 *WHY IS STRONG THE NEW SEXY?*

Good question! The answer is that for many years women have been persuaded to do types of exercise that simply don't work. Long distance cardio, two pound dumbbells, tiny trampolines, etc., etc. The list of fads and gimmicks is almost never ending when it comes to fitness, and especially fitness for women.

We're here to change all of that. Let us say it plainly; gimmicks and fads do NOT give you results. Your body will respond to work, and if you want results you have to work! Doing easier exercises will not force your body to change shape, or help you lose body fat, or raise your metabolism.

You might think that being strong has nothing to do with being sexy, but again you would be wrong. It's your muscles that give your body shape, and if you want to improve your shape then you have to work on your muscles, and to work on your muscles you have to improve your strength!

1.2 *I DON'T WANT TO GET BIG!*

You won't! Many women are terrified of their muscles getting bigger if they introduce resistance training into their exercise routine. People see bodybuilders and assume they will look like that if they pick up a heavy weight, or start doing resistance training.

In reality, nothing could be further from the truth. Resistance training will NOT make you big, but will in fact make you lose body fat, increase strength, perfect your muscle tone, and get you in better shape than any amount of cardio or aerobics classes will.

So, why won't resistance training make you big?

First, gender has a huge role to play. Men have lots of testosterone flowing around their bodies, which is the male sex hormone. This hormone is responsible for all the male traits, like hair growth, muscle growth, aggression, and so on (we're also sure it affects remembering anniversary dates, the ability to buy flowers, leaving the toilet seat up, etc.). Simply put, it is much, much harder for women to build muscle, even if they want to! This is why female bodybuilders have to resort to drugs to build lots of muscle, and even then, they are nowhere near as big as the men.

Second, to get big requires years and years of concentrated training and eating. We cannot overstate this; the people you see that are big have spent years training with very heavy weights and eat as much every week as the average family.

Third, women's muscles work differently to men's. Whereas men can lift a large amount of weight for a single rep by using lots of muscular force, women struggle to do this. Again, this affects the ability of women to build muscle.

Lastly, women have different physiology than men. This is why many women struggle to perform pull-ups, but do well with squats. The reason for this is that men have disproportionately strong upper bodies compared to their lower bodies, and women have disproportionately strong lower bodies compared to their upper bodies.

In summary, don't worry about getting "big". You really won't, and the benefits seen from resistance training far outweigh any possible negatives that may come from it.

1.3 *WHY DOESN'T CARDIO WORK?*

We've already said that cardio doesn't work well for getting in shape, but why is this?

First, cardiovascular training breaks down muscle tissue and reduces the amount of muscle that you have. If you're trying to lose weight this is a disaster! Your muscle is your engine, burning calories both when you are resting and exercising. The worst thing you can possibly do if you're trying to lose weight is to lose muscle!

Second, cardio is boring. Running on the treadmill, sitting on the bike, or doing any other form of cardio takes a long time, and involves doing the same thing over and over again. This is why there are televisions in the cardio area of your gym, but not the weights area! If you have to do boring exercise every time you go to the gym, then you will stop going to the gym. If you don't go to the gym, you won't get results!

Third, cardio only burns calories when you're actually doing the exercise. You might burn 500 calories at the gym if you run for 90 minutes on the treadmill, but as soon as you step off you stop burning calories. This is not true with resistance training, and high intensity exercise, as you will continue to burn calories long after you leave the gym.

So, is there any type of cardio that does work? Yes, but it's very different from the normal cardio exercise that you see most people doing. High Intensity Training, or HIT for short, is short duration, very high intensity exercise, designed to require massive effort. An example would be hill sprints (running up a hill as fast as possible), burpees, or anything else that raises the heart rate and requires lots of effort.

We have a section on High Intensity Cardio Exercise later in the book, but our type of cardio is nothing like what you think!

1.4 *WHY SHOULD I DO RESISTANCE TRAINING?*

There are many reasons, but first we should make clear what resistance training is. Resistance training is where your muscles work against a resistance. This resistance can be your own body weight, a dumbbell, or a weight on a machine.

So, why is resistance training good for you?

First, resistance training builds and maintains muscle. This is important because muscle is the only body tissue that uses calories. So, if you have more muscle, you burn more calories, even when you are sitting on your couch. This is very useful if you are trying to lose weight!

Second, resistance training increases the density of muscle tissue. This means that you will have better muscle tone, and better muscle shape as well.

Third, resistance training makes you stronger! Being strong is not just for men, and being strong simply means you will be able to do more physical things, like jumping, hiking, playing sports, or even running around after your children.

1.5 *SHOULD I LOSE WEIGHT, OR BODY FAT?*

Body fat! When people say that they want to lose weight, they want the number on the scale to be lower. But, to get in shape and to look in shape, you must reduce the amount of body fat you have.

But what is body fat? Body fat is the layer of fat that sits above the muscle and below the skin. All of us have toned abs, legs, and bums; they're just not visible because we just have too much body fat on top of the muscles!

So, to get in shape you need to do two things:

1. Strengthen and shape your muscles

2. Reduce the amount of fat on top of your muscles

To strengthen and shape your muscles you need to perform resistance training, and to reduce the amount of body fat you have you need to eat a good diet (and do some high intensity cardio). And that's it! As long you do these two things consistently, you will have the body you want, for as long you want it.

This naturally means that looking at the number on the scales is not really the best way to track progress. The reason for this is that as you get stronger and your muscles become more toned and better shaped you may even put on some weight as muscle. This is because muscle is heavier than fat. So, ignore the number on the scales! What you really should be looking at is your body fat percentage, and how you look. As long as your body looks the way you want, what does it matter what the scales say?

So, are there ways to monitor your body fat? Yes, there are! The most common method these days is to measure body composition with a machine (you may have seen some of these in doctor's surgeries, or even in some gyms). These machines allow you to measure your body fat percentage in a reliable and accurate way, and will tell you much more information than a simple number on a scale. You may see a number such as 25% body fat, or 22% body fat, and so on. This number shows how much body fat you have. Most women who are in shape have body fat levels of around 15% to 20%. This gives a toned, strong, athletic look, whilst keeping health and wellbeing at a high level.

1.6 *I HAVE A SLOW METABOLISM!*

This is a very common complaint, but if you've been doing lots and lots of cardio for years on end this might be true! If you have very little muscle then your metabolic engine will be tiny, and your metabolism will be slow. Your metabolism is simply the rate and efficiency that you use energy, and if you have a small engine you won't use much energy. You need a big engine!

So, what are the best ways of speeding up your metabolism? Well, you need to drop all of the long slow cardio exercise, and start resistance training now. This is non-negotiable, and is the key feature of this book. To get a faster metabolism you need to increase the amount and quality of the muscle that you have, and the only way to do that is to use resistance training.

To get scientific for a second; each pound of extra muscle that you have will burn 70 calories a day, for nothing! This is because muscle requires blood, oxygen, and other nutrients to be sent to it. If you do exercise then that pound of muscle will burn even more than 70 calories, and this is exactly why putting on muscle, or at least maintaining the muscle that you already have, is the best way of losing body fat. Imagine if you put on 10 pounds of muscle; that is 700 calories you will burn, every day, without any extra effort whatsoever! And then when you do get to the weight or body fat level that you want, it will be much easier to maintain that weight and body fat level, because your metabolism will be faster, and you will burn more energy, even at rest. It's a no lose scenario!

1.7 THE WEIGHTS AREA IS SCARY!

We get it! The weights and resistance training areas can be intimidating, but in reality these parts of the gym are full of energy and encouragement. Weights areas are often home to experienced people who will be happy to help if you have a question or need some assistance.

One thing to note is that the weights area can be slightly different from the rest of the gym. There may be people making noises, but this is because they are putting in a lot of effort, and should be interpreted as them making progress!

Also, those deadlifting or doing other exercises might drop the weight, or allow the weight to hit the floor. We know the sound can be a bit much, but think of it this way; if the noise is loud it means a lot of work is being done, and results come from work! If you need any further proof, take a look at the cardio area, and then take a look at the weights area. Which group looks like they are doing more work? Which group looks like they are going to get better results?

If you are still reluctant to go into the weights area, then try taking along your partner or a friend; preferably one that does resistance training. They will be able to soothe any fears you might have, and also help you out if you get stuck or demotivated!

We understand. In fact, as being consistent is the most important thing when it comes to exercising and eating right, staying motivated is the one thing that will decide if you succeed or fail!

We also know it can be hard to get motivated in the first place. But, if you're reading this sentence then you have taken the most difficult step, which was deciding to do something about it!

So, what can you do to become and stay motivated?

SET A GOAL

First, you need to have a realistic goal. After all, if your goal is to have the body of your dreams in 3 weeks, then this is extremely unlikely to happen. However, if you give yourself two years to reach this goal, and make a little progress every time you go to the gym, then this goal is not only possible, it becomes very likely to happen. The first thing is to decide what goal you are trying to achieve. Only you will know what this is. Some possible goals might be to lose 20 pounds, to drop a dress size, to squat your own body weight, to get ready for your wedding, to be able to run a mile in 15 minutes, to recover from injury, or to get fitter for a partner or your kids. Whatever your goal is, make sure that you give yourself enough time to achieve it. Obviously the time it takes you to reach your goal will be specific to you, and unfortunately we cannot tell you exactly how long it will take (although you can contact us via email, and we will try to help you as much as possible!).

FOCUS ON THE SMALL THINGS

If you concentrate on the huge things, or your major goal (like losing 50 pounds, or being able to perform 3 pull-ups, etc.), then it may get a little overwhelming. To avoid this try and concentrate on the small things that you can control in the moment, such as the exercise you are performing, what food you are eating that day, and a single workout at a time. Focusing on these small things will make it much easier to reach your overall goal.

FOLLOW THE 80:20 RULE

Many people think that in order to get in shape and stay in shape you need to be 100% committed. This is true, but it doesn't mean that you need to follow the rules rigidly 100% of the time. This goes for both exercise and diet!

If you want results but do not want to live like a nun, then a great method to follow is the 80:20 rule. This simply means that as long as you follow your exercise plan and diet for 80% of the time, then the other 20% really won't have much of a negative impact. For example, in a week you will be eating approximately 25 meals. As long as 20 of these meals follow your diet and nutrition plan, then you do not need to be so strict with the other 5 meals.

HAVE FUN!

The last rule is to enjoy yourself! Fitness and getting healthy should be fun, and if it isn't, then you're much more likely to give up or become demotivated. The exercises we've put in this book are not all fun (we're looking at you, squats and burpees), but they are all varied and beneficial. Likewise with our approach to diet; we're not going to make you eat boring food and force you into eating a certain way or giving up your favourite treats. Life is for living, and you need to live it!

1.9 PROGRESSION AND REGRESSION

We know, the title of this section sounds like jargon, but progression and regression simply mean making things more difficult and less difficult.

Making exercises more or less difficult is very important, as it means each exercise can be adjusted to your ability. For example, the barbell squat can be made very easy or very hard, simply by reducing or increasing the weight that you use. The push-up can be made very easy or very hard, by altering the angle of your body. The plank can be made very easy or very hard by supporting your body on your toes or knees.

Basically, you progress an exercise when you want to make it more difficult, and regress an exercise when you want to make it less difficult. Throughout the book we will give hints and tips on how to progress and regress all of the exercises, so that whatever your ability, you will be able to take part!

1.10 TERMINOLOGY

OK, so we hate jargon as much as you probably do, but there are a few words and phrases that you should learn, as it will make your fitness journey much easier! We'll keep this section short, and only tell you what you need to know.

REPS

Rep is short for "repetition" and simply means the number of times that you do an exercise. For example, "squat for 10 reps" means to perform 10 squats in a row without stopping. "Do 20 push-ups" means to do 20 push-ups in a row without stopping.

Sometimes you may also see exercises that are not performed for reps, but are instead held for a certain amount of time. An example of this is the plank. Instead of doing reps you hold the plank for 30 seconds.

The number of reps that you do in each set affects how your body will change and adapt. Lots of reps will increase the ability of your muscles to perform the same movement over and over again. This is also called muscular endurance, and is useful if you are interested in doing sports, or need some stamina for some other purpose. Doing a small number of reps is used when you need to get strong. This is because 2 to 5 reps will place a huge stress on your body (if the exercise is hard enough of course), and make the muscles respond in a specific way.

The number of reps that we recommend most commonly in this book is somewhere in the middle. 8 to 12 reps will build some strength, some muscle, and also help with muscular endurance as well. We are not concerned with building just pure strength (although getting strong is a good thing!), and nor do we want to focus purely on endurance. We want to shape the muscles so that they look better, and we have found 8 to 12 reps works for this.

SETS

Sets means the number of times you do a group of reps. For example, you may see "3 sets of 10 reps". This means that you would do 10 reps of an exercise (the first set), then do another 10 reps (the second set), and then do another 10 reps (the third set).

Sets and reps will almost always be written together, and you will see things like, "3 sets of 5 reps" or "10 sets of 10 reps" and so on. They are also written as 1 x 20, or

3 x 15, or 5 x 5, and so on, where the first value is the number of sets, and the second value is the number of reps in each set.

The number of sets that we recommend is anywhere from 3 to 6. Lower numbers of sets are good for beginners, or when you are pressed for time and need to get a quick workout in, and more sets are better for more advanced readers.

REST

When you see the word rest, it means to take a break from the exercise. For example, you may perform 10 push-ups and then rest for 60 seconds, before doing another 10 push-ups, and resting for another 60 seconds, and so on. When you rest it is a good chance to get your breath back, allow your muscles to recover, and prepare for the next set!

RANGE OF MOTION

Range Of Motion, often shortened to ROM, refers to the amount of movement your joints can do in an exercise. To understand this, picture a push-up: someone lowering themselves to the floor only halfway would be a small range of motion, and someone lowering themselves all the way down to the floor would be a large range of motion.

Almost always, a smaller range of motion will be easier, and a bigger range of motion will be harder. We can use this to progress and regress exercises as well, which makes ROM a very useful tool!

2. DIET

Now we come to the big one: diet and nutrition. Before you run away yelling about never going on another diet again, rest assured that our approach to diet and nutrition is as simple as we could possibly make it, whilst still giving great results. We're not going to recommend any radical diet habits, but rather we're going to give you good, solid, common sense information and guidance so that you can eat properly without worrying too much about it.

We know how confusing it is these days to know what to eat, how much to eat, when to eat, and a million other variables that fitness gurus seem to talk about constantly. But, eating well, both for fitness and for getting in shape, isn't difficult. It just requires a little bit of knowledge about how you gain weight, how you lose weight, and how you maintain your weight.

NOTE: *Obviously, we can only cover so much ground here, and if you really want to know more about diet, then check out Dr Rhonda Patrick, a leading figure in the nutritional field.*

So, what does a diet or nutrition plan have to do? In our eyes it has to do three things:

IT MUST BE EASY TO FOLLOW

You can have the best diet plan in the world, that's guaranteed to deliver incredible results, but if it's impossible for a normal person to follow then it isn't worth anything! A diet or nutrition plan must be easy to follow, and not require huge amounts of time in the preparation, cooking, or eating stages. If it's easy to follow then you're much more likely to stick to it, and if you stick to it, you'll get results! It really is that simple.

IT MUST PROVIDE ENERGY FOR LIFE AND EXERCISE

Lots of diets have fasting elements, days where certain foods are eaten and some aren't, and lots of other strange rules. Well, if you're trying to work, live, look after your kids, exercise, and do everything else a modern women does, then you need enough energy to do all of these things! A diet where you feel hungry, or where you feel lethargic because you haven't eaten enough, is just as bad as one in which you eat too much. You will become run down, you will pick up injuries more easily, and you will not see the results that you want.

A diet must give you all of your nutrients as well, to ensure that your overall health is maintained or improved. You don't need to know the details of every single nutrient that your body needs, or which foods each of those nutrients is found in, but just enough to know what foods to eat and in what quantities.

IT MUST MAINTAIN YOUR MUSCLE MASS

This point is extremely important! Doing resistance training is the best way to get in shape and stay in shape, but all of that hard work will be wasted if you don't eat the right foods to maintain the muscle mass that you have or gain. If you don't maintain your muscle mass your metabolic rate will *decrease*, and you will find losing weight and maintaining your weight much, much harder.

To maintain muscle mass is pretty easy; you need to eat protein. Protein is the building block of muscle, and if you don't eat enough of it, then your muscle will start to break down. That's why skipping breakfast, eating meat free salads, and many other bad nutritional habits have got to stop.

So what foods is protein found in? Well, it is mainly found in meat, fish, eggs, and a little is found in dairy. There are some vegetable proteins found in legumes, beans, and other vegetables, but these are inferior to animal protein, mainly because animal protein contains all of the essential amino acids that the human body needs.

So, the best way to get protein into your diet is to eat animal protein. If you are a vegetarian or vegan then try and eat as much protein as you can from various sources, to ensure that you get as many essential amino acids as possible. This book is not specifically aimed at vegetarians or vegans, so if you need specialist advice on those types of diets, there are many excellent resources that are available.

THE 80:20 RULE

It goes without saying that if you want maximum results you have to put in maximum effort, and for your diet this would mean eating cleanly and healthily all the time.

However, for the vast majority of people this simply isn't possible, and the extreme discipline it takes is not realistic. So, instead of eating like a saint 100% of the time you can follow the *80:20 rule*. This means that as long as you eat well for 80% of the time, the other 20% can be a little more liberal.

For example, if you eat 3 meals a day, over a week this adds up to 21 meals. Using the 80:20 rule would mean eating 17 healthy, all natural meals, and 4 meals that "cheat" a little. This is a great way of doing things, as it makes you look forward to your cheat meals, takes away a little of the monotony, and means you don't have to worry about being ultra strict all of the time. This means that you can have the odd desert, or go out with friends and family a few times per month, and not worry about all losing all your progress.

If you take anything away from this section on diet, please take away the 80:20 rule! It will make your journey to getting and staying in shape much more enjoyable!

HOW MUCH PROTEIN DO I NEED?

Now that you know how important protein is for getting and staying in shape, you need to know how much protein to eat! The general rule is that you should eat 2 grams of protein for every kilogram of body weight (or 1 gram of protein for every pound of body weight) per day.

So, if you weigh 60 kilograms, or 130 pounds, then you should aim to eat between 120 and 130 grams of protein every day. This will make sure that you get enough protein to both enable muscle growth and maintain the muscle that you already have. However, the last thing we want you doing is counting out calories or grams of protein each day, so we've made this table showing how many grams of protein there are in the most commonly eaten foods.

FOOD TYPE	AMOUNT	GRAMS OF PROTEIN
Egg	1 Whole	6
Beef Steak	8 oz / 1 Steak	40
Chicken	5 oz / 1 Breast	60
Turkey	5 oz	41
Pork	5 oz	37
Lamb	5 oz	38
Salmon	5 oz	37
Tuna	5 oz	37
Nuts (Peanuts, Cashews, Walnuts, Almonds, etc.)	1 oz / Small Handful	6
Lentils	1/2 Cup / 100 grams	9
Kidney Beans	1/2 Cup / 100 grams	8
Milk (Skimmed)	1/2 Pint / 250 ml	8
Cheese	1 oz	7
Greek Yogurt	6 oz / 200 ml	18

ARE CARBS REALLY THE ENEMY?

This is a tough subject, and the answer to the question is both yes and no. For years we've been told that eating lots of carbs is good for us, and that the majority of our calories should come from carbs. However, carbs (from a scientific viewpoint) are simply sugars (in varying degrees of complexity), and they will breakdown in the body as such. Eating lots of carbs, even the good, complex variety, is a bad idea if you are trying to lose body fat and get in shape.

So, what's the difference between "better" carbs and "worse" carbs. The best types are the more complex variety, that have many other nutrients tied up with them. These are foods like sweet potato, brown rice, beans, pulses, legumes, and non-starchy vegetables like carrots and broccoli.

Worse carbs (the simple variety) are things like white bread, pasta, sugar, and refined grains. These will contribute towards unwanted weight gain if they are consumed too much, especially if you have a sedentary job or lifestyle.

So, the right approach is to eat the more complex carb types, but not too many of them! You need to eat enough to fuel your daily life and workouts, but not so much that you start to gain weight from eating them.

DOESN'T FRUIT CONTAIN LOTS OF SUGAR?

Yes, but it's miles away from the refined table sugar that goes in your coffee, or that's found in processed food, or soda drinks. The sugar in fruit is tied up with fibre and many other nutrients, and is not digested in the same way that refined sugar is.

Some fruit, like dried apricots, cranberries, and other types can contain refined sugar, but this has been added after the fact, and should be avoided if possible. Fruit is full of beneficial nutrients and minerals, so eating it is never really a negative!

ISN'T FAT BAD?

No, absolutely not! Fat is a vital nutrient, responsible for many of the most important functions and structures in the body. Part of the problem is that the word for the nutrient and the derogatory term about overweight people is the same: fat. We should all try and distance ourselves from the thought that eating fat will make you fat; it doesn't work like that!

In the modern world we have all sorts of ways to produce food, and many of them are not what nature intended. Cold pressing olives yields olive oil, but cold pressing other foodstuffs does not. When this is the case, all sorts of chemical processes have to happen to get oil and fat out of the raw ingredient. This is not what nature intended, and we can say no more than stay away from those types of fats (and foods) as much as possible. What are these types of fat? Margarine, vegetable oils, trans fats, and anything that you are likely to find in processed foods. The low fat brigade and their approach is based on very shaky science, and there is lots of new research that shows natural fats are much more beneficial than it was once thought. Go natural all the way!

So, what fats are good? Simply put, any fat that is natural, and unprocessed in any way. Just make sure that you have a good amount of the following foods in your diet, and everything will keep running smoothly!

• Avocados
• Olive Oil (cold pressed if possible)!
• Coconut Oil
• Butter
• Oily Fish
• Milk (if you aren't lactose intolerant)
• Meat (and the fat that goes with it)
• Eggs (with the yolk)

DO I NEED SUPPLEMENTS?

No! Unless you have a specific medical need, there is no requirement to use supplements. Lots of women might think they need protein powder, BCAA's, and other supplements to get in shape, but you should easily be able to get all of the nutrients that your body needs just through normal food.

Not only are supplements expensive for what they are, they are inferior when it comes to actual nutritional value that they provide. Natural, unprocessed food is much better, and cheaper, and will give a greater benefit to you.

Other downsides to supplements are that many of the protein powders contain lots of carbohydrates, which is great if you are training for a Strongman competition, but no so great if you are a woman trying to get in shape!

SHOULD I EAT LOW FAT FOODS?

Probably not! Most packaged foods that are labeled as low fat are filled with sugar or sugar substitutes, and will no doubt do more harm than good if you eat them. If you are unsure if a food contains hidden sugar, simply don't buy it. This is very easy if you stick to the rule of only buying natural, unprocessed foods. This way, you're extremely unlikely to eat anything that has any added sugar in it.

HOW MANY MEALS SHOULD I EAT?

No doubt you've already heard that breakfast is the most important meal, and that it's best to eat a number of smaller meals throughout the day, but in reality many of these rules are either hard to follow for the average working person, or don't do what they advertise to do. So, how many meals should you eat during the day? In an ideal world it would be better if you could eat five or six smaller meals spread out evenly throughout the day, but unless you work from home or have lots of breaks at work this is almost impossible.

For the average woman that has to balance work, kids, family, friends, and everything else, three meals a day is the perfect balance. Make sure not to skip any meals, otherwise you'll just be tempted to snack on junk late at night, or when you do get a chance to eat. Remember, our goal is to get you into the best shape of your life taking your own individual circumstances into account.

HOW MUCH WATER SHOULD I DRINK?

We can't overstate the importance of staying hydrated, especially if you live in a hot and dry climate, or if you do lots of exercise. Water makes up a huge part of your body, and it's needed for lots of important processes. We're not going to bore you with all of them, but it's safe to say that drinking enough water is key if you wish to stay in shape. It will also help in other unexpected ways. Feeling irritable or unable to concentrate at work? Drink more water!

"But I drink plenty of coffee. Doesn't that count?"

No, it doesn't! Coffee and other hot drinks will not hydrate you anywhere near as effectively as water will, and some actually cause you to lose water (they can act as a diuretic). Limit your coffee and tea intake if you can!

To make it as easy as possible for you to know how much water you should be drinking, we have included this handy chart showing how much water should be drunk according to your body weight. Just find your weight in the left hand column, and read across to find out how many litres you should be drinking. Note that this amount will need to be adjusted up or down depending on other factors, such as humidity, activity level, training history, and other things.

YOUR WEIGHT (LBS)	YOUR WEIGHT (KGS)	WATER INTAKE (L)
100	45.5	1.5
110	50	1.7
120	54.5	1.8
130	59	2
140	64	2.1
150	68	2.3
160	73	2.4
170	77	2.6
180	82	2.7
190	86	2.9
200	91	3
210	95.5	3.2
220	100	3.3
230	104.5	3.5
240	109	3.6
250	113.5	3.8
260	118	3.9
270	122.5	4.1
280	127	4.2
290	132	4.4
300	136.5	4.5

To make things simple, in this chapter we will list all of the foods that you can and should eat. We've included as many different whole, natural foods as possible, so if you stick to just these then you'll be well on your way to meeting your goals! If something isn't on this list, it doesn't mean that you shouldn't eat it, but that it should be eaten in very limited quantities. Remember the 80:20 rule!

MEAT AND FISH

This group of foods will be your main source of protein and fats (unless you're a vegetarian or vegan), and so it is a good idea to get a mixture of these. You don't have to eat meat or fish at every meal of course, but just as long as at least one of your meals contains something from this list.

- Beef (steak is especially good; very nutrient dense)
- Chicken (try higher welfare if possible)
- Pork
- Lamb
- Fish (all types)
- Eggs (choose higher welfare if possible)

DAIRY

These days many people have sworn off dairy, but it still has its place if you eat it in moderation. Lactose intolerance is one possible downside (which affects one of the authors), but there are plenty of lactose free options out there if you must consume dairy.

- Milk (avoid the low fat options! Full fat is best for health and training)
- Cheese (things like feta and mozzarella are great in salads)
- Butter (despite all the scaremongering, butter is much better for you than processed margarine)

FRUIT

Basically any fruit is OK, as long as it's natural, raw, and unprocessed. Be careful when looking at things like dried fruit, as this can contain oils and sweeteners, even sugar, to make it more palatable. This is especially true with things like dried cranberries, which are often sweetened. Shown next are some fruits that are great to eat, but there are many more also!

• Apples (sliced up with peanut butter is a great snack)!
• Oranges (a good shot of vitamin C)
• Bananas (great for both pre and post workout)
• Pears
• Grapes
• Strawberries
• Kiwi fruit
• Melon
• Grapefruit

VEGETABLES

Vegetables provide tons of minerals, vitamins, and other nutrients like fibre, so get as many of these into your diet as possible! There are lots of inventive ways to cook them as well, so don't ever think that eating them should be boring. Also, don't worry about getting millions of different types into your diet. There will undoubtedly be some vegetables (and fruits, meats, fish, etc.) that you don't like, so if you don't like them, don't eat them! You should still get all of the nutrients that you need even with moderate variety.

• Sweet potato (better for you than normal potato)
• Broccoli (full of good vitamins and minerals)
• Peas
• Sweet corn
• Squash (these can be roasted)!
• Celery (great as a base in stews and casseroles)
• Tomatoes (perfect with salads)
• Kale
• Spinach (goes great with scrambled eggs in the morning)
• Peppers
• Onions
• Cucumber
• Lettuce

NUTS AND LEGUMES

Nuts and legumes are good sources of protein and fat, and it is well worth you including them in your diet (as long as you are not allergic of course)!. Pick the unsalted, raw versions wherever possible, as these will likely be cheaper, and better for you as well. Mixing them with dried fruit like raisins, sultanas, cranberries, etc., is a great way of making a quick snack.

Nut butters are also a great way of getting nuts into your diet. These days you can get peanut, cashew, almond, and many other types of nut butter, so you should be able to find one that you like. If you can, try and avoid the types that have palm oil and sugar in them. You should be looking for the raw nut butters, which have the minimal amount of ingredients in them.

• Peanuts (avoid the salted variety)
• Brazil nuts
• Cashews (these are especially tasty with raisins)
• Almonds (almond milk is OK, but check it doesn't have sugar in it)!
• Hazelnuts (no, Nutella doesn't count)!
• Macadamia nuts

FATS

Although fats are in lots of foods, it is worth mentioning some of the more common foods that they can be found in here. Make sure you don't avoid fat! It's vital for your cell structure and proper brain function, and if you're training you'll need the energy and nutrients that it provides!

• Olive oil (good for cooking with and for dressings)
• Butter (much better for you than margarine)
• Avocados (can be used as a spread substitute)
• Coconut Oil (great for cooking again)
• Nuts (any kind, but make sure they are of the unprocessed, raw variety)
• Animal fat (again, make sure that the meat you're eating is unprocessed for better quality nutrients)

2.2 SAMPLE MEALS

In this section we're going to look at an actual day in the life of Abbie, our co-author and exercise model, and show you exactly what she eats.

BREAKFAST

For breakfast Abbie had two poached eggs, salmon, and whole-wheat toast with avocado. She also had sea salt and pepper, and water as a drink. Note that there's protein and fat from the eggs, protein and fat from the salmon, fat from the avocado, and complex carbs from the toast. This is a perfect breakfast for someone looking to maintain or build their muscle mass, lose weight, and keep feeling full until lunch time.

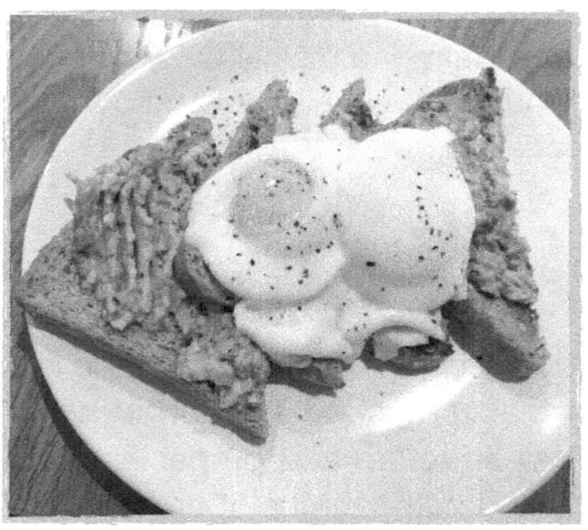

LUNCH

For lunch Abbie had a salad, with feta cheese (protein and some fat), roasted peppers, tomatoes, sweet corn, salad leaves like lettuce and spinach, and some balsamic vinegar dressing. This is a great lunch as it has all of the nutrients that the body needs, is quick to prepare, and is quick to digest.

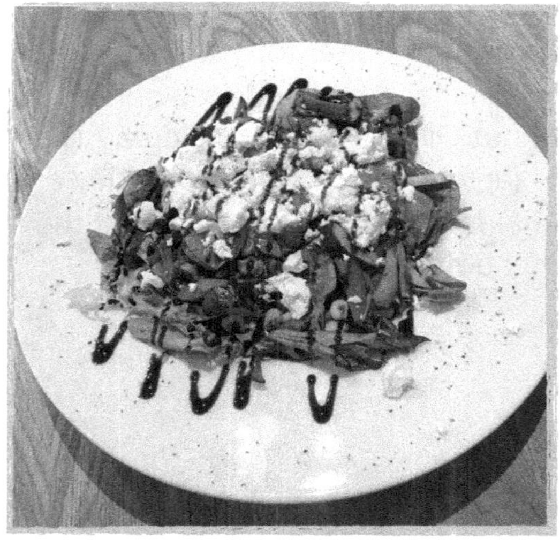

DINNER

For dinner Abbie had some steak with sauce, couscous, raw celery, broccoli, and a small salad of roasted peppers. Again this is perfect for those looking to get in shape and lose body fat. The steak will provide protein, fat, and other nutrients to help the body recover from workouts, the couscous and peppers will provide some good carbs, and there is a good spread of minerals and nutrients here.

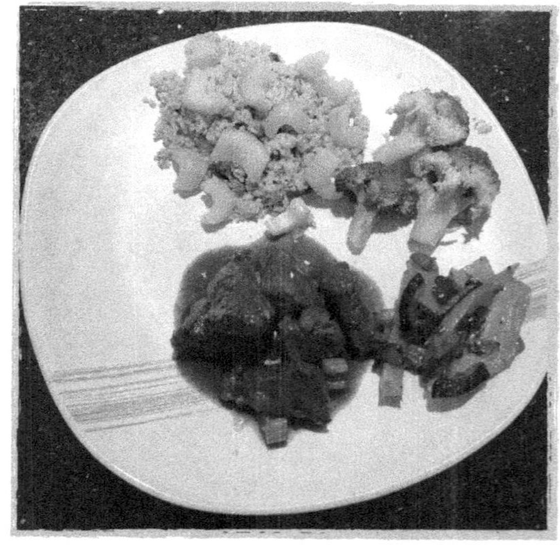

3. EQUIPMENT

When doing the exercises in this book you will come across various pieces of equipment that will help you get the results you want. Some of these are simple and some are more complex, but all of them are useful. Note that some pieces of equipment are more readily found in gyms, and to get the most out of this book you will likely need a gym membership. Many forms of exercise can be performed without any equipment (in fact, Ashley has written a number of books solely on body weight exercise), but exercises that use barbells, assisted machines, and other pieces of equipment, can obviously only be performed in a gym, or in a very well equipped home gym.

3.1 FLOOR SPACE

Never underestimate the humble floor! Many of the body weight exercises can be performed with no equipment whatsoever, and so a good piece of floor space is all you need for some workouts. Obviously you want the space to be free of debris, small children, and other obstacles, and also be comfortable enough to rest the knees and hands on. An exercise mat will cushion hard floors, and make certain exercises more comfortable.

3.2 EXERCISE STEP

An exercise step is a pretty common piece of equipment, but it can be used for much more than just step aerobics. The step is useful for any exercises that require you to support your weight, or step up onto something. Most exercise steps in gyms come with blocks that allow them to be raised or lowered. These are very useful, especially as in some of the exercises (the push-up, for example), raising or lowering the box relates to the difficulty of the exercise. If at home you can also use stairs, the edge of the couch, a sturdy box, or anything else that is strong enough and stable enough to use for the purpose.

3.3 PULL-UP BARS

Pull-up bars are another feature of modern gyms that can be used for more than just pull-ups. You will see them in the weights area, or functional training area, or even on their own station. A pull-up bar is a very basic piece of equipment, designed for you to grab onto and perform pulling exercises.

Pull-up bars for home use can also be found in sports shops and on the Internet, but you will need somewhere suitable to mount them, like a sturdy wall on the outside of your house, or in your garage. Door mounted pull-up bars are available, but these are less sturdy than wall mounted ones, and require a doorframe that is compatible.

3.4 BARBELLS

Barbells (also just called bars), are almost essential for the squat, deadlift, and other multi joint movements. They come in a few different types, so we'll let you know about them here.

The first type of barbell is the exercise class barbell. These are quite short, light, and are designed for small weights that you find in exercise classes all around the world. These bars are OK for some exercises, like light weight squats and lunges, and pressing overhead, but unsuitable for things like deadlifts.

The second type of barbell is the Olympic Barbell. These are fairly uniform, and come in either 15 kilogram (30 pound) or 20 kilogram (45 pound) variations. The 20 kilogram barbell is perhaps more common, and your local gym will likely have a few of these lying around. They can be found on flat benches (where you do bench presses), as well as on the squat rack, or just freely in the gym.

3.5 DUMBBELLS

Dumbbells are like mini barbells. They are typically short in length, with handles a few inches long, and have a weight on each end. They range in size and weight from small and light to large and very heavy. In this book we use them for some of the strength exercises. Note that unless you have some sort of injury or weakness, you will not be using extremely light dumbbells, for any exercise. We know it's fashionable in some celebrity circles to use 1 or 2 pound dumbbells, but this is basically pointless. Such light weight will elicit almost no response from the body, and if there is no response, your body will not change! As we said in the earlier sections, resistance training has to put enough of a stress on the body to make it change. Using very light weights will not accomplish this task.

3.6 SQUAT RACK

We know squat racks look like the kind of place that body builders hang out and chat about themselves, but they are in fact an amazing piece of equipment that make certain exercises (the overhead press, squat, lunge, etc.) much easier and safer to perform. They are normally made from steel, are very rugged and strong, and will hold barbells securely to allow you to safely get into position.

The best ones will have adjustable hooks, so that you can adjust the height that the bar sits at, to make sure you can remove and replace the bar safely. If you are unsure how to use the particular squat rack that is in your gym, then make sure to ask a trainer. They will only be too happy to assist you, and it is very important that you know how to use the equipment properly!

3.7 AB WHEEL

The ab wheel is only used for one exercise (the rollout) but it's so effective that it's worth including in this book. Luckily, ab wheels are very cheap (if you want to buy one of your own), and most gyms will have one. They come in a few different types but basically have a short bar that goes through the middle of a wheel, with foam or plastic handles on the bar to cushion the hands.

3.8 DIP BARS

Dip bars are used for the triceps dip, and you'll find these in most gyms around the world. They are sometimes part of a bigger piece of equipment, with a pull-up bar and sometimes a weight stack in a single unit. In fact, these larger units are better, as they also allow assisted triceps dips and pull-ups to take place, which allow you to progress steadily and get stronger and fitter over time.

3.9 EXERCISE BANDS

Another piece of useful equipment are exercise bands. These can provide resistance or assistance when you need it. They are actually really useful for assisted versions of the pull-up and dip, and can also be used for making many exercises harder. They come in lots of different types and strengths, and are fairly inexpensive.

4. WARMING UP

Warming up is one thing that has to be done, or injury can happen. Think about warming up like leaving your car running on a cold winter's morning; the engine needs to time to warm up and for everything to get up to temperature. Just like with your car, your body also needs to warm up as well. Your joints, muscles, and other tissues work much better when they are warm and supple!

So, how should you warm up? Basically, any cardiovascular or repetitive exercise is good for this, as it ticks all of the boxes that need to be ticked. You need your heart rate to increase, your blood flow to increase, your core temperature to rise, your muscles to warm up, and your ligaments and tendons to become more flexible. Personally, we recommend running, cycling, rowing, and other cardiovascular exercises to get started, and then easier versions of the exercise you are going to perform.

Also, when you are doing you workout it is also advisable to perform a number of simpler, easier, or lighter movements of the same type that you will be performing. For example, if you are doing barbell squats, you will want to do a few shallow body weight squats, then some full body weight squats, and then some squats with just the bar to get fully warmed up.

5. FLEXIBILITY

Is flexibility really that important? Yes, it is! Flexibility means being able to move into positions that require your muscles to stretch, like touching your toes or even doing the splits. Obviously you don't need to do the splits for the exercises in this book, but some of the exercises require more flexibility than movements in daily life.

For example, the squat actually requires good flexibility in the hips, knees, and ankles in order to perform it correctly, and to get deep enough for it to benefit you. Working on your overall flexibility is not something you need to do separately, but it's going to be part of the workouts that we give you at the end of the book.

In this section we're going to show you only the stretching exercises that really matter. Most of the large muscles groups can be stretched properly with a handful of exercises, and they are the ones that we are going to look at here. Note that the flexibility exercises can be done at the start and at the end of your workout. In the program section we have put them at the end of the session, as this is the most time effective method. However, if you feel that parts of your body need to be more flexible feel free to spend more time on doing stretches, even on rest days.

5.1 SHOULDER STRETCH

Tight shoulders can stop you from doing some great exercises, such as the dip, pull-up, and even the squat. Taking a few minutes to stretch the shoulders before and after your workout can help you in this area!

1. To stretch your shoulders kneel down and place your hands on the ground, arms straight.

2. Push your hips back and up, and allow your chest to sink towards the ground.

3. Keep descending until you feel the stretch. Hold for 30 seconds, and relax.

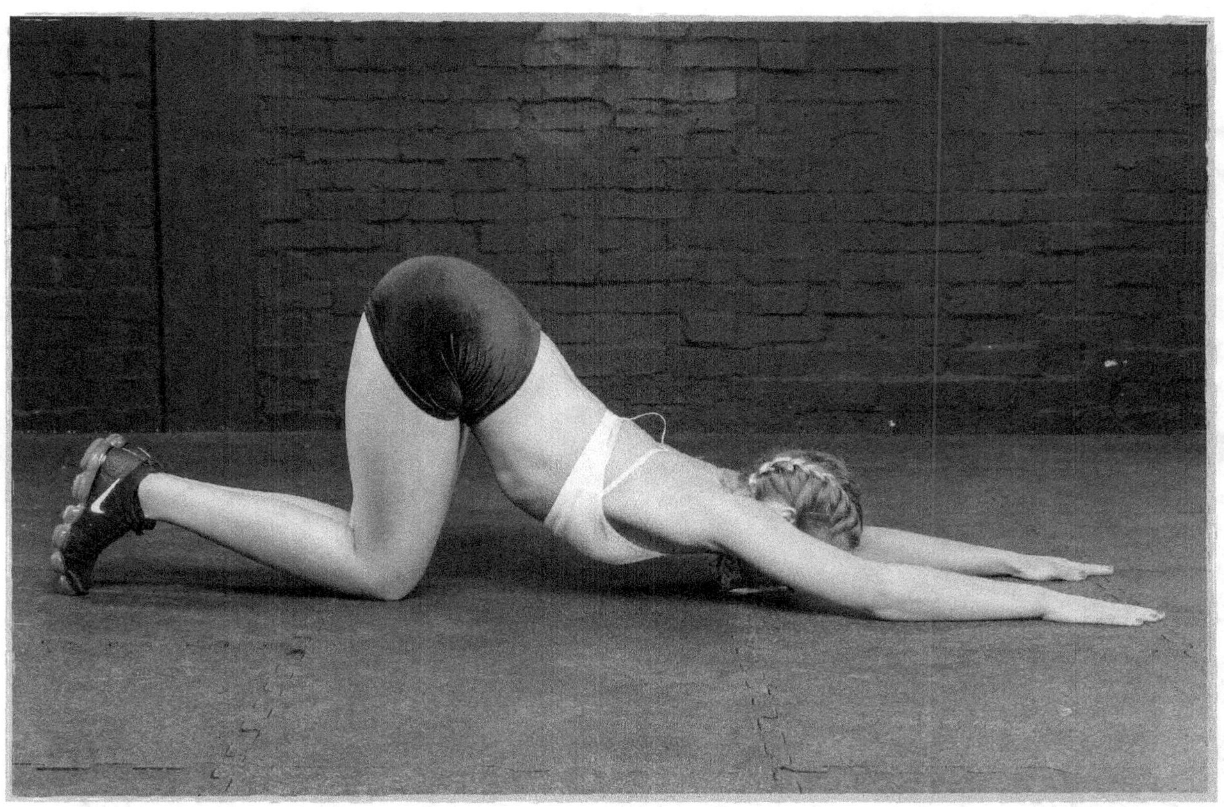

5.2 CHEST STRETCH

The bench press, push-up, and even the dip all use the muscles of the chest, and so stretching this area is a good habit to get into, to avoid any tightness or potential injury. To stretch the chest you will need a wall or other solid object. A squat rack is ideal!

1. Stand up straight and place one hand on the wall or solid object.

2. Make sure that your hand is level with your shoulder, and that your elbow is straight.

3. Turn away from your arm until you feel the stretch on your chest.

4. Hold the position for 30 seconds, and then change arms and repeat.

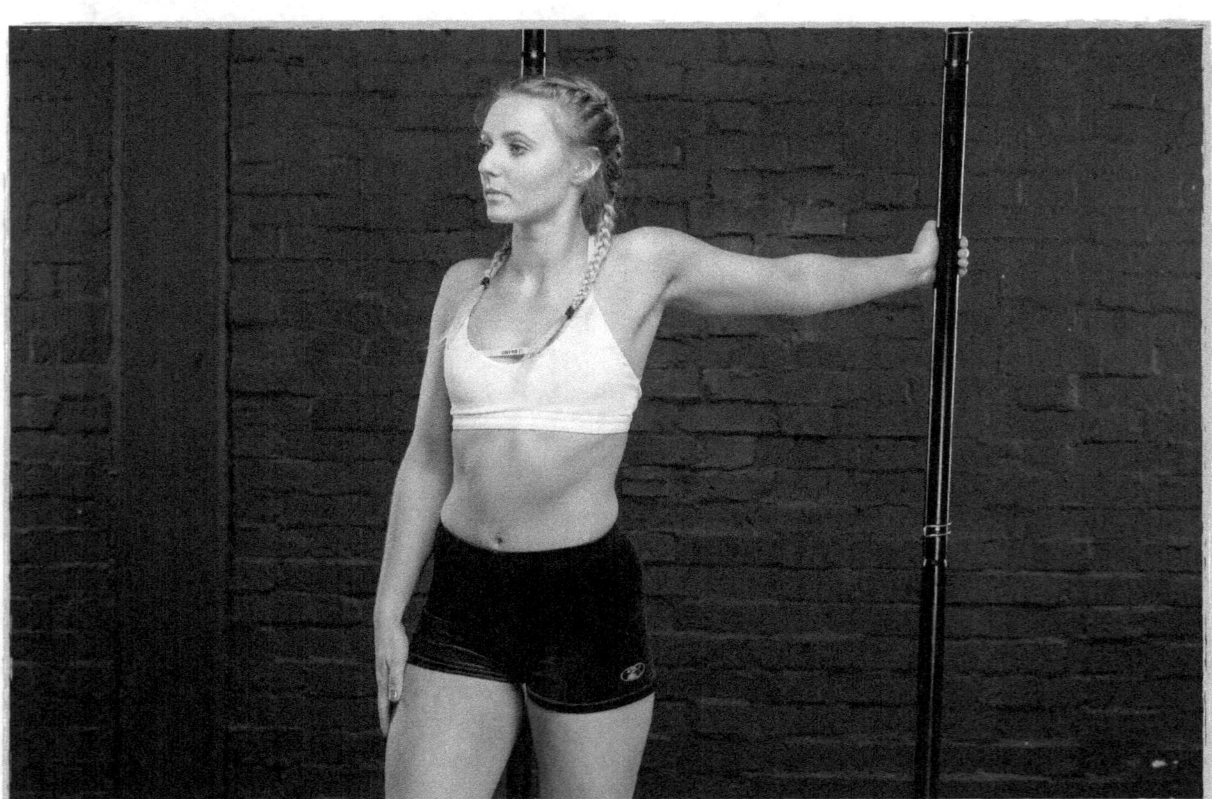

5.3 UPPER BACK STRETCH

The back is another large muscle group, and as such it needs to be stretched! The exercises that work the back (deadlift, pull-up, barbell row, etc.) are demanding, and so keeping the back supple and pain free is key.

1. To stretch the back crouch down and get onto your hands and knees.

2. Push down into the floor with your hands, and push your shoulder blades up and apart. Imagine trying to raise a heavy weight up into the air with your spine and you should activate the right muscles.

3. Keep pushing up until your spine is arched, with the muscles of the upper and middle back stretched.

4. Hold this position for 30 seconds, and then relax.

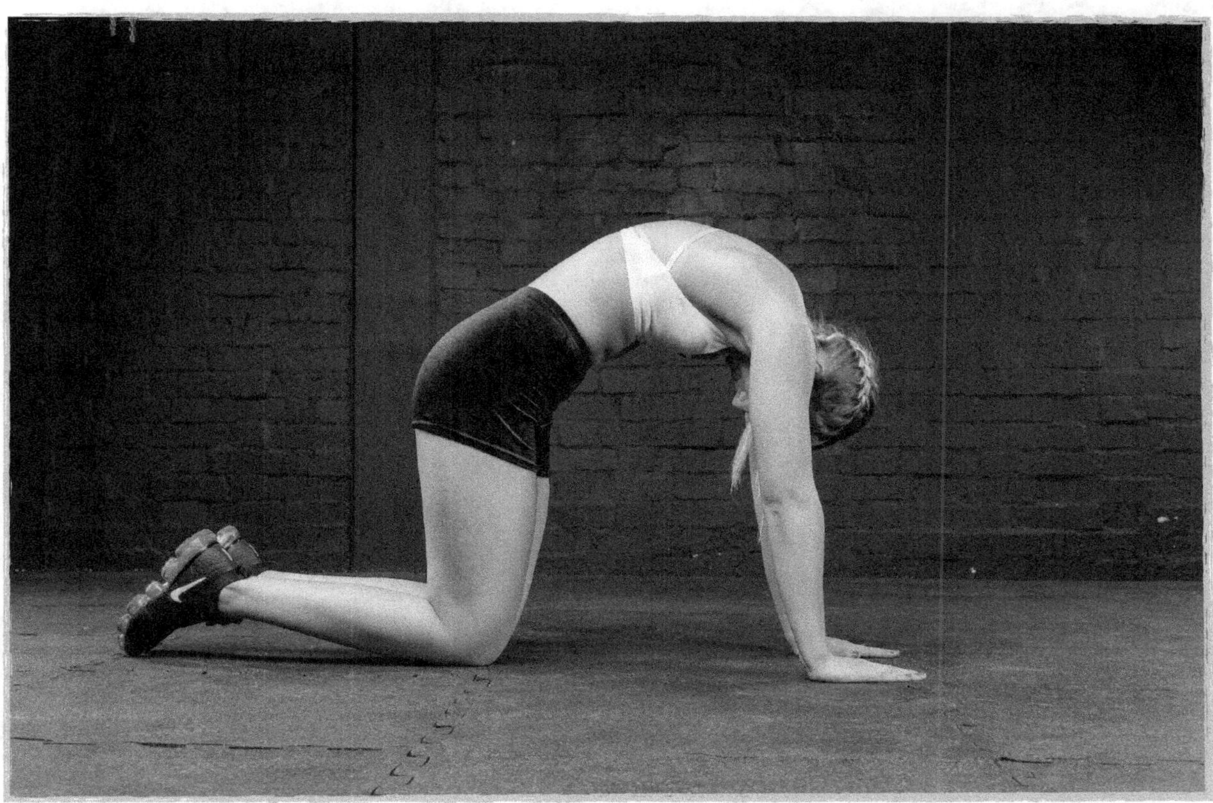

5.4 C*ORE STRETCH*

Exercises like the rollout, plank, and dish all put tremendous stress on the abs, and so stretching this area of the body is important to keep any cramps from happening, and to make sure you don't get too tight.

1. To stretch the core lie down and press your hands into the floor.

2. Push down into the floor with your hands, and raise your upper body off the ground. Keep your hips pushed into the floor.

3. Keep pushing up until your spine is arched, and you should feel a good stretch in the front of your core, or your abs.

4. Hold this position for 30 seconds, and then relax.

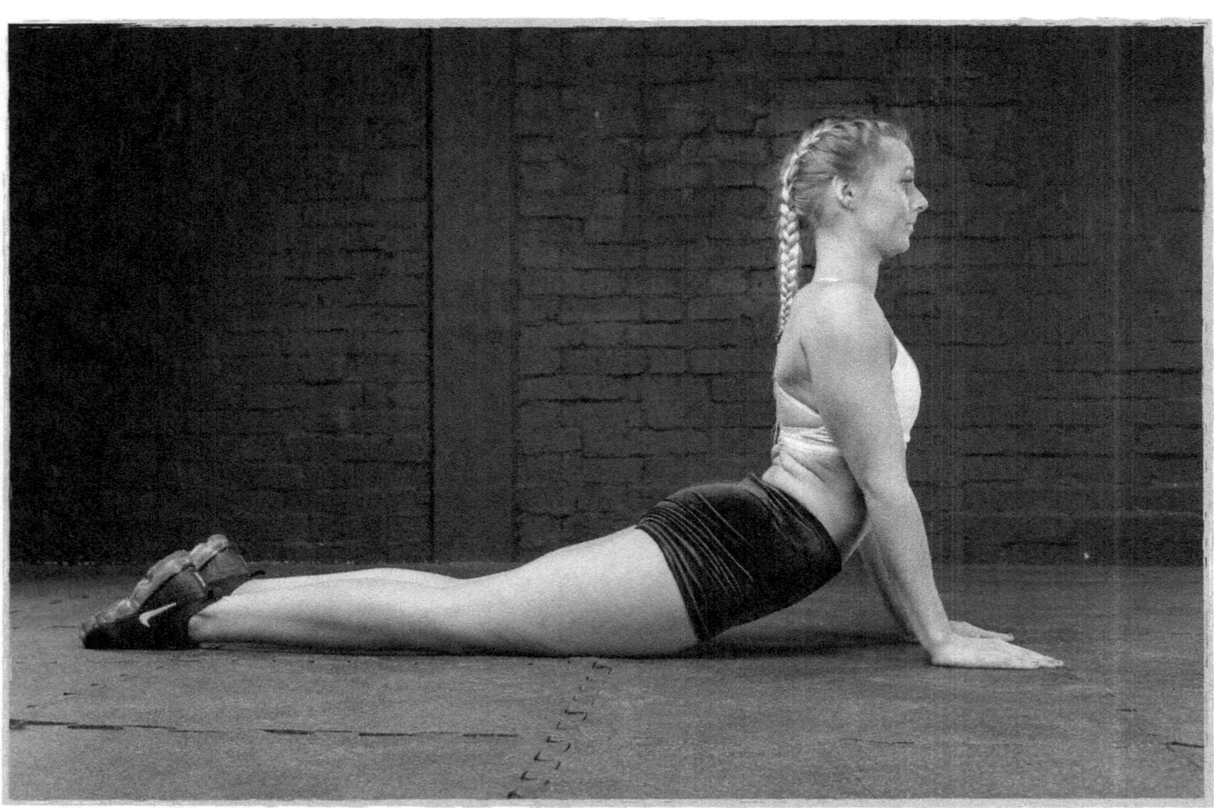

5.5 HAMSTRING STRETCH

The hamstrings are the big muscles at the back of the thigh. In the modern world most people have tight hamstrings, and they can really affect your ability to get into certain exercise positions, like the squat, for example. Making sure your hamstrings are flexible is a very good idea, and the simple method we show next can be used before, during, and after workouts.

1. Sit down and stretch one leg out in front of you, with the other tucked up into your groin.

2. Keeping your back straight, bend from the hips and reach forward, attempting to reach your toes with your hand.

3. Move forward until you can feel the stretch in the back of you upper leg (your hamstring).

4. Hold this position for 30 seconds, change legs, and repeat.

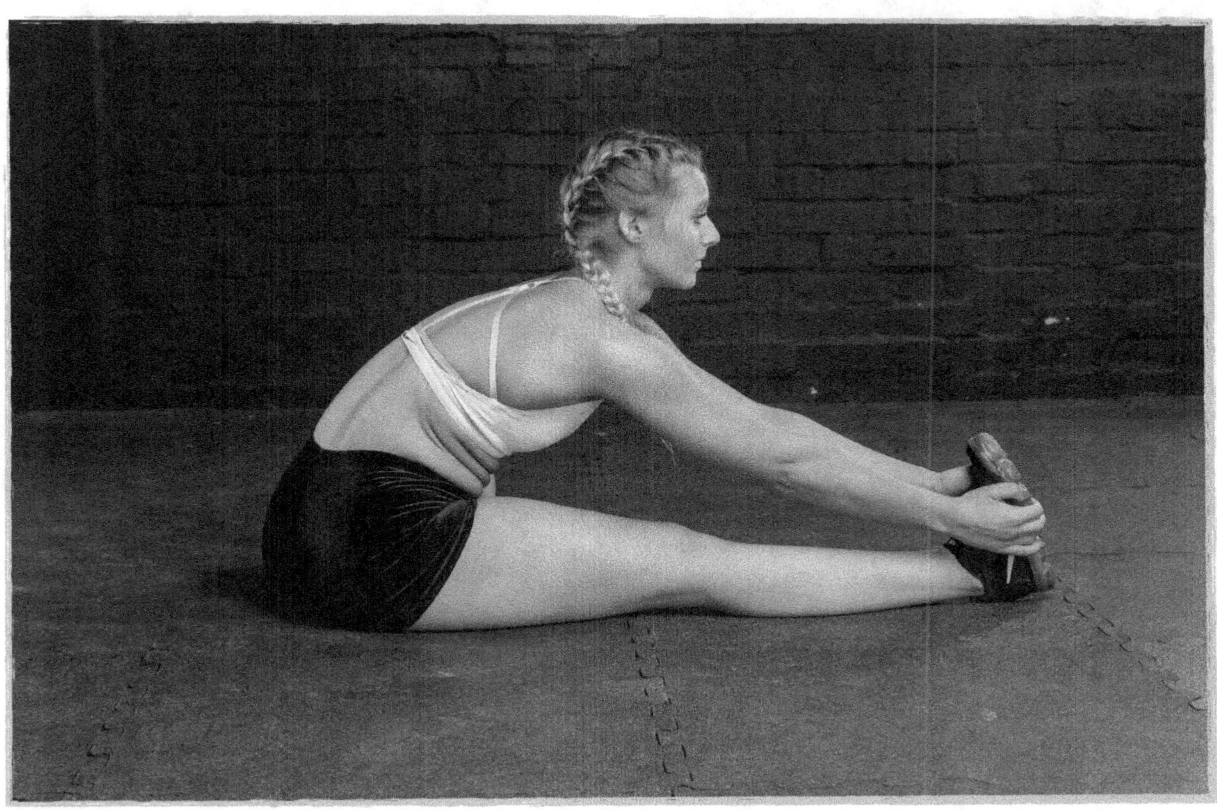

5.6 GROIN STRETCH

By the groin we really mean the insides of your legs (actually called your adductor muscles), and these are actually very important for overall hip flexibility. Again, we've gone with simplicity here, and included a stretch that is easy but effective.

1. Sit down and tuck both legs up into your groin.

2. Place the soles of your feet together and pull them as close to your butt as possible.

3. Keep your back straight, and allow your knees to drop towards the floor. You should feel the stretch on the insides of your thighs (adductor muscles).

4. For an extra stretch push down on your knees with your arms. Hold the stretch for 30 seconds, and then release.

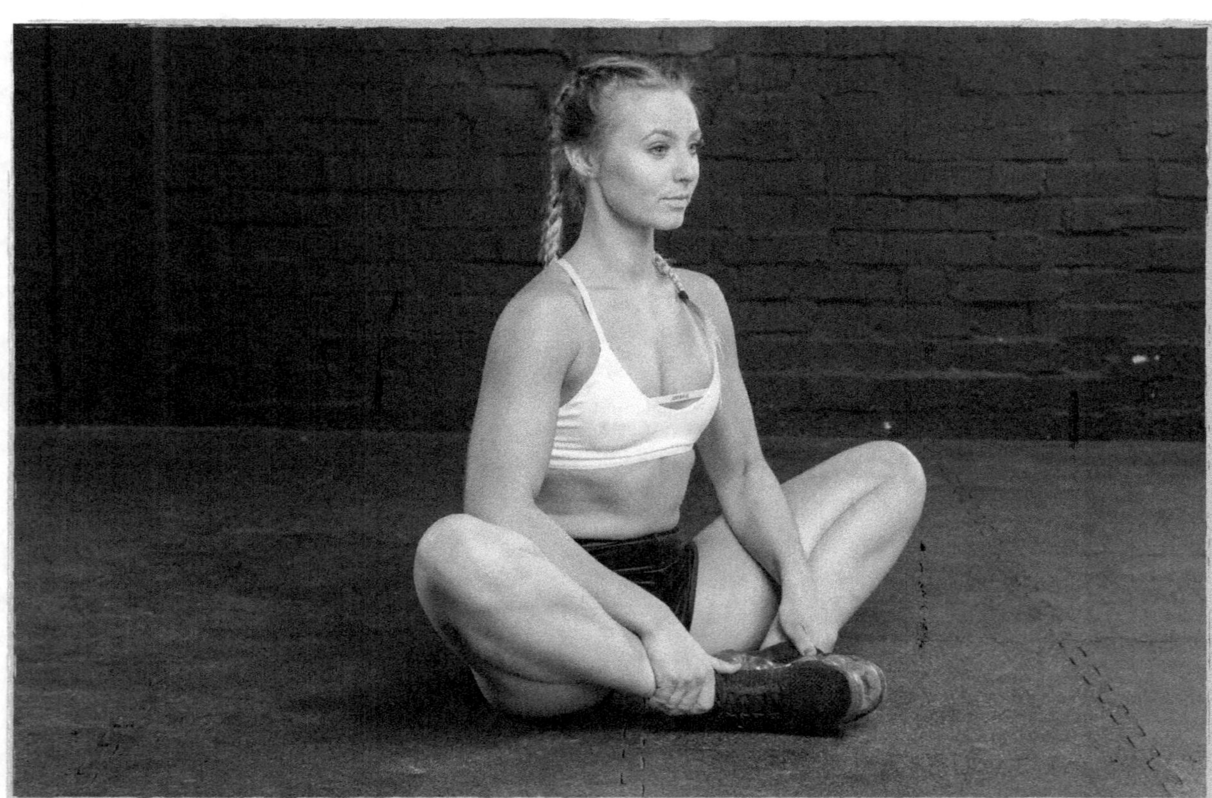

5.7 GLUTE STRETCH

Another set of large lower body muscles are the glutes, or butt muscles. The glutes are all about power; and are used when running, jumping, squatting, lunging, and when moving using the legs. As you'll be doing lots of leg work it makes sense to stretch the glutes!

1. To stretch the glutes sit down on with one leg straight and the other bent.

2. Put one foot on the outside of the opposite knee, and hold your thigh.

3. Push your bent knee towards the straight leg and turn away, and you should feel the stretch in the glute of the bent leg.

4. Hold this position for 30 seconds, and then change legs and repeat.

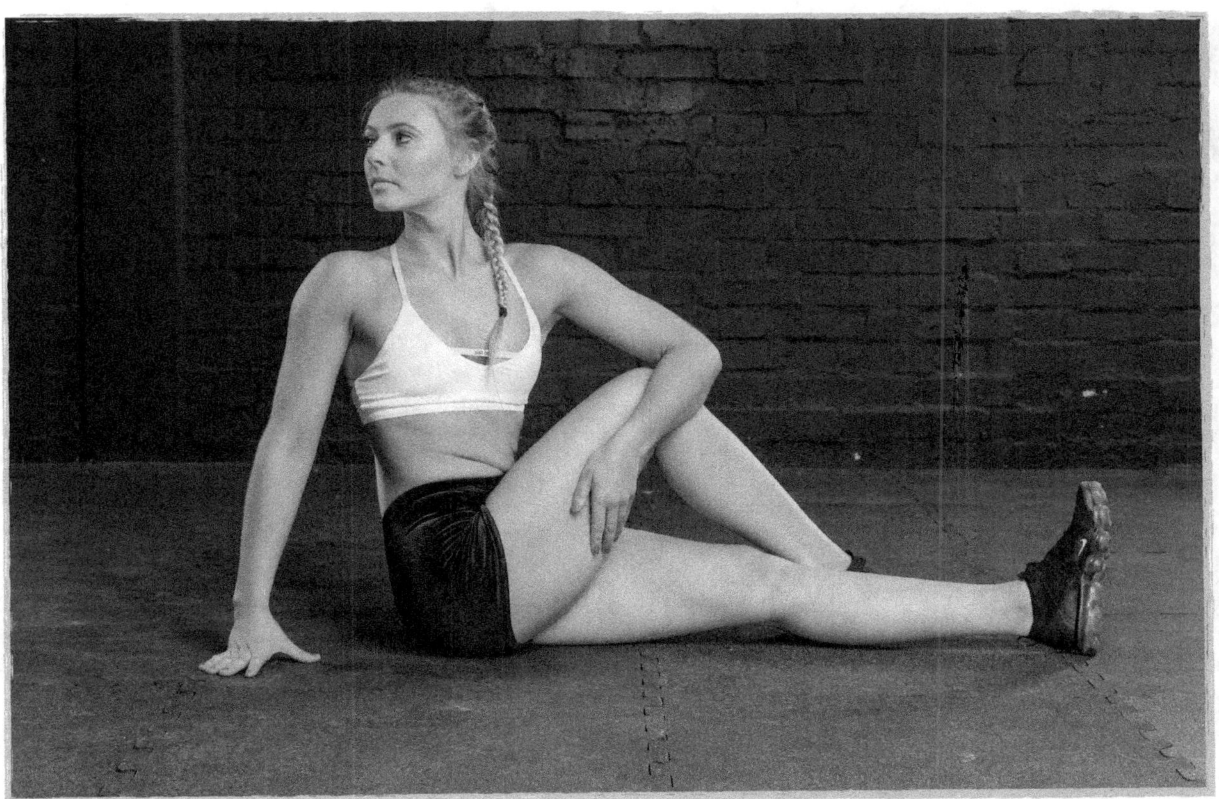

5.8 Calf stretch

Tight calves can affect squatting ability (and therefore the ability to build your glutes)!, so it's vital that you make sure that your calves are flexible. This is easily done, and our stretching exercise for the calves can be done anywhere.

1. Get into a push-up position, with your hands on the floor and your legs stretched out behind you.

2. Place one foot over the other, pressing down so that your heel is pushed backwards.

3. Keeping your legs straight, push your heel down until you feel a stretch in the back of your lower legs (the calves).

4. Hold this position for 30 seconds, change legs, and then repeat.

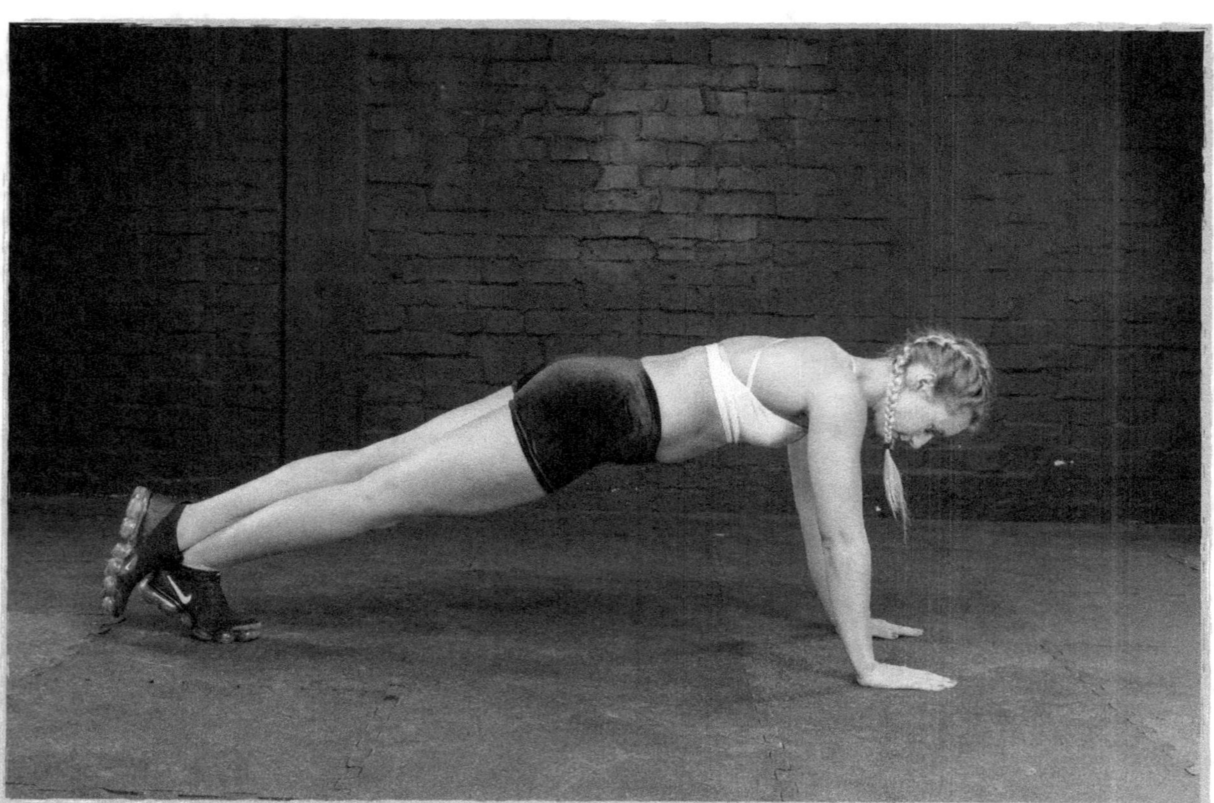

5.9 QUAD STRETCH

As important as stretching the back of your thigh (hamstrings) is, stretching the front of your thigh is also important. Doing squats, step-ups, lunges, and other leg heavy exercise will really work the front of the thighs, and so stretching them will keep them supple and pain free.

1. The easiest way to stretch the quads is to lie face down, with one leg straight and the other bent.

2. Use one hand and support your front, and use the other to pull the foot of the bent leg towards your butt.

3. Keep bending your leg until you feel a stretch in the front of your thigh, whilst keeping your hips pushed into the ground.

4. Hold this position for 30 seconds, then change legs and repeat.

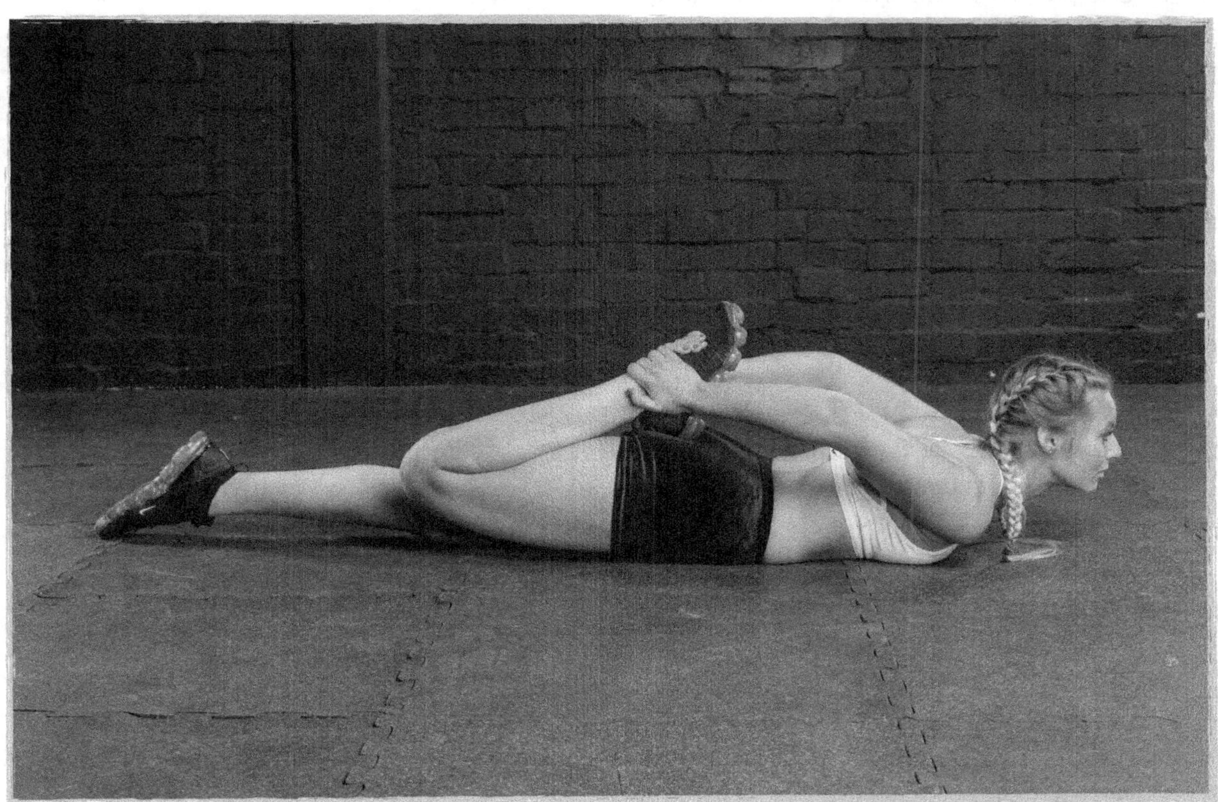

6. TYPES OF EXERCISE

If you have ever visited a gym we're sure that you saw many different types of exercise being performed. Body weight exercise, classes, weights, machines, cardio, and so on. There are literally dozens of different ways of training; so why have we included only two? The answer is that some forms of exercise work better than others, and those forms of exercise are the ones we have picked. It's a sad fact that the fitness industry is plagued by fads and gimmicks, which makes it easy to fall for the marketing hype behind a new form or type of exercise.

Both body weight exercise and weighted exercise are three dimensional movements. This simply means that they require the movement of lots of body joints at the same time, in lots of different planes of movement, at different speeds, and at different intensities.

This rule is the most important! Your body is an adaptive machine, and will change if you put enough stress upon it. For example, walking up a hill very slowly will not do much for your fitness, because walking up a hill slowly does not place a huge stress on the body. However, if you were to sprint up the hill, as fast as possible, then that would be enough to force the body to change. The same rule applies to all exercise: if it claims to make things easier it's no good!

6.1 BODY WEIGHT EXERCISE

Body weight exercise is the easiest to do and to describe; it's exercise that uses your own body weight as the resistance. This is awesome for a number of reasons! First, it requires almost no equipment, which means you can do it at home, when travelling, or when you are away from the gym. Second, it is very easy to progress and regress for different abilities, making it perfect for beginner and advanced exercisers alike. Third, it builds a very solid foundation of physical ability. In other words, it makes you good at moving, pushing, pulling, running, jumping, and just moving in general. This is why gymnasts do so well when they move into other sports; their balance, poise, and ability to move is much better than other people's!

6.2 BARBELL AND DUMBBELL EXERCISE

Barbells and dumbbells have long been thought of as men's equipment; but not anymore. Women are becoming more switched on with what works and what doesn't when it comes to exercise and results, and barbell and dumbbell training definitely does work! Loading a bar with weight and squatting, deadlifting, or lunging with it burns huge amounts of calories, strengthens, builds, and firms muscles, and puts curves in all the right places.

7. THE EXERCISES

Finally! The next part of the book will show you all of the exercises that will help you get the body you want. We have broken down the exercises into four sections:

SECTION ONE: *ARMS AND SHOULDERS* – This contains exercises that target the arms, shoulders, chest, and upper body.

SECTION TWO: *ABS AND CORE* – This contains exercises that target the abs, obliques, lower and middle back, and all the muscles of the core.

SECTION THREE: *LEGS AND BUM* – This contains exercises that target the bum, thighs, calves, and the muscles of the lower body.

SECTION FOUR: *HIGH INTENSITY CARDIO* – This contains exercises that blast the cardiovascular system, and help to melt fat from the body.

SECTION ONE: *ARMS, CHEST, AND SHOULDERS*

The first areas that we are going to look at are the arms, chest, and shoulders. These muscles make up the upper body, which helps with pushing, pulling, grasping, and other movements. Your arms, shoulders and chest are home to many different muscle groups: you don't need to know the names of all of them, but a few are worth knowing. The chest muscles are also called the pectorals (or pecs), the shoulders are called the deltoids, and the upper arm is home to the biceps and triceps.

The exercises in this section all work these muscles, and will help to strengthen, shape, and tone the entire upper body! We are going to look at body weight exercises first, and then the barbell and dumbbell exercises.

7.1 PUSH-UP

The push-up is a classic exercise, but one that many of us women find difficult. We naturally have weaker upper bodies than men, but this doesn't mean that we can't do them! To work up to proper push-ups requires three stages, but each stage will still work the correct muscles, and you will still see benefits, regardless of what level you start at.

In terms of the muscles they work, the chest (pectorals) and backs of the arms (triceps) are the main muscles targeted here. The core will also get a workout (as it holds the hips up) and so will the legs as they have to remain tight and strong.

STAGE 1: KNEELING PUSH-UP

The first stage in learning the push-up is to do a kneeling version. This is basically the starting point, and makes sure you learn proper technique whilst still using the correct muscles.

HOW DO I SET THE EQUIPMENT UP?

You will need a space on the floor, preferably with an exercise mat to cushion your knees. If you need to make it easier you will also need an exercise step, or platform, that you can place your hands on.

HOW DO I DO IT?

1. Kneel down on the floor and let your feet rest on the ground. Place your hands on the ground or a raised platform, with your hands shoulder width apart.

2. Make sure that your body and legs are in a straight line, and that your head is neutral.

3. Bend your elbows and lower your chest to your hands. Your elbows should move out a little, at 45 degrees if possible.

4. Keep going until your chest nearly touches the ground or platform, or you reach the limit of your strength or mobility.

5. Pause for a second, and then push back up under control. This is one rep.

HOW MANY SETS AND REPS?

You should be looking to perform 3 to 5 sets of 8 to 12 reps. If you cannot perform this number then raise the height of the platform that you are placing your hands on. If you can perform this number easily then lower the height of the platform that you are resting your hands on, until you can perform them with your hands on the floor.

HOW DO I ADJUST THE DIFFICULTY?

Even though the kneeling push-up is the easiest version of the push-up that we have, it can still be too difficult for a lot of people. To make the kneeling push-up easier it is best to place your hands on a raised platform, so that the hands are higher than the knees. This puts less stress on the upper body, and makes the exercise easier! As you feel yourself getting stronger and fitter you can lower the height of the platform until you can perform them on the floor.

WHEN DO I MOVE ON?

You should move onto the next stage when you can perform 15 to 20 kneeling push-ups in one set, without stopping. The chest should nearly touch the ground on each rep, and the form should be as perfect as possible.

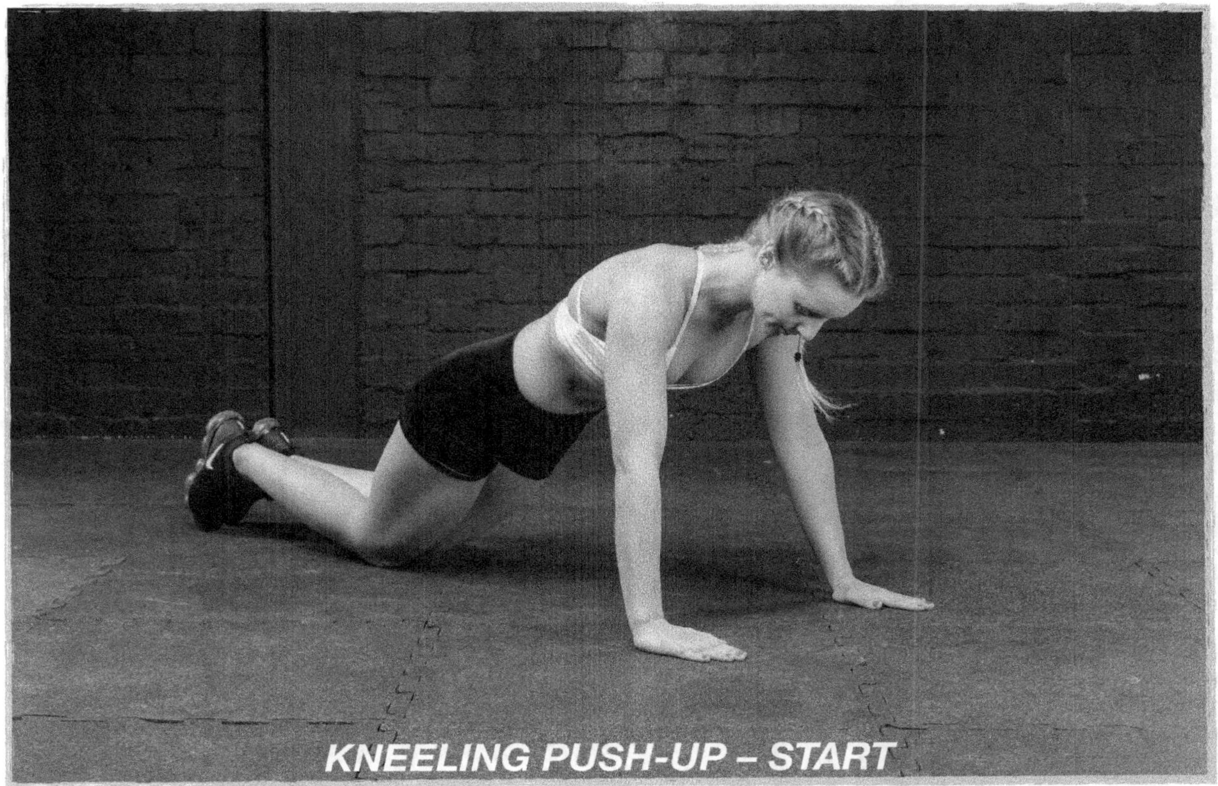

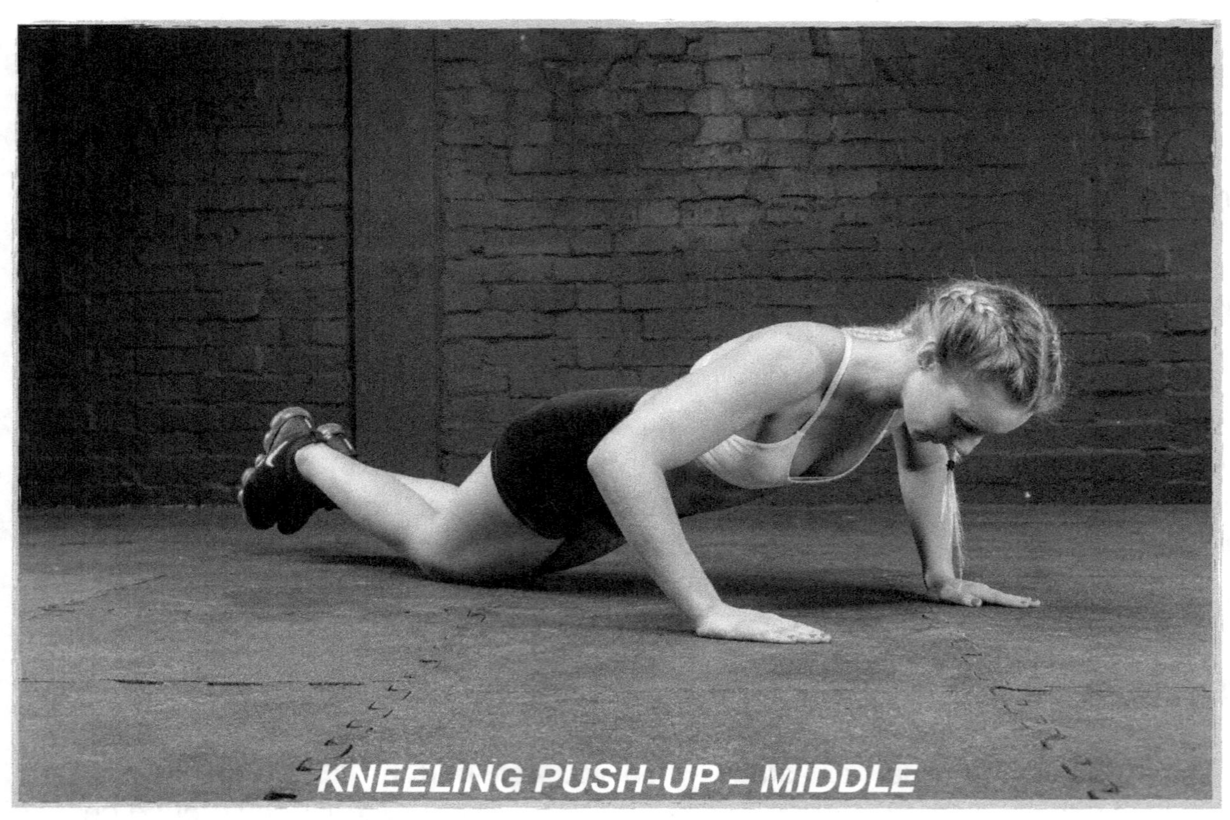

KNEELING PUSH-UP – MIDDLE

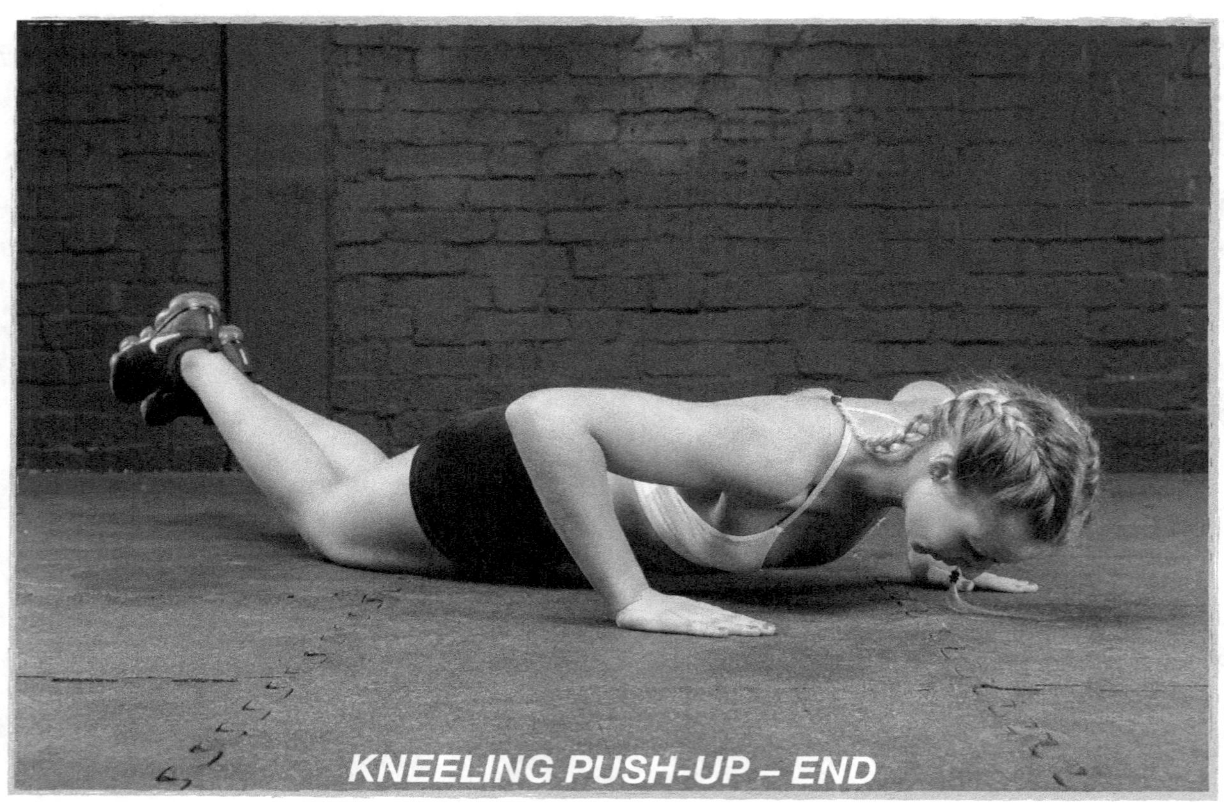

KNEELING PUSH-UP – END

STAGE 2: PLATFORM PUSH-UP

The second stage in learning the push-up is the platform push-up. The difficulty is changed in the same way as the kneeling push-up: making the body more vertical (using a higher platform) makes the movement easier, and making the body more horizontal (using a lower platform) makes the movement harder.

HOW DO I SET THE EQUIPMENT UP?

When starting the platform push-up ideally you'll want to start with the platform at a decent height (waist high, for example), as this will make the exercise easier. To set the step or platform up properly is easy; simply make sure that it is sturdy, will not move when you push on it, and is wide enough for you to place your hands on.

HOW DO I DO IT?

1. Place your hands on the platform, shoulder width apart, with your fingers facing forwards. Move your feet backwards and balance on your toes, making sure that your shoulders, hips, and feet are in line.

2. Now bend your elbows and allow your chest to move towards the ground. Your elbows will move out to the sides slightly, but this is fine. Keep your core tight and your hips in line with your shoulders and feet as you descend.

3. Keep going until your chest touches the edge of the platform, or you reach the limits of your mobility.

4. Pause for a second, and then push back up to the start position, making sure to straighten your arms completely. This counts as one rep.

HOW MANY SETS AND REPS?

You should be looking to perform 3 to 5 sets of 8 to 12 reps. If you cannot perform this number then raise the height of the platform you are using. If you can perform this number easily then lower the height of the platform until it starts to test your ability.

HOW DO I ADJUST THE DIFFICULTY?

Very easily! To make the platform push-up easier simply raise the height of the platform. To make the platform push-up more difficult lower the height of the platform.

You should move on to the next stage when you can perform 10 to 15 reps with a platform that is anywhere from 6 to 12 inches high.

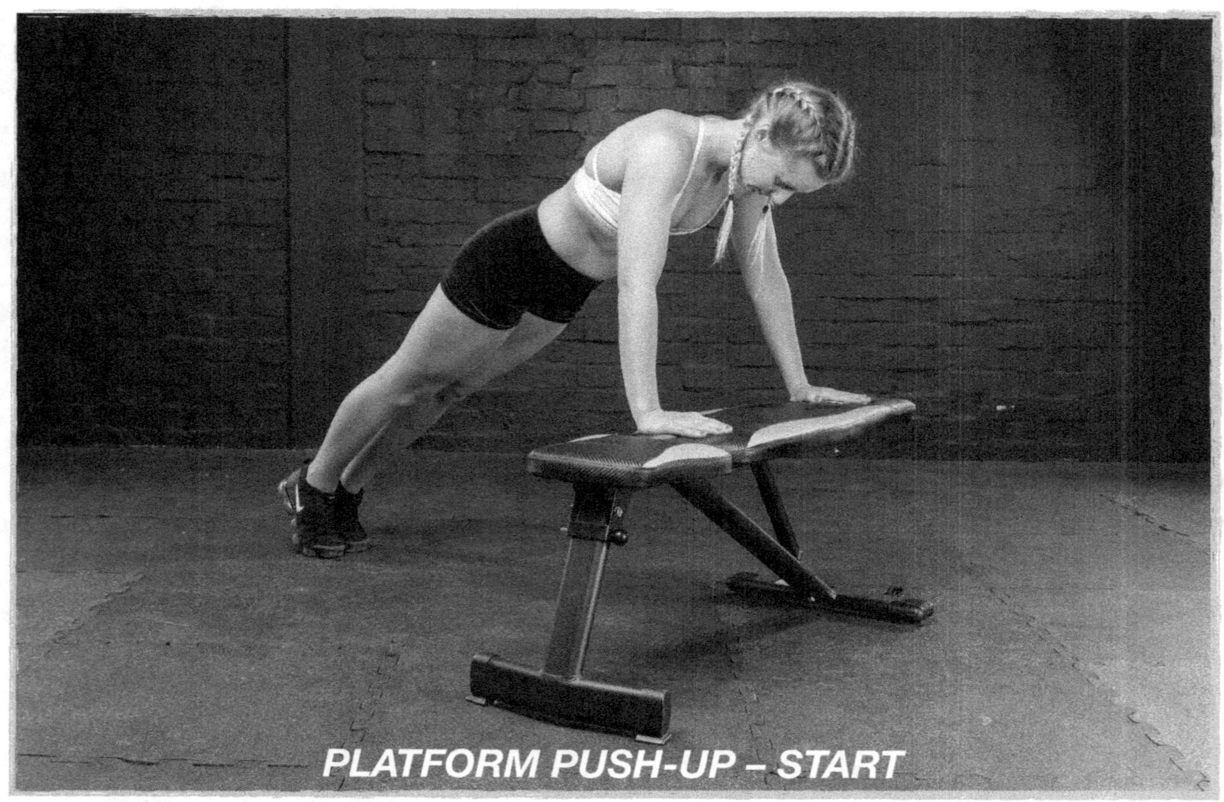

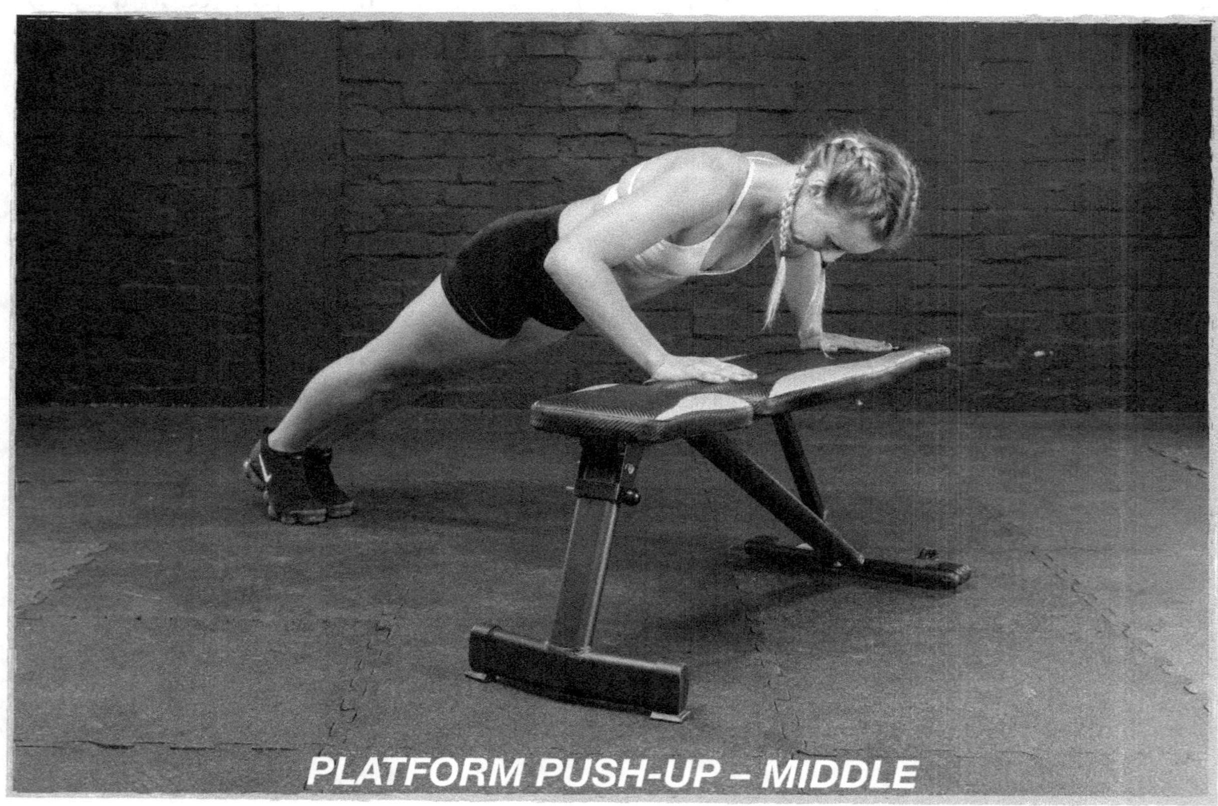

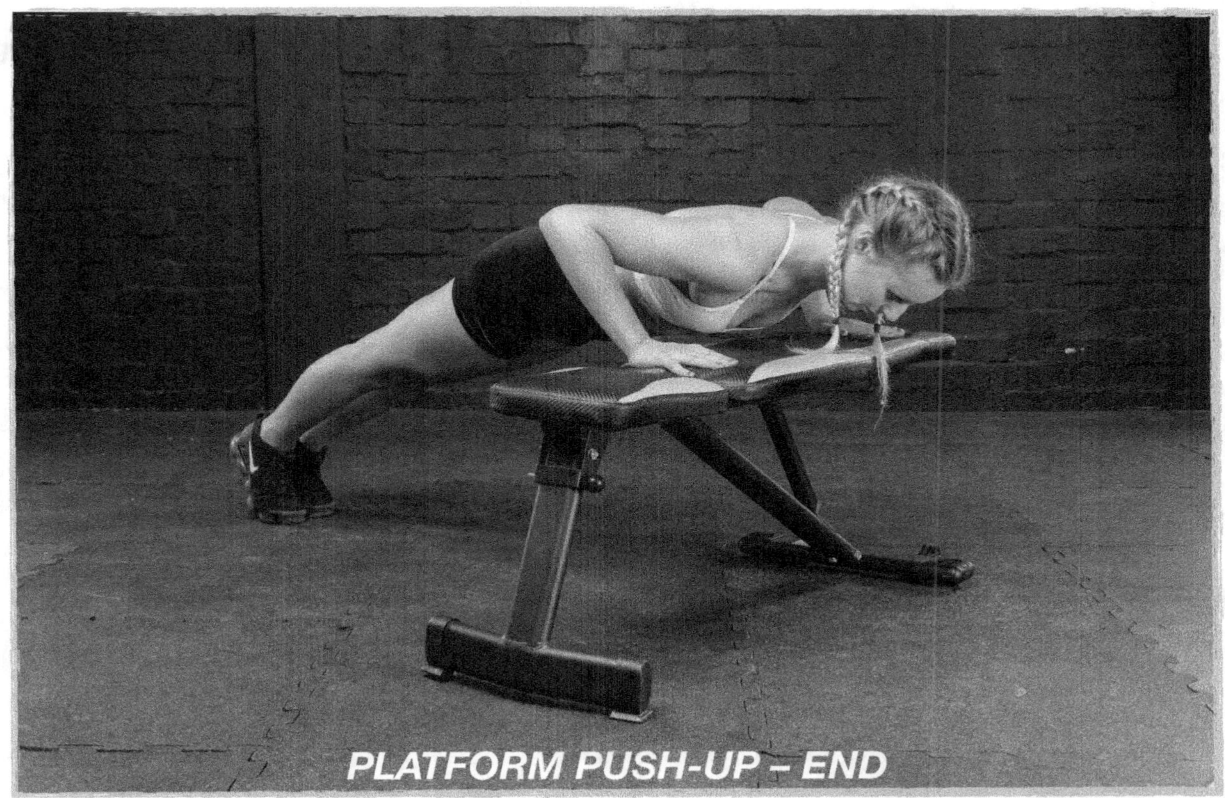

STAGE 3: PUSH-UP

Nearly there! This stage is the proper movement, with no platform, no reduced range of motion, and no other adjustments. If you've gotten to this stage then now's the time to put it all together and work on increasing the number of reps you can perform, and concentrating on perfecting your form.

HOW DO I SET THE EQUIPMENT UP?

You will require some floor space and a mat for your knees if needed.

HOW DO I DO IT?

1. To perform the push-up, place your hands on the floor, shoulder width apart. Stretch your legs out behind you and balance on your toes, with your torso and legs in a straight line.

2. Start to bend your elbows and allow them to move out to the sides, around 45 degrees.

3. Keep bending your elbows until your chest reaches the floor, or as far as your strength and mobility allow. The goal is for your chest to nearly touch the ground!

4. Pause for a second at the bottom, then push back up until your arms are straight.

HOW MANY SETS AND REPS?

You should be looking to perform 3 to 5 sets of 8 to 12 reps. If you cannot perform this number consistently then move back to the platform push-up.

HOW DO I ADJUST THE DIFFICULTY?

If you find the push-up too difficult, but can do the other stages no problem, then you will want to make the exercise easier. To do this you reduce the range of motion, so that you only bend your elbows a little way. As you get stronger you can increase the range of motion, and progress steadily!

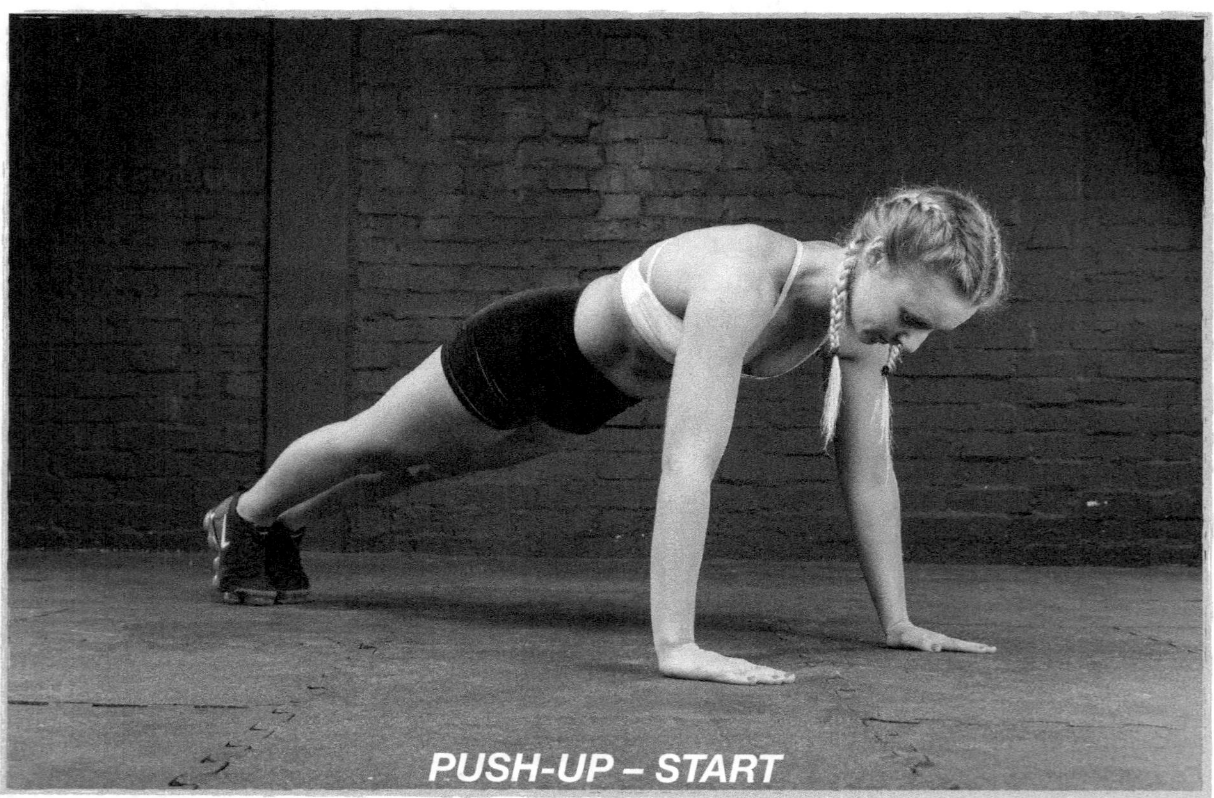

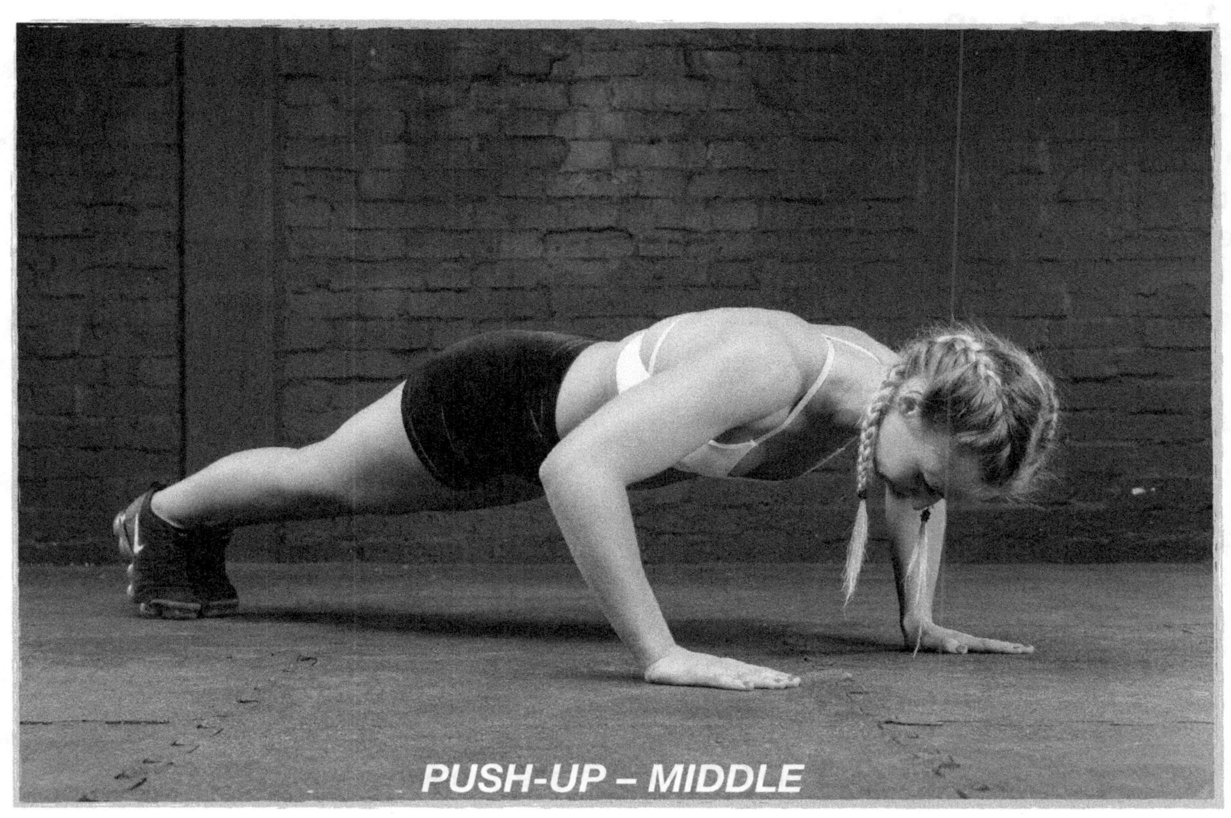

PUSH-UP – MIDDLE

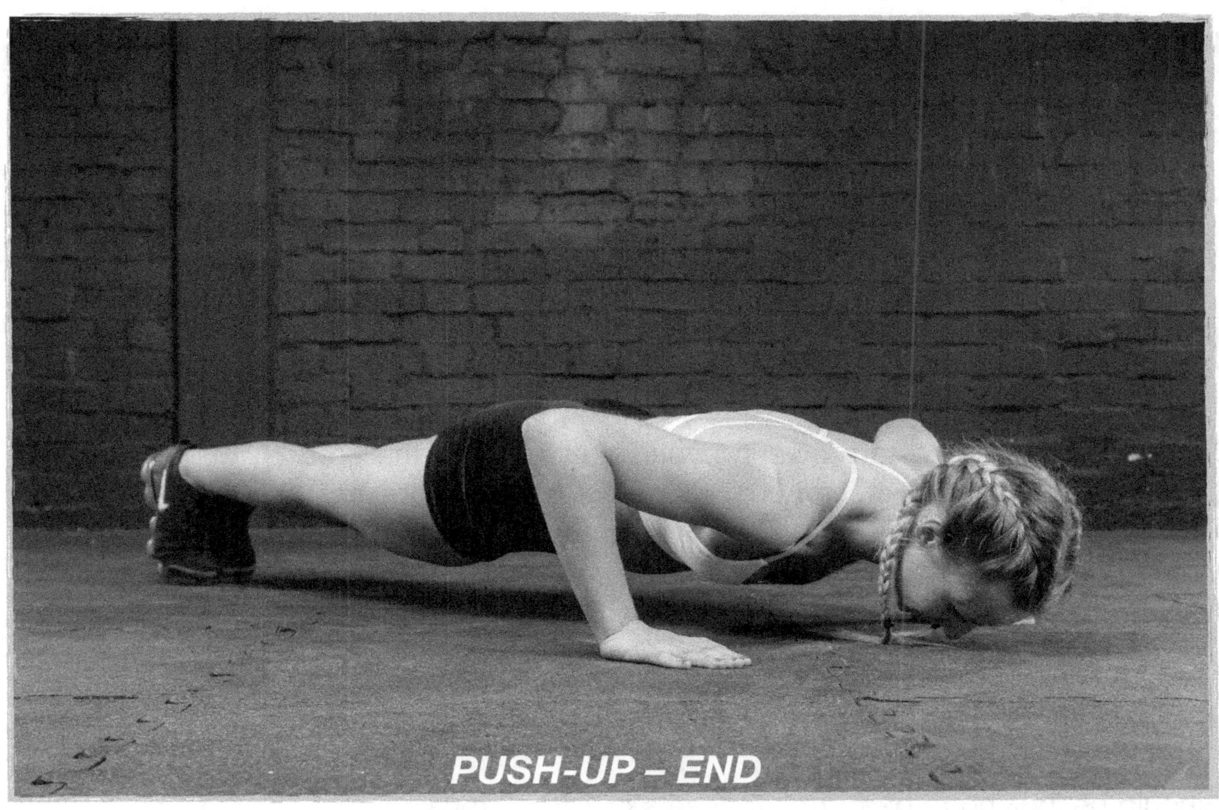

PUSH-UP – END

7.2 TRICEPS DIP

The dip is like the squat for the upper body; it builds great shape in the arms, gets rid of any bingo wings, and will tone and firm the entire upper body. The full on triceps dip is a difficult exercise, and like the push-up, there are a few stages to learning the exercise, each one more challenging than the last, enabling you to progress at a good rate and see results from day one.

STAGE 1: LEDGE DIP

We know that the Triceps dip (the proper version where you support your entire body weight) is a tough exercise, so we're going to start with the ledge dip, which is a simpler and easier version.

HOW DO I SET THE EQUIPMENT UP?

You will need an exercise step or platform for this one, preferably about knee high.

HOW DO I DO IT?

1. Crouch down with the exercise step behind you.

2. Place your hands flat on the step, with your fingers facing forwards, curled over the edge.

3. Now stretch your legs out in front of you and balance on your heels. Your torso should be upright, your legs straight, and your head in a neutral position.

4. Bend your elbows to start lowering your bum towards the ground. Keep going until you cannot go any further, or until your elbows are bent at least 90 degrees.

5. Pause for a second, and then push back up to the start position. This counts as one rep.

HOW MANY SETS AND REPS?

You should be looking to perform 3 to 5 sets of 8 to 12 reps.

HOW DO I ADJUST THE DIFFICULTY?

To make the ledge dip easier you can bend the knees and bring your feet closer to the step. This will reduce the resistance felt by the upper body, and allow your legs to help out if they need to. To make them harder straighten the legs, or dip down lower. You can see the difference between the two versions in the pictures that follow!

WHEN DO I MOVE ON?

You should move on when you can perform 3 sets of at least 15 reps, with straight legs and a 90-degree bend in the elbows.

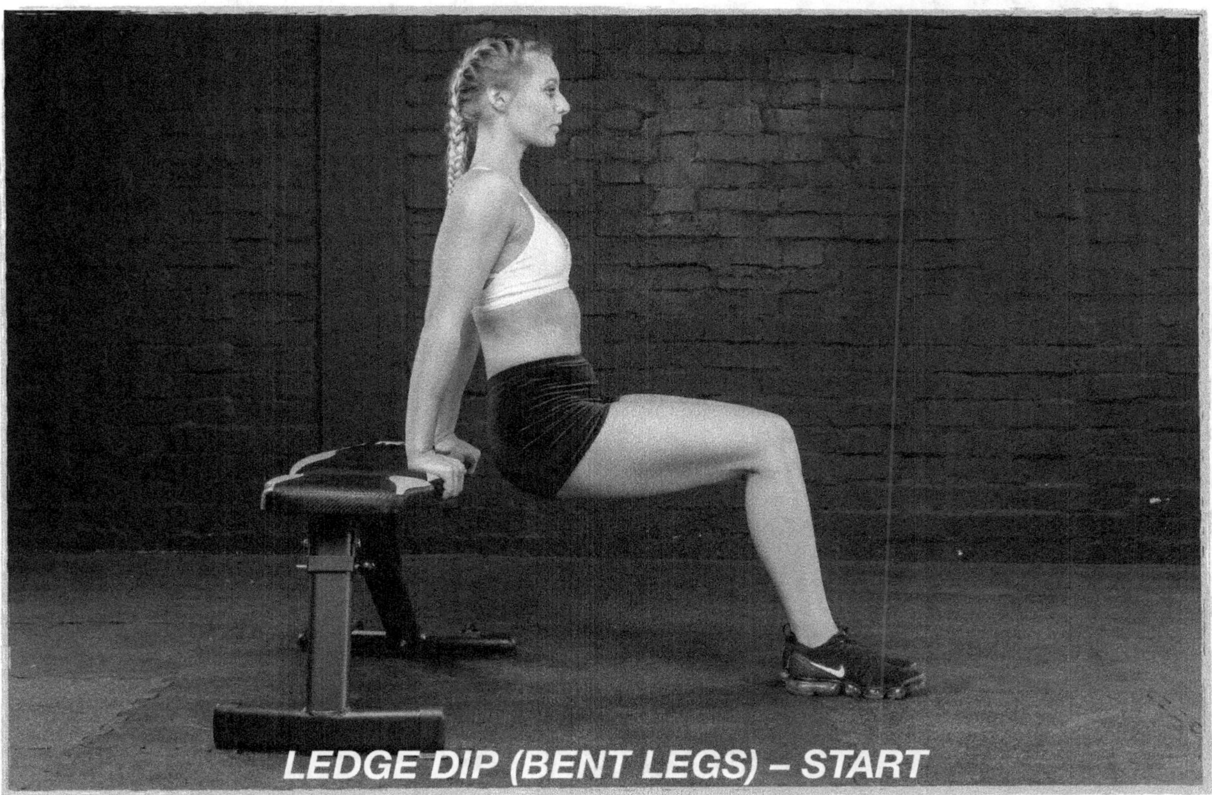

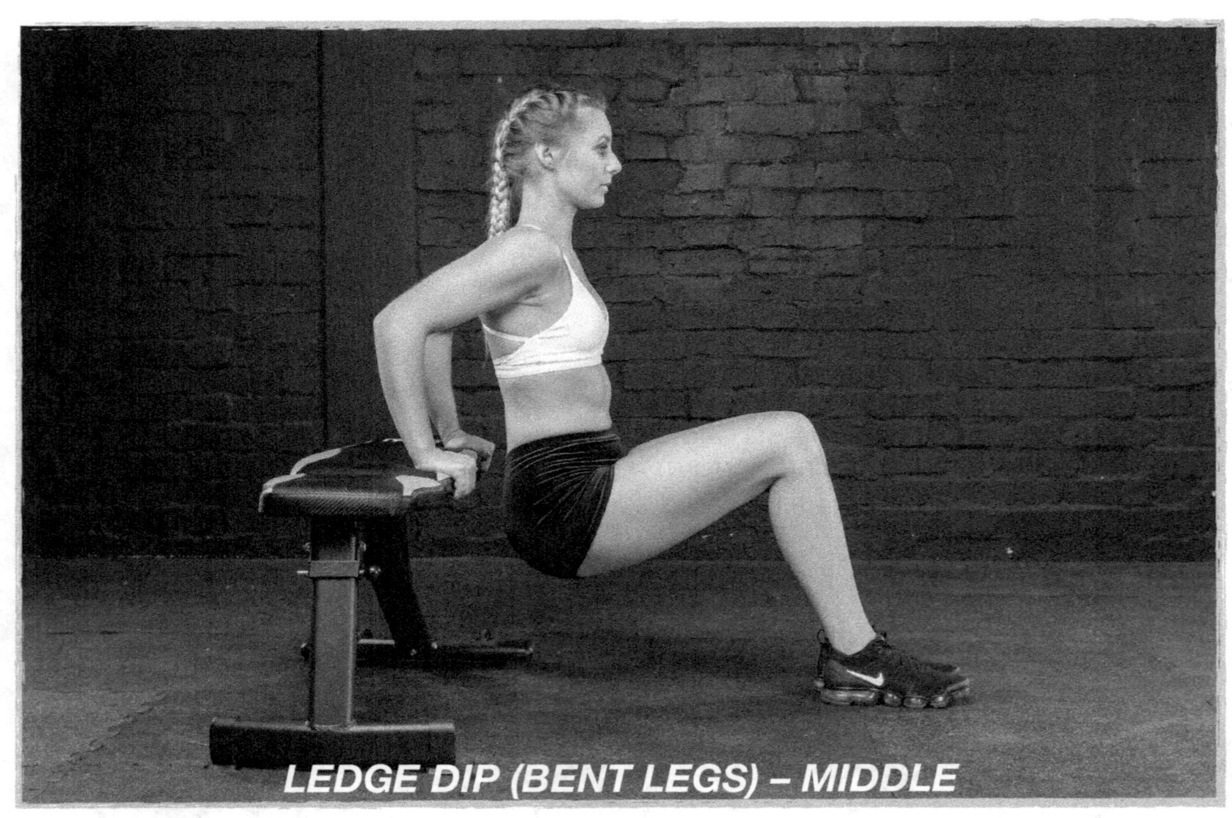

LEDGE DIP (BENT LEGS) – MIDDLE

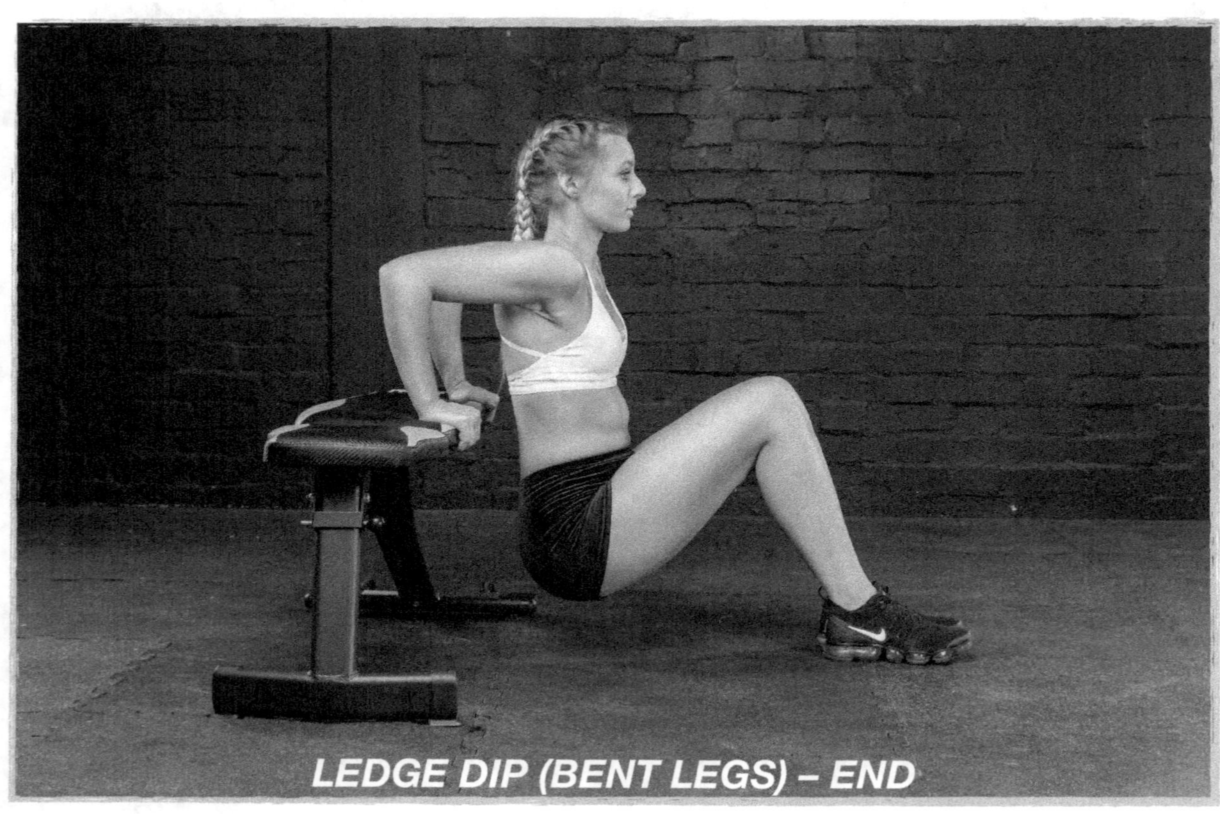

LEDGE DIP (BENT LEGS) – END

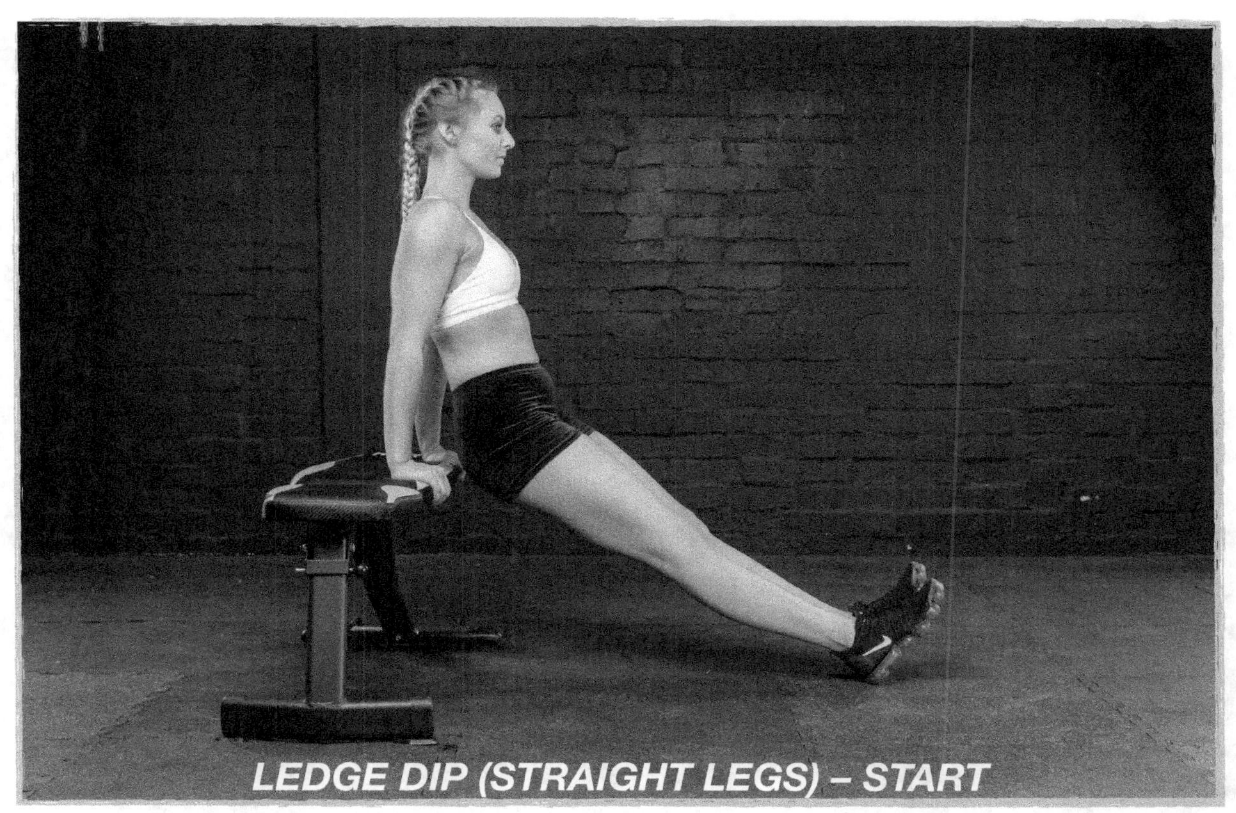

LEDGE DIP (STRAIGHT LEGS) – START

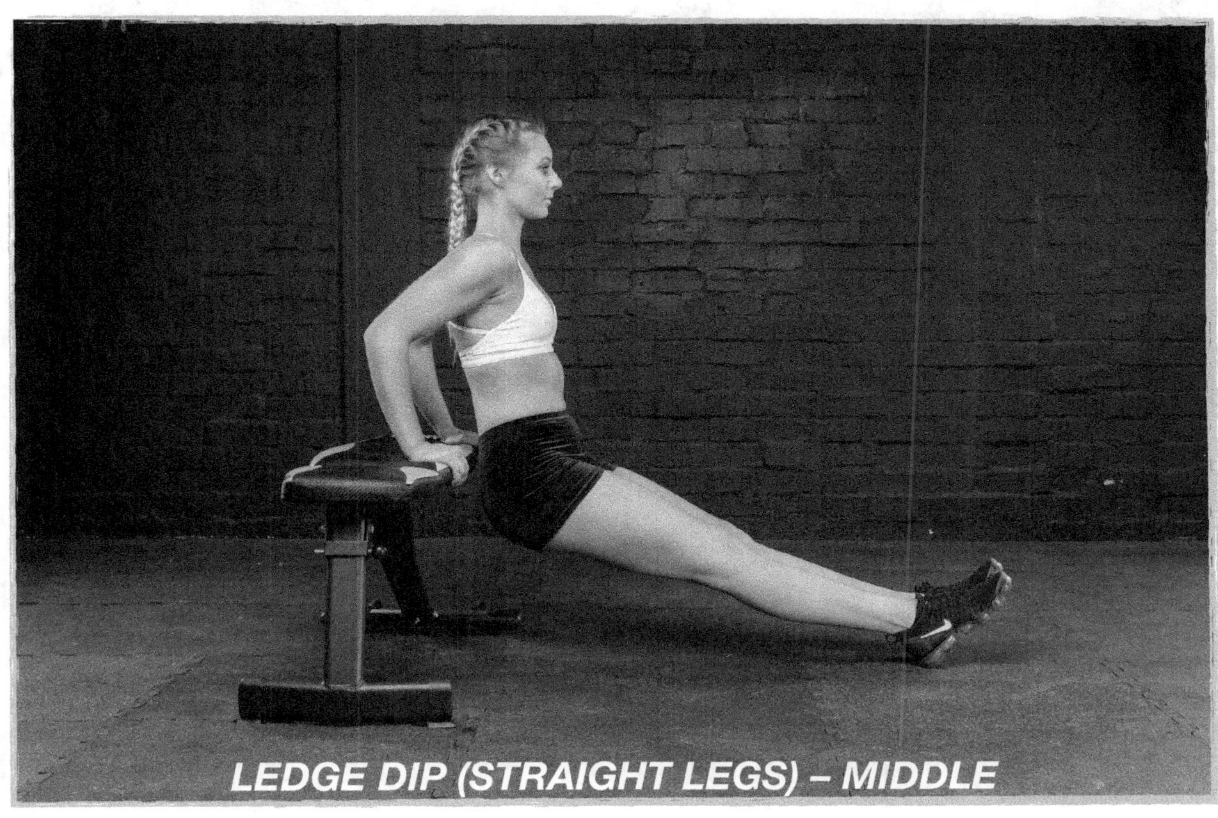

LEDGE DIP (STRAIGHT LEGS) – MIDDLE

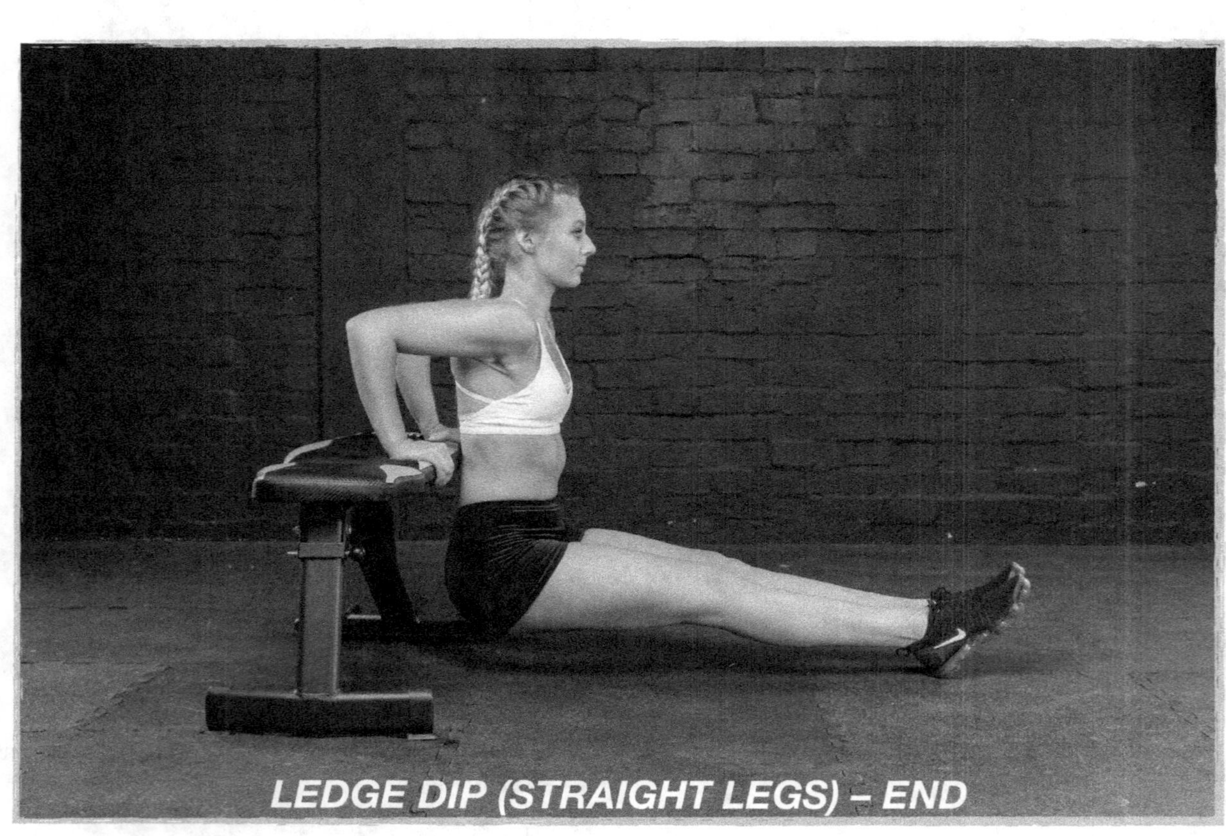

LEDGE DIP (STRAIGHT LEGS) – END

STAGE 2: NEGATIVE DIP

Once you're comfortable with the ledge dip you can move onto this stage, which is the negative dip. This exercise really works the muscles, like any other negative, and requires a good amount of strength to perform.

HOW DO I SET THE EQUIPMENT UP?

You will need access to a set of dip bars, preferably ones that you can reach without jumping or having to push yourself up. If they are high, then use a step or box to allow you to have straight arms before you take up your body weight.

HOW DO I DO IT?

1. Grab the dip bars with your palms facing inwards, and your arms straight. Remove your feet from the step or floor, or tuck them up so that your upper body takes your entire weight.

2. Now bend your elbows and start to lower yourself down towards the floor slowly. Keep your head and neck in a neutral position.

3. Keep bending your elbows until they reach a 90-degree position (or more if you have the strength), and then drop off the bars. This counts as one rep.

HOW MANY SETS AND REPS?

As with the other negative type exercises, the number of sets and reps you need to perform is lower as the muscles are under tension for a longer period of time for each rep. Try 3 to 5 sets of 1 to 2 reps, with at least 60 seconds rest between each rep.

HOW DO I ADJUST THE DIFFICULTY?

To make the negative dip easier you can lower yourself down faster. To make it more difficult you can take longer to lower yourself down. You can also work with a decreased range of motion to make them easier, or an increased range of motion to make them harder!

WHEN DO I MOVE ON?

You should move on when it takes you 15 to 20 seconds to go from the start position to the bottom position of the dip. The slower you can go, the stronger you are, so don't be afraid to spend a little time on this exercise until you can get it right!

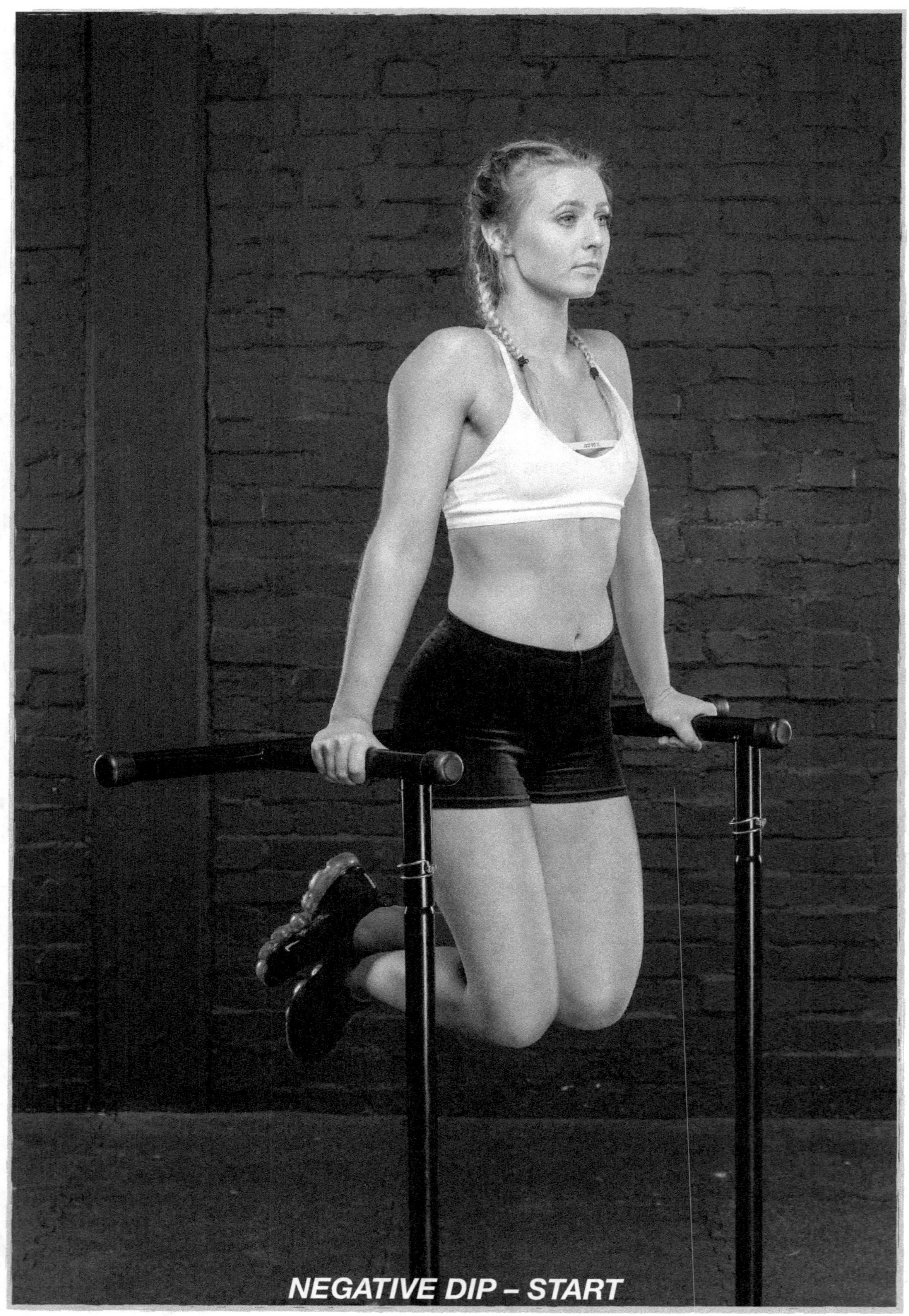

NEGATIVE DIP – START

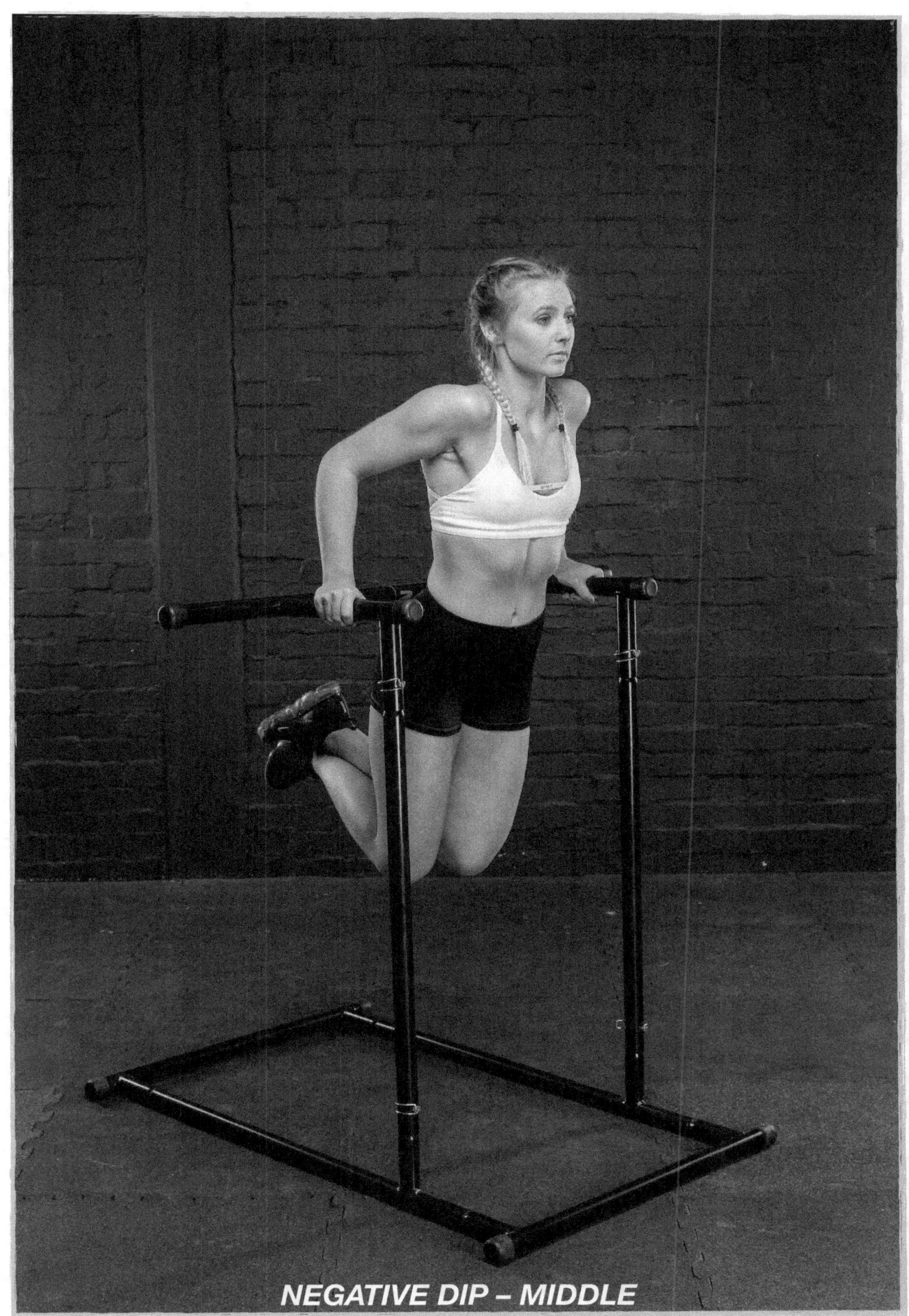

NEGATIVE DIP – MIDDLE

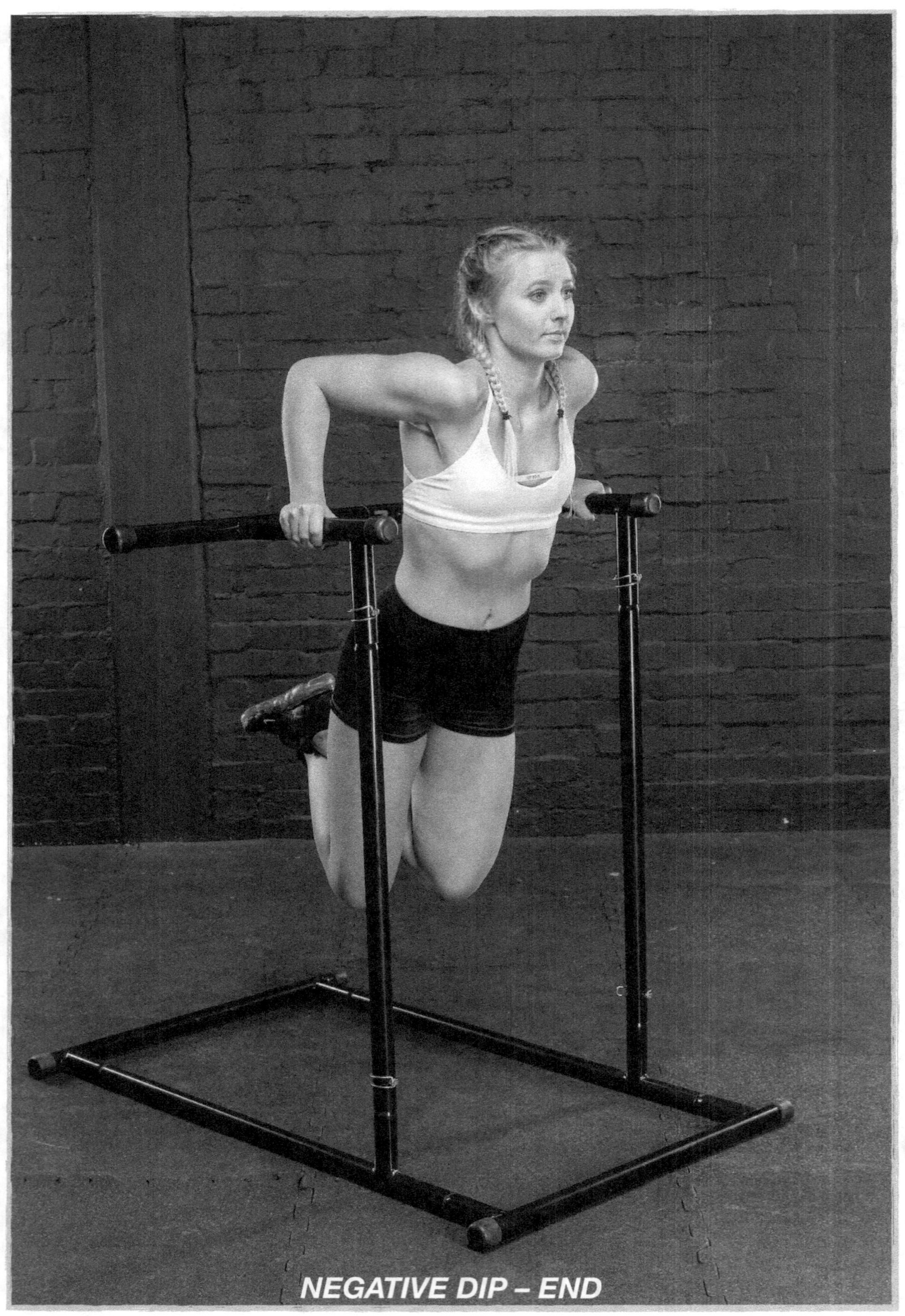

NEGATIVE DIP – END

STAGE 3: TRICEPS DIP

Nearly there! This last stage is where you will be attempting the proper version of the triceps dip, with no assistance, and your full body weight being supported by your upper body.

HOW DO I SET THE EQUIPMENT UP?

You will need access to a triceps dip bar for this exercise. These do not normally require any setting up, although some do allow the height to be adjusted.

HOW DO I DO IT?

1. Grab the bar with both hands, palms facing inwards.

2. Jump into the air, or push yourself up until your arms are straight and your feet leave the ground.

3. Take a movement to settle yourself here. Your arms should be straight, your torso upright, and your head in a neutral position. If the dip bars are low, then cross your feet and bend your knees to avoid hitting the floor when you descend.

4. Bend your elbows and start to descend. Allow your elbows to flare out as is comfortable.

5. Keep the core tight and lower under control, until your elbows are at 90-degrees, or as far as your strength and mobility allow.

6. Pause for a second, then push back up to the start position. This counts as one rep.

HOW MANY SETS AND REPS?

You should be looking to perform 3 to 5 sets of 8 to 12 reps.

HOW DO I ADJUST THE DIFFICULTY?

To adjust the difficulty of the triceps dip is simple. To make them easier reduce the range of motion by bending your elbows less. To make them harder increase the range of motion by bending your elbows more.

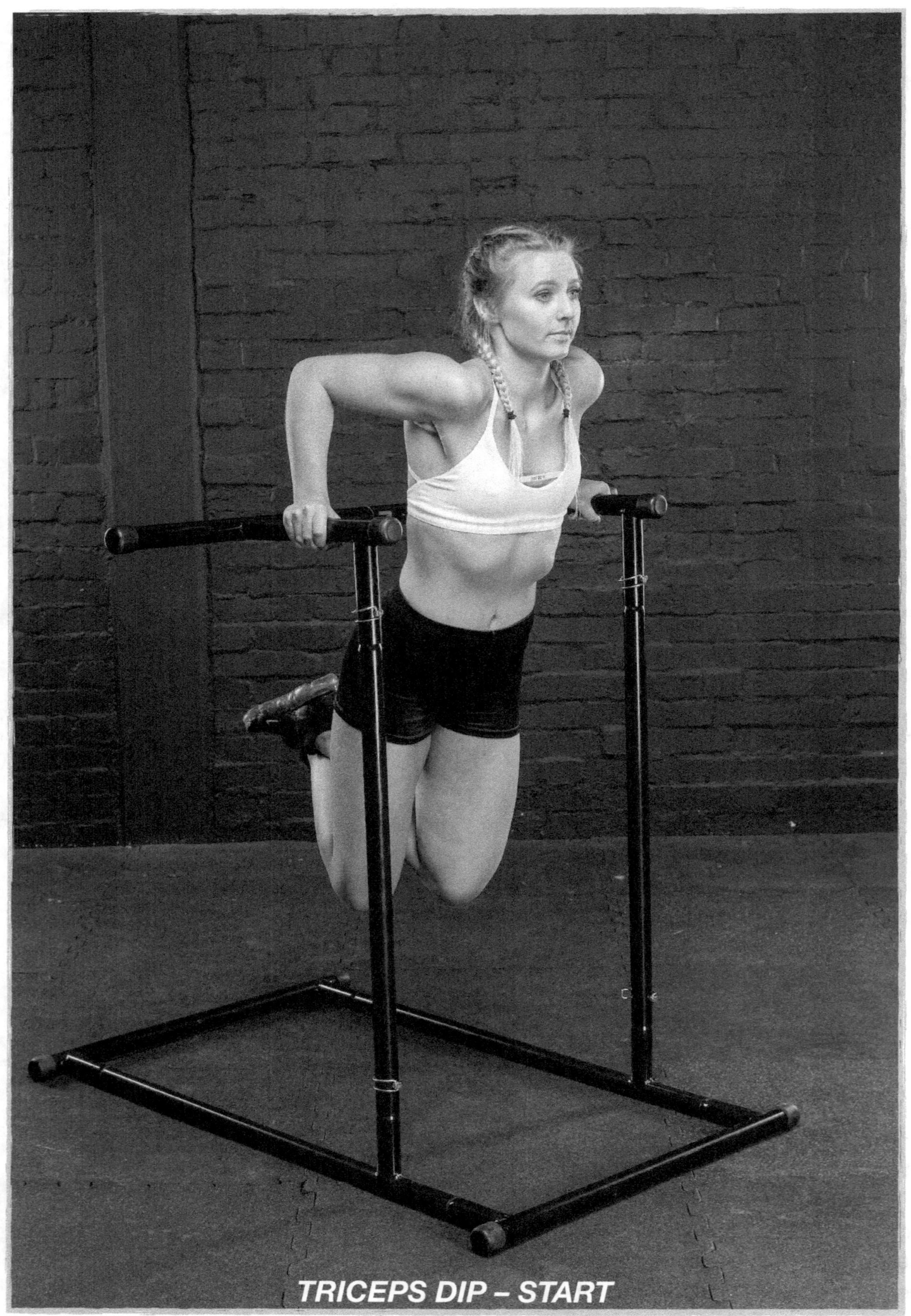

TRICEPS DIP – START

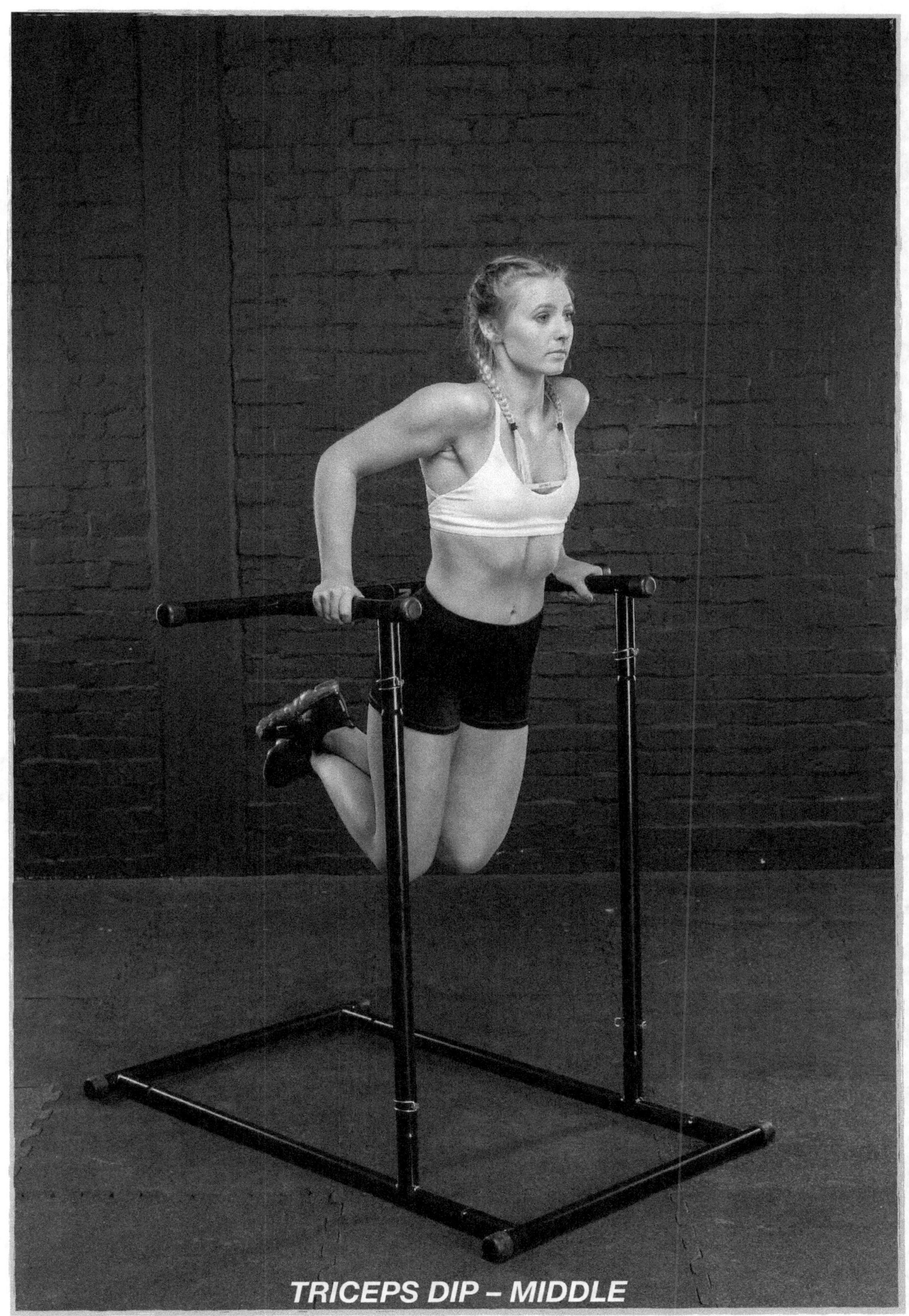

TRICEPS DIP – MIDDLE

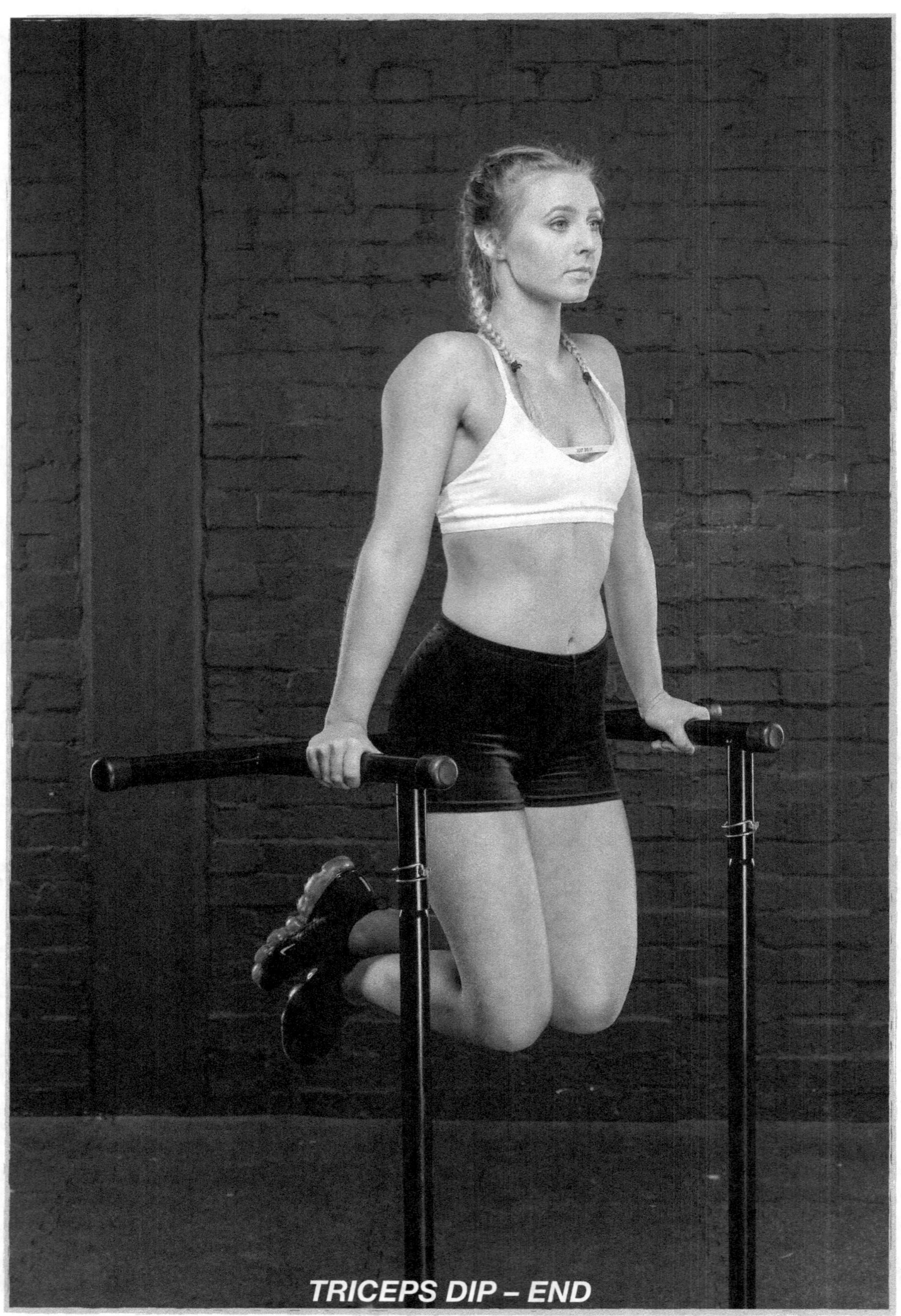

TRICEPS DIP – END

We now come to the first of two pulling exercises, which is the chin-up (the other being the pull-up). The chin-up and the pull-up are almost identical at first glance, but they differ in the hand position. This difference in hand position makes the chin-up noticeably easier than the pull-up, which is why they are both featured, and why the chin-up is examined first.

One last thing; we show five different stages in learning the chin-up and pull-up, starting with a very easy version and ending with the hardest version. Make sure to start at the beginning and go through each stage in turn. This way you will gain strength and fitness gradually, and progress steadily!

STAGE 1: ROW (SUPINE)

The first stage in learning the chin-up is the supine row. "Supine" might sound complicated but it simply means to face up. The great thing about the supine row is that it can be adapted for different levels of ability, from complete beginners to gym bunnies who live and breathe exercise. You'll need access to a bar that can be raised and lowered, such as a squat rack, a smith machine, suspension trainer, or other piece of equipment that allows the same thing.

HOW DO I SET THE EQUIPMENT UP?

As said in the intro, you will need a bar that can be adjusted in height, preferably on a squat rack, smith machine, or suspension trainer. To begin, set the bar at shoulder height. Make sure that everything is secure, and that the bar cannot move when you pull on it.

HOW DO I DO IT?

1. To perform the supinated row stand in front of the bar and grab it with both hands. Your grip should be shoulder width apart, and your palms should be facing the ceiling.

2. Position your feet under the bar to start then move them forward by a few inches.

3. From here pull on the bar until your chest touches it, or you cannot pull any further. Keep your body straight and head in a neutral position.

4. Pause for a second, and then return to the starting position. This counts as one rep.

HOW MANY SETS AND REPS?

You should be looking to perform 3 to 5 sets of 8 to 12 reps.

HOW DO I ADJUST THE DIFFICULTY?

To make the row easier raise the height of the bar and make your body position more vertical. This will move more weight off the arms and onto the legs. To make the supine row harder lower the height of the bar and move you feet forwards. This will move more weight onto the upper body.

WHEN DO I MOVE ON?

The goal with the supine row is to move on when you can perform 3 sets of 8 reps with your body positioned at an angle of 45 degrees. You can keep coming back to tis exercise as well as doing the next one (dead hang) to keep building strength.

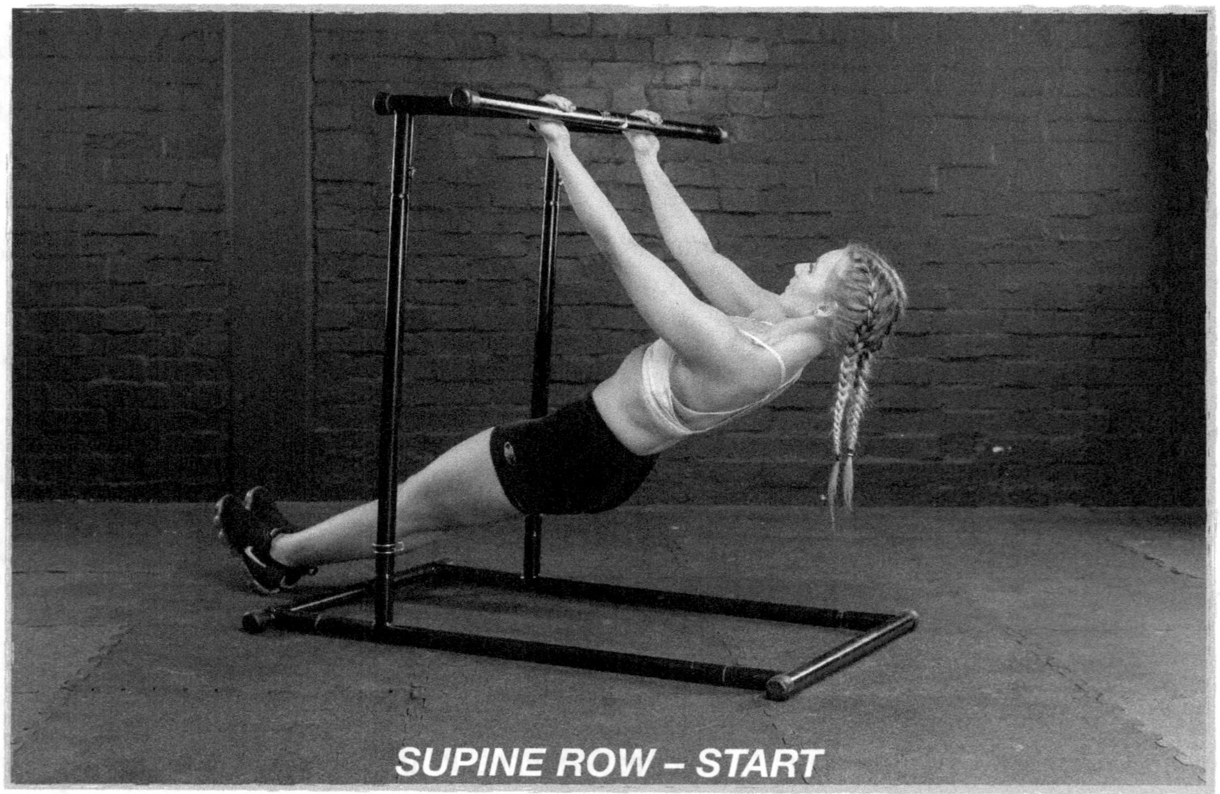

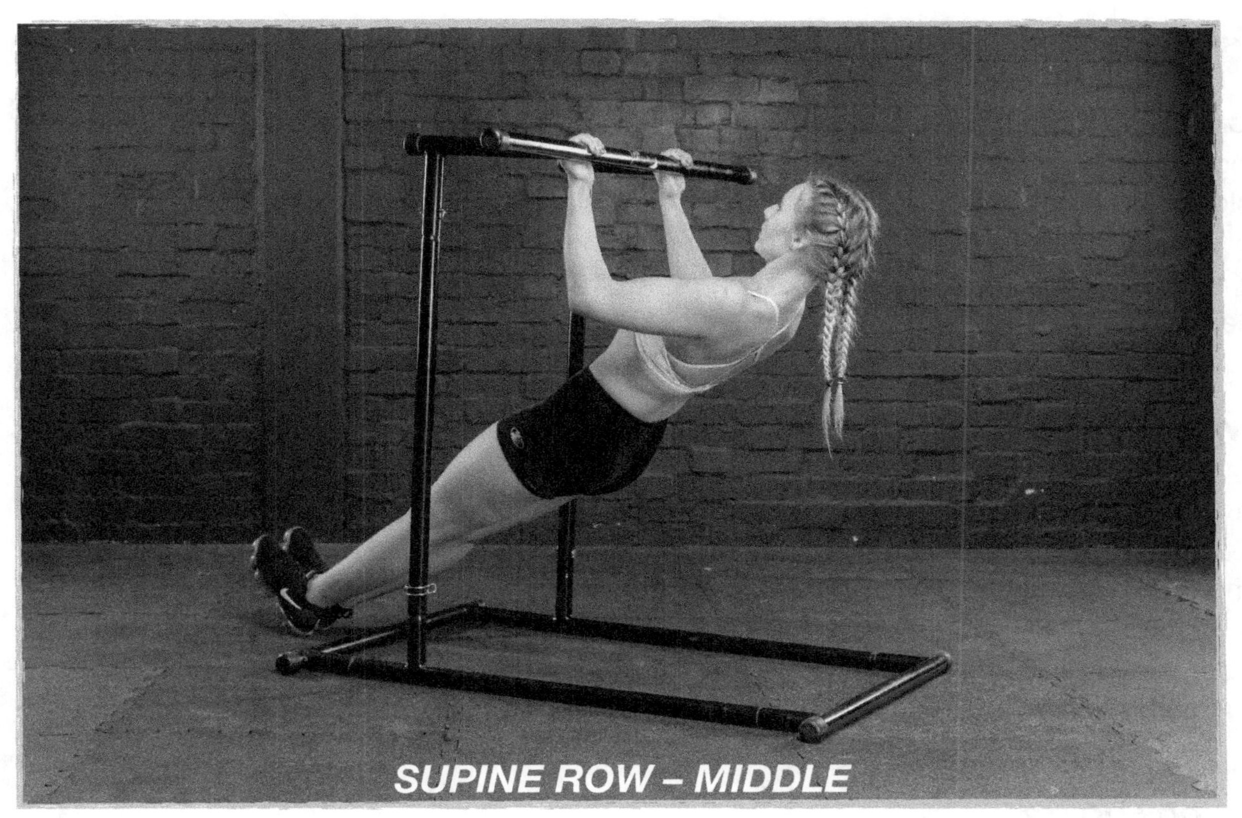

SUPINE ROW – MIDDLE

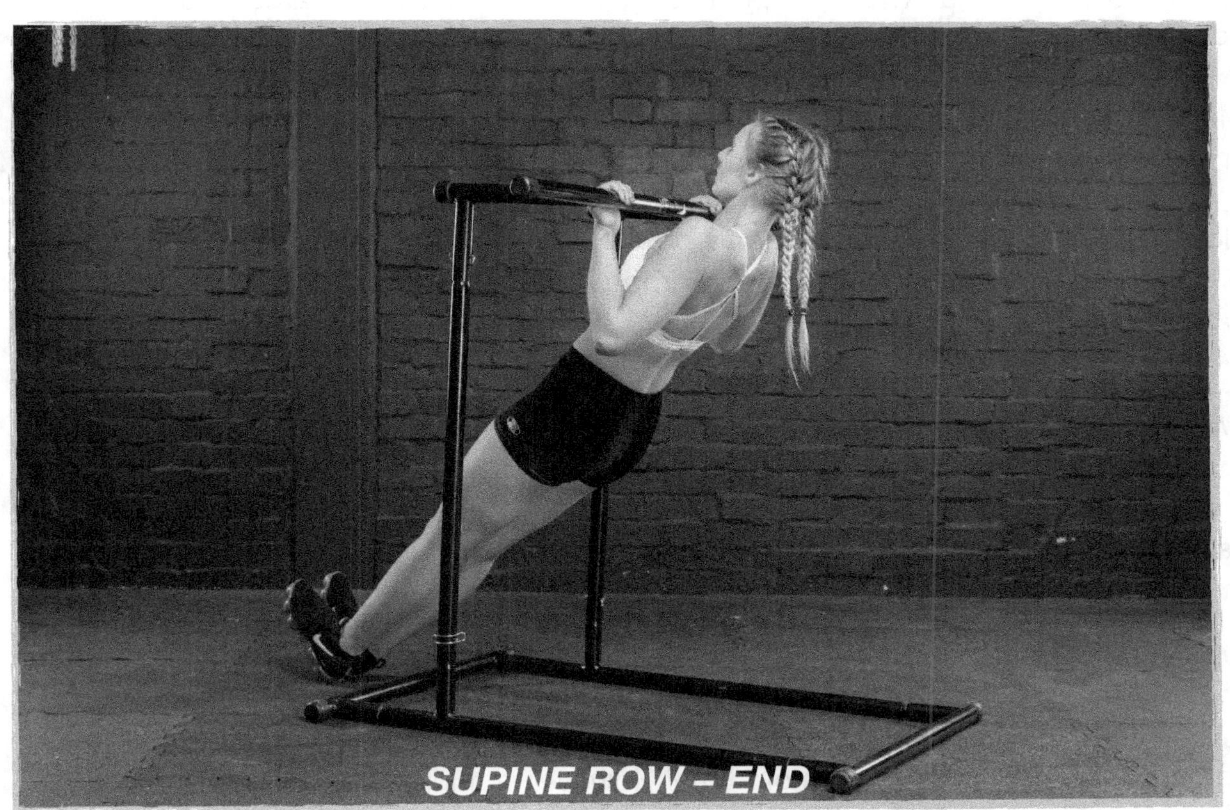

SUPINE ROW – END

STAGE 2: DEAD HANG (SUPINE)

This stage is where you actually get to grips with the pull-up bar, literally! The Dead Hang is where you hang from the bar for as long as possible. This exercise is designed to increase your grip strength, so that when you come to performing chin-ups you can hold on to the bar long enough to knock out some reps. Needless to say this can be quite tough on the hands, so if you need to wear gloves then go ahead.

HOW DO I SET THE EQUIPMENT UP?

The pull-up bar should be set up already; if it's a stand-alone bar then it will be fixed to the wall or other piece of equipment. If the pull-up bar is part of a larger gym frame then this will also be fixed in place. If none of these are available then you can use a smith machine bar. This bar will be adjustable, so in this case make sure that the bar is high enough to allow you to hang from it without hitting your knees on the ground (you can tuck your feet up to avoid them fouling the ground).

HOW DO I DO IT?

1. Grab the pull-up bar with a supinated grip (palms facing towards you). Your hands should be about shoulder width apart.

2. Make sure that your elbows are straight and your head is in a neutral position, lift your feet off the ground, either by bending your knees or lifting your legs up.

3. Now hang onto the bar for as long as possible! As soon as you start to feel your grip loosen, or feel that you are going to drop off the bar, then let go and rest. This counts as one rep.

HOW MANY SETS AND REPS?

You should be looking to perform 5 sets of 1 rep. So, hang on to the bar as long as possible, drop off and rest, and then repeat this four more times.

HOW DO I ADJUST THE DIFFICULTY?

Adjusting the difficulty of the dead hang is not really possible, as you can either hang on the bar for less time or more time! However, a thicker bar will be harder to hold on to, and a thinner bar will be easier to hold on to.

WHEN DO I MOVE ON?

You should move on to the next stage when you can do a dead hang for at least 20 seconds without dropping off the bar.

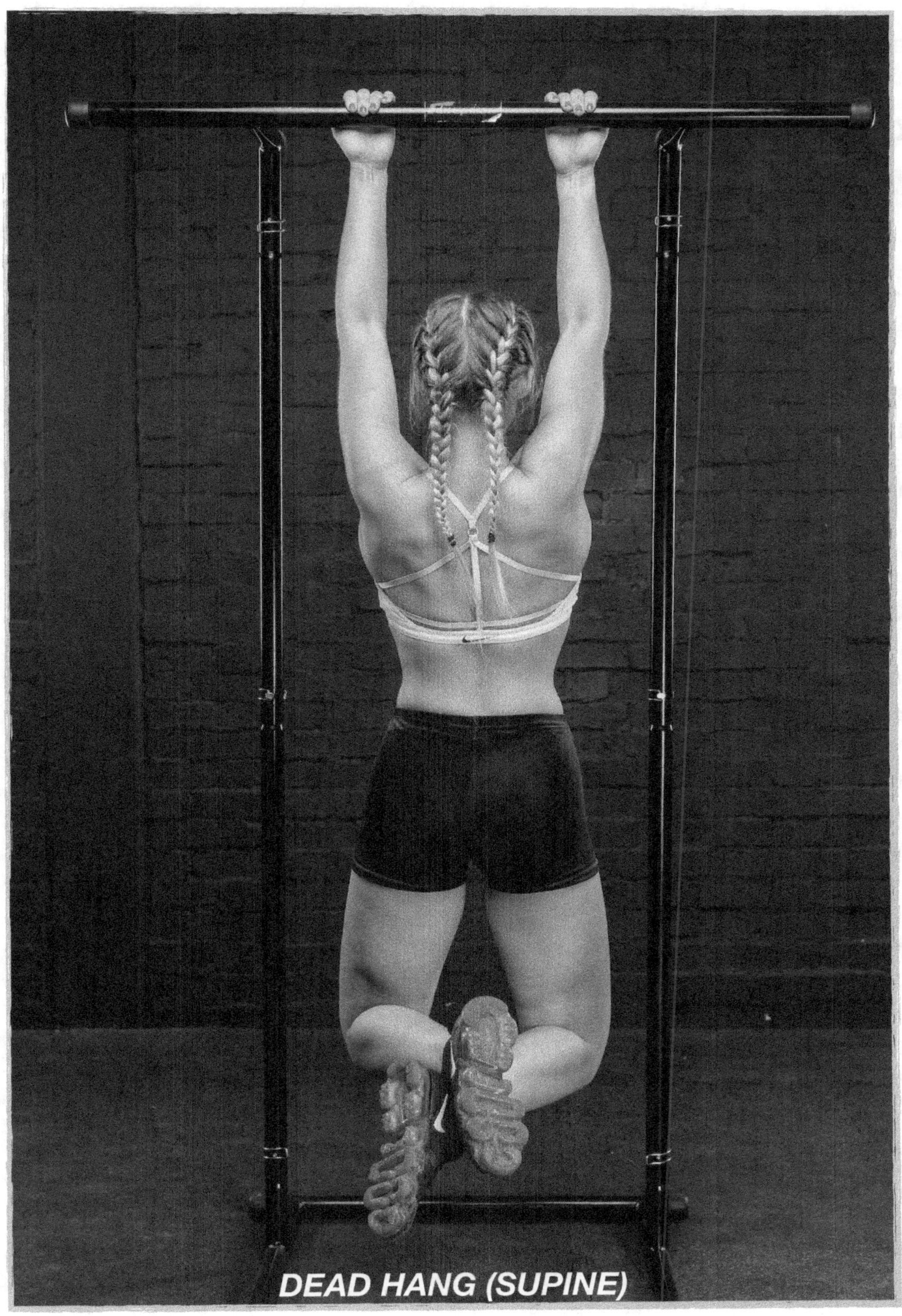

STAGE 3: ASSISTED CHIN-UP

The next stage in learning the chin-up is the assisted chin-up. This stage is basically the entire chin-up exercise, but you will be assisted in some way (usually an exercise band, or assisted machine). Although the assisted machines are good (basically a pull-up/dip station with a weighted mechanism), we prefer using bands. Using bands allows the movement to be more "real" and will prepare you better for the full exercise.

HOW DO I SET THE EQUIPMENT UP?

To use the elastic exercise band you will need to first secure it to the pull-up bar. You can do this by looping one end over the bar and then threading the other end through the loop, and pulling tight. Check that it secure before using it! Then, when you are ready to go, put a foot (or a knee) in the bottom loop of the band, and you will be ready to go.

If you use an assisted pull-up station, these work by offsetting some of your weight, meaning that you are pulling a fraction of your body weight. Begin by setting up with at least 75% of your body weight on the machine. For example, if you weigh 60 kilograms (130 pounds), then put 45 kilograms (100 pounds) on the machine. Remember, the more weight that is on the machine the *easier* the exercise will be!

HOW DO I DO IT?

For the exercise band version:

1. Secure the band on the pull-up bar as detailed earlier. If the pull-up bar is too high to reach without jumping, place a step or box underneath as well.

2. Place your foot or knee (depending on how long the band is), in the loop, and grab the bar with both hands in an underhand (supinated) grip.

3. Hang with your arms straight, allowing the band to stretch and build up resistance.

4. Now pull up hard, keeping your leg straight so that the band can give assistance. Keep pulling until your chin rises above the bar.

5. Pause for a second, and then lower down to the start position. This counts as one rep.

__For the assisted machine version:__

1. To get started, set up the machine so that you can reach the bars, your knees or feet can reach the support pad easily, and there is plenty of weight on the machine (you can reduce the assistance later, but make it easy to start with!).

2. Now get into position. Your hands should be gripping the bars with your palms facing you, your knees or feet should be in contact with the support pad, and your torso should be vertical.

3. Make sure your arms are completely straight, and then start to pull-up slowly and strongly. Keep going until you chin goes over or is level with the bar.

4. Pause for a second, and then lower yourself down to the start position. And that's it!

HOW MANY SETS AND REPS?

You should be looking to perform 3 to 5 sets of 5 to 8 reps.

HOW DO I ADJUST THE DIFFICULTY?

To adjust the difficulty of the assisted chin-up is easy. If you are using exercise bands then using a heavier band will make the exercise easier, and using a lighter band will make the exercise harder.

If you are using an assisted machine, add more weight to the machine to make the exercise easier, and take weight off the machine to make the exercise harder.

WHEN DO I MOVE ON?

If you are using an exercise band, then you should move onto the next stage when you can perform 3 sets of 5 to 8 reps with a light band. Many bands are different, so it is impossible to give an exact estimate here, but you should be looking at pulling at least 50% of your body weight.

If you are using an assisted machine, you should move on to the next stage when you can perform 3 sets of 5 to 8 reps with 25% of your body weight on the machine. For example, if you weigh 60 kilograms (130 pounds), then you need to have 15 kilograms (37 pounds) on the machine.

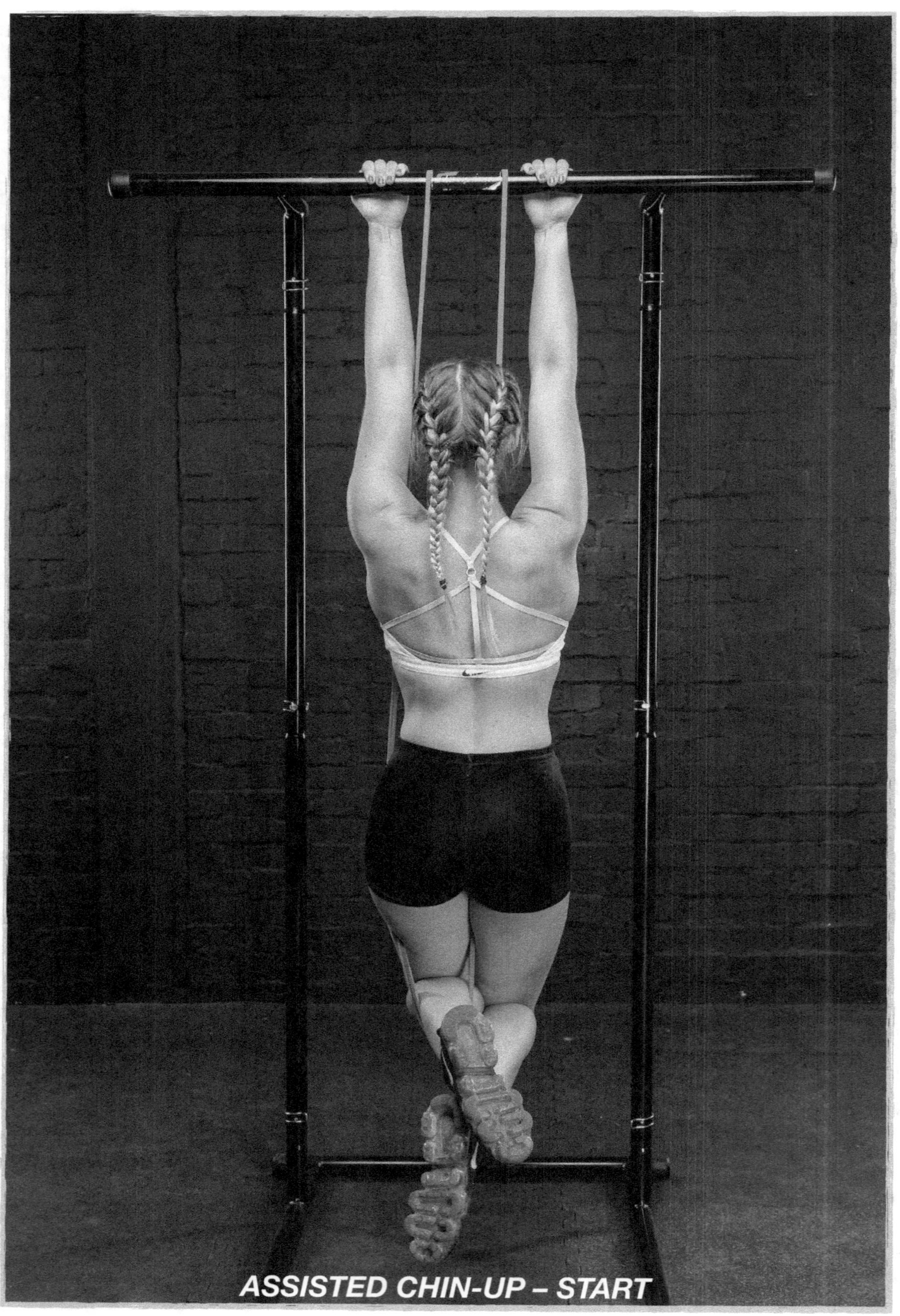
ASSISTED CHIN-UP – START

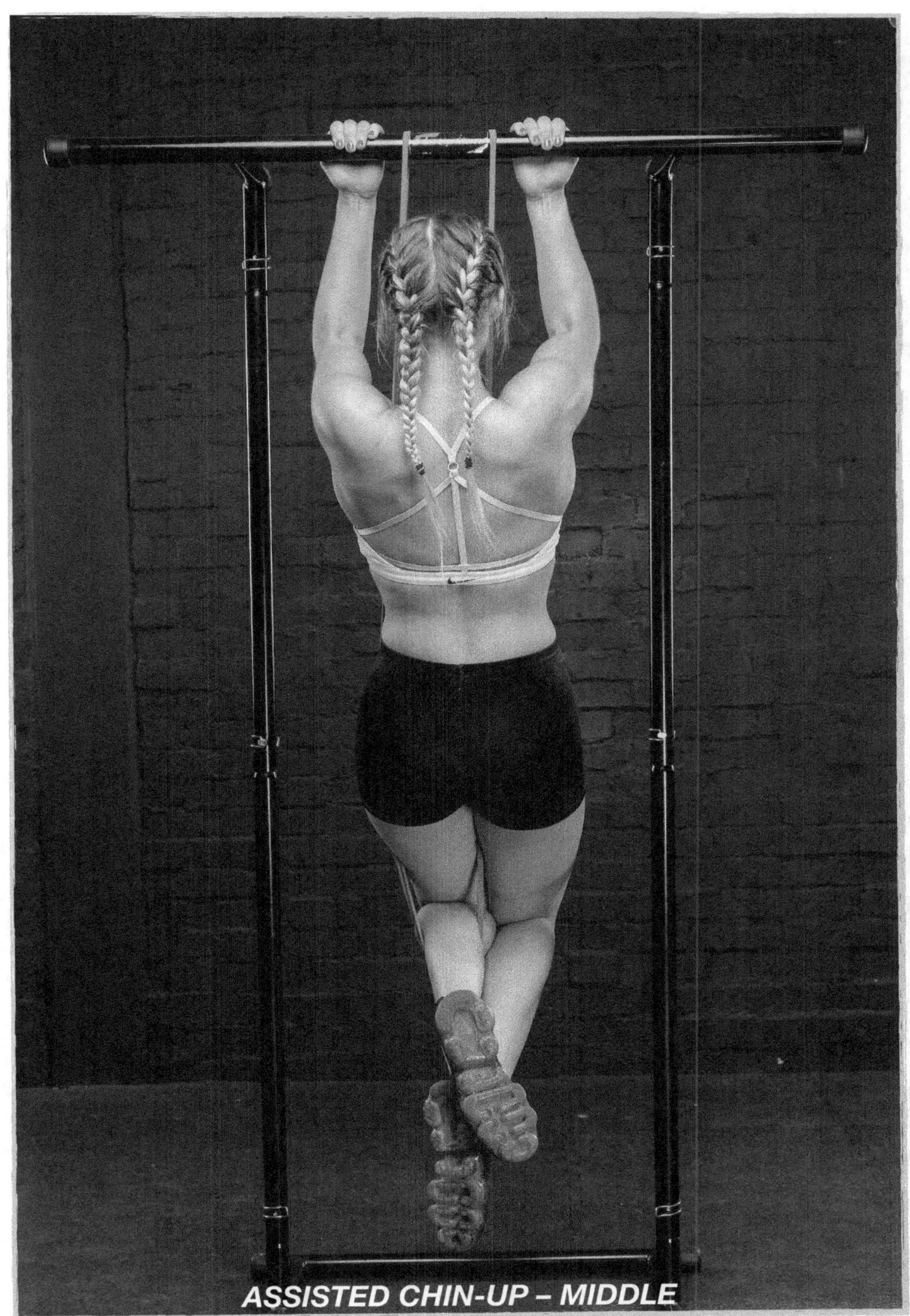

ASSISTED CHIN-UP – MIDDLE

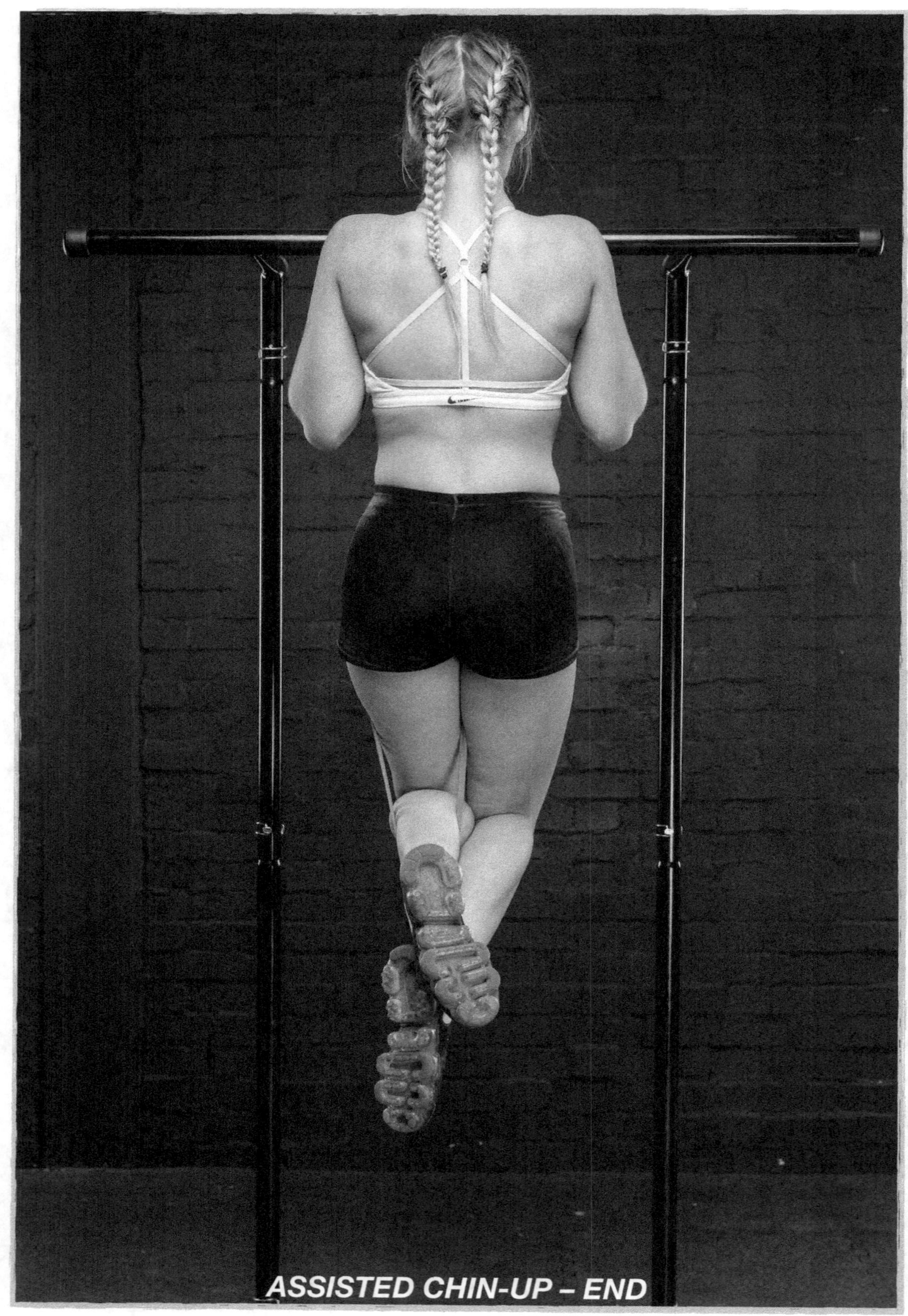

ASSISTED CHIN-UP – END

STAGE 4: NEGATIVE CHIN-UP

The negative chin-up is a great stage, and is in fact one of the best ways of building strength. You start at the top of the chin-up movement, and then lower yourself down as slowly as possible. Your muscles will be under tension the whole time, and although you're moving in the opposite direction to the pull, you'll still get stronger!

HOW DO I SET THE EQUIPMENT UP?

You'll need access to a pull-up bar, and enough space below and behind for you to drop off the bar when needed. You will also need a step or platform of some kind, to allow you to start the exercise with your chin above the bar.

HOW DO I DO IT?

1. Grab the pull-up bar with both hands in an underhand (supine) grip, hands about shoulder width apart.

2. Step onto the platform and stand up straight, so that your chin is over the bar (if your bar is low then you may be able to stand on the floor and get into this position).

3. Contract your muscles hard and pull down. Now take your feet off the box (or lift them off the ground if your bar is low) and hold yourself at the top of the position.

4. Now start to lower yourself as slowly as possible. Pull on the bar very hard, but let your muscles lengthen as gravity pulls you down.

5. Keep going all the way until your arms are completely straight, then drop off or let go of the bar, and rest. This counts as one rep.

HOW MANY SETS AND REPS?

As the negative chin-up works differently to the other exercises, you should be looking to do 3 to 5 sets of 1. So, you would do 1 rep, taking as long as possible to lower yourself to the bottom position, then rest, and then repeat 2 to 4 more times.

HOW DO I ADJUST THE DIFFICULTY?

To make the negative chin-up more difficult simply take longer to lower yourself down to the bottom position. To make it easier take less time to lower yourself down to the bottom position.

The idea of the negative chin-up is to increase the amount of time that it takes you to reach the bottom. Ideally you should move on to the next stage when it takes you at least 15 to 20 seconds to do a single rep.

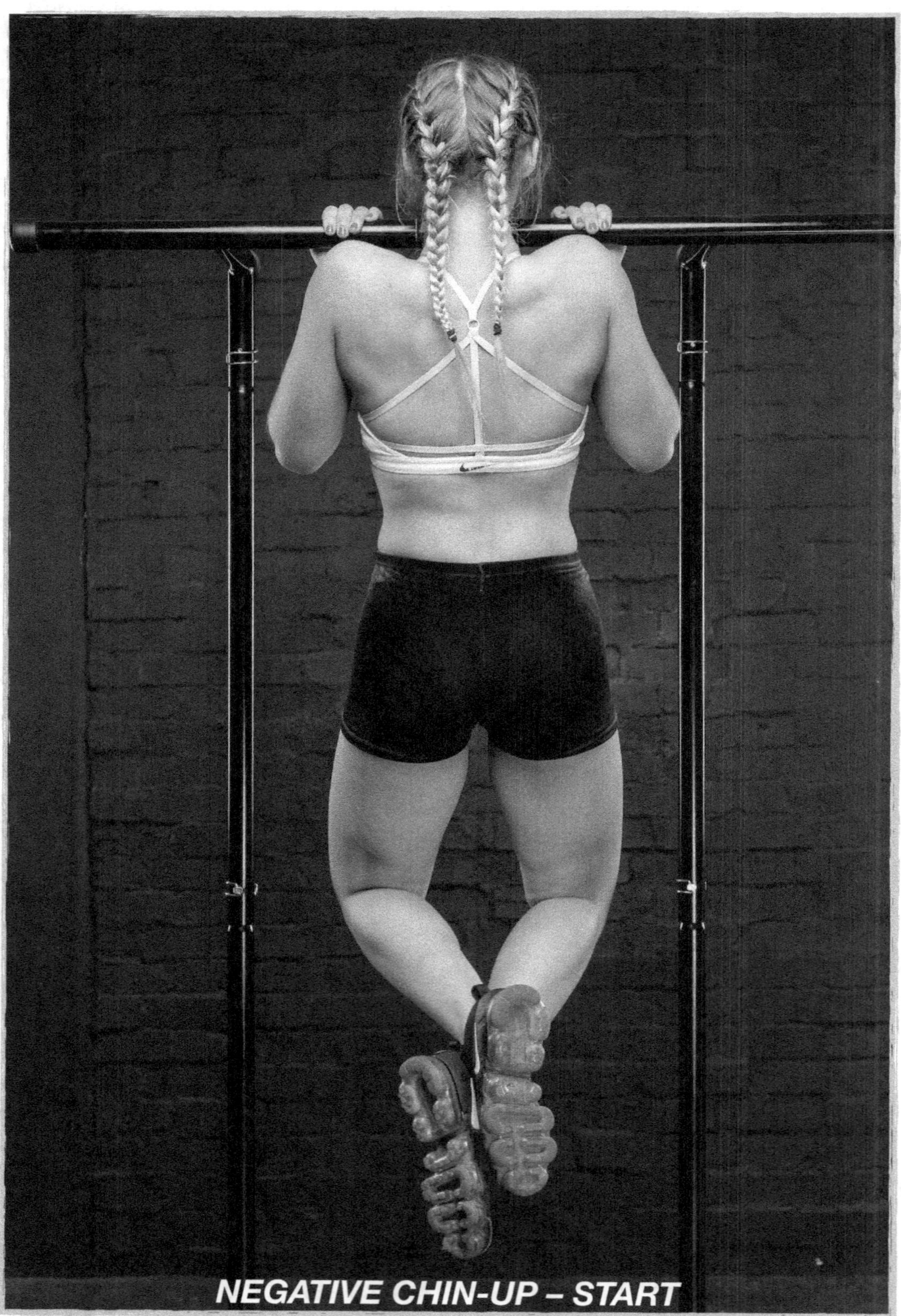

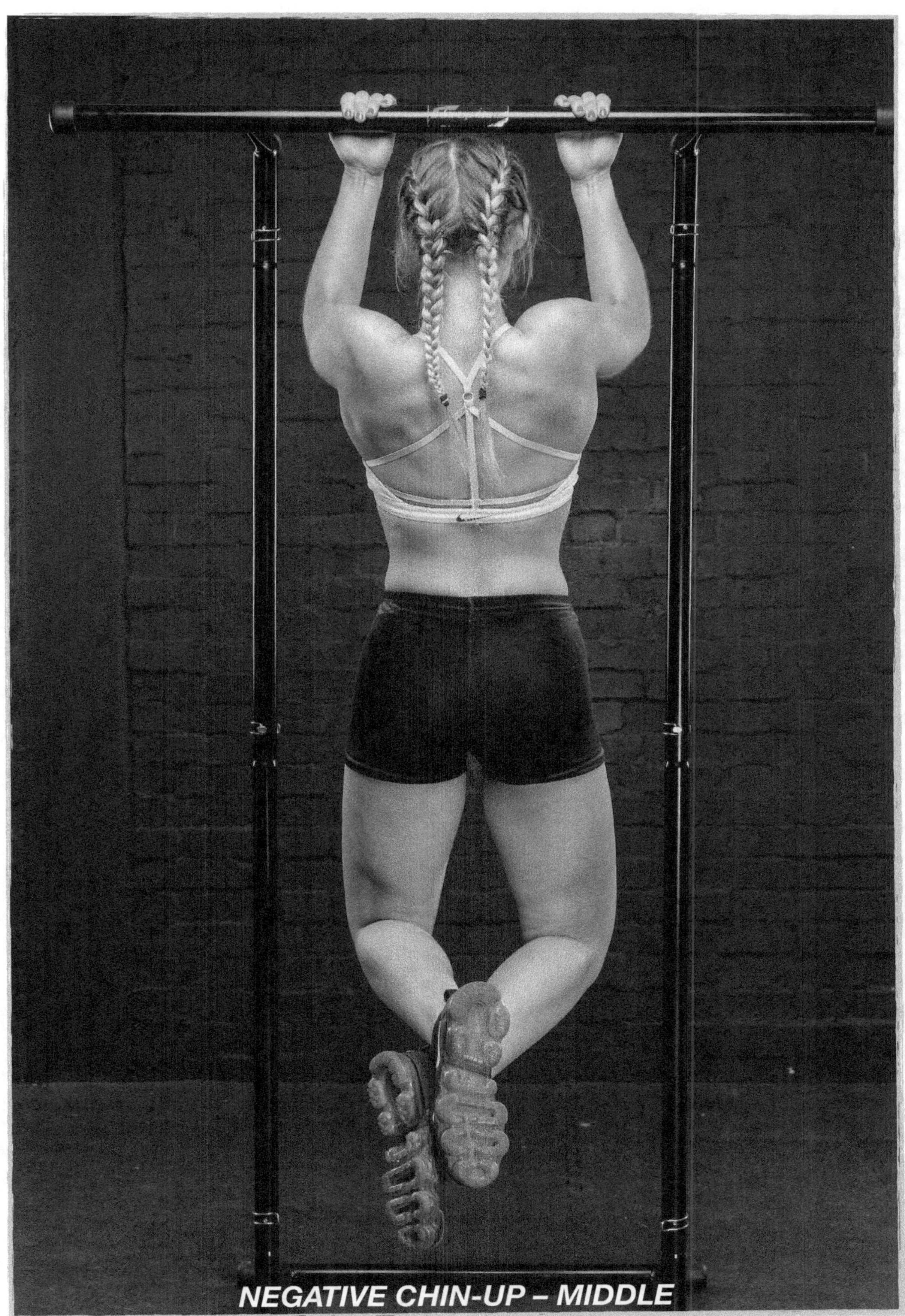

NEGATIVE CHIN-UP – MIDDLE

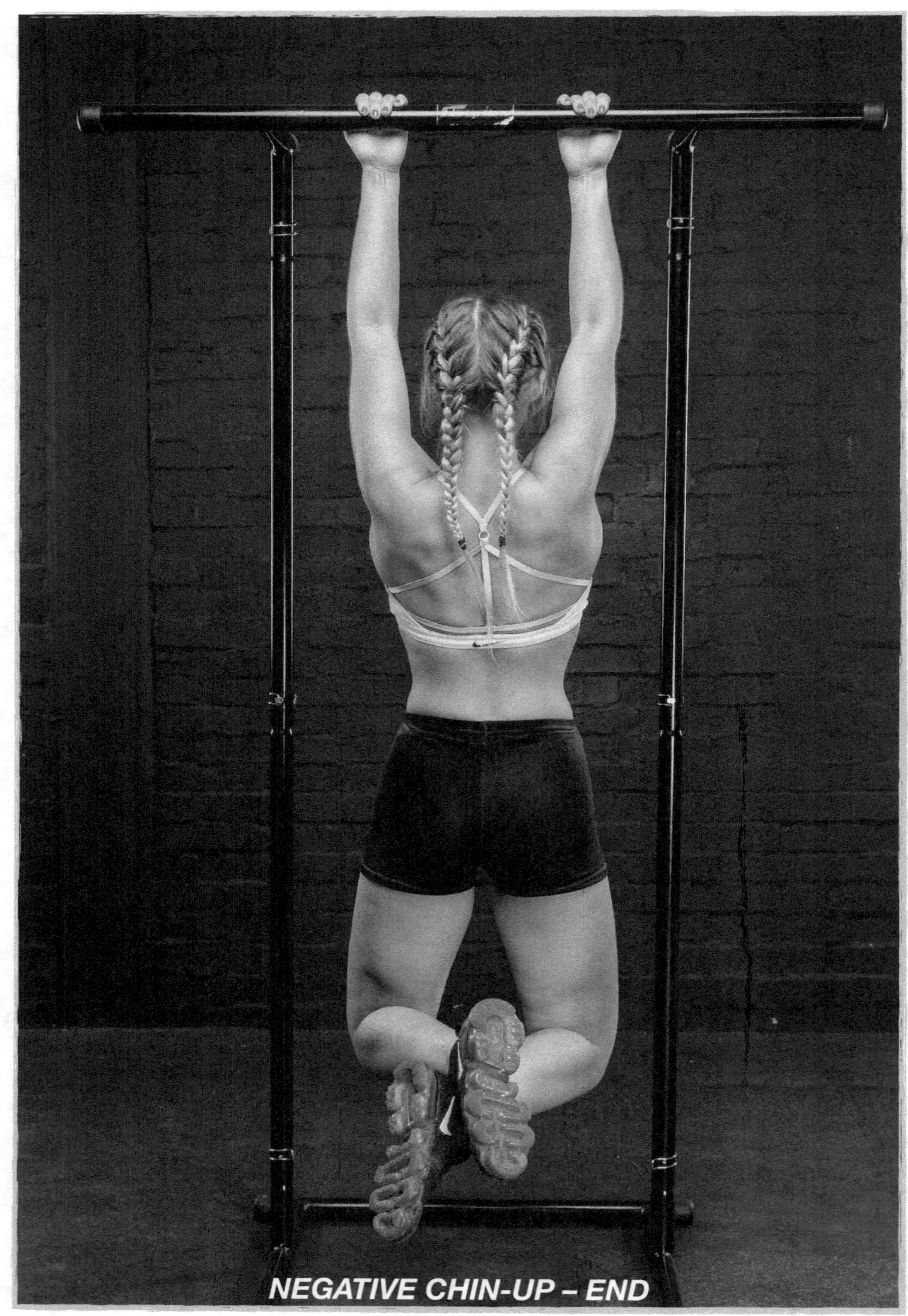

NEGATIVE CHIN-UP – END

STAGE 5: CHIN-UP

You've almost made it! This last stage is where you put it all together and start to practice real chin-ups. It is likely that even if you have followed all of the stages so far, performing perfect reps will take a little practice, so don't be surprised if you can't do them immediately. Take your time, make sure to concentrate on the fundamentals, and you will see amazing strength and physique gains.

HOW DO I SET THE EQUIPMENT UP?

You will need a pull-up bar that is preferably just above your reaching height, so that you can relax your legs and not have your feet foul on the floor.

HOW DO I DO IT?

1. Grab the pull-up bar in an overhand grip. Your hands should be about shoulder width apart.

2. Hang with your legs straight, and allow your shoulders to rise up to meet your ears. This is the starting position.

3. Start to pull with your arms and back. Your elbows will bend as you do this; allow them to flare out to the sides as is comfortable.

4. Keep pulling until your chin reaches over or is level with the bar. Pause for a second, and then lower yourself down to the starting position. This counts as one rep.

HOW MANY SETS AND REPS?

As chin-ups are difficult, you should be looking to perform 3 to 5 sets of 3 to 5 reps.

HOW DO I ADJUST THE DIFFICULTY?

Out of all of the exercises in this book the chin-up is the one that may give you the most trouble. We understand this however, and have a few pointers to give you to help you out.

First, don't rush the previous stages, and only move onto this stage once you are ready. If you move too quickly then you will not have built the basics enough to perform the exercise properly.

Second, do not cheat! Make sure that your arms are fully straight when you reach the bottom position, and do not be tempted to kick or lift the legs when pulling up.

Lastly, squeeze the bar as tightly as possible. This will help to focus your strength and make you feel as though your connection to the bar is stronger.

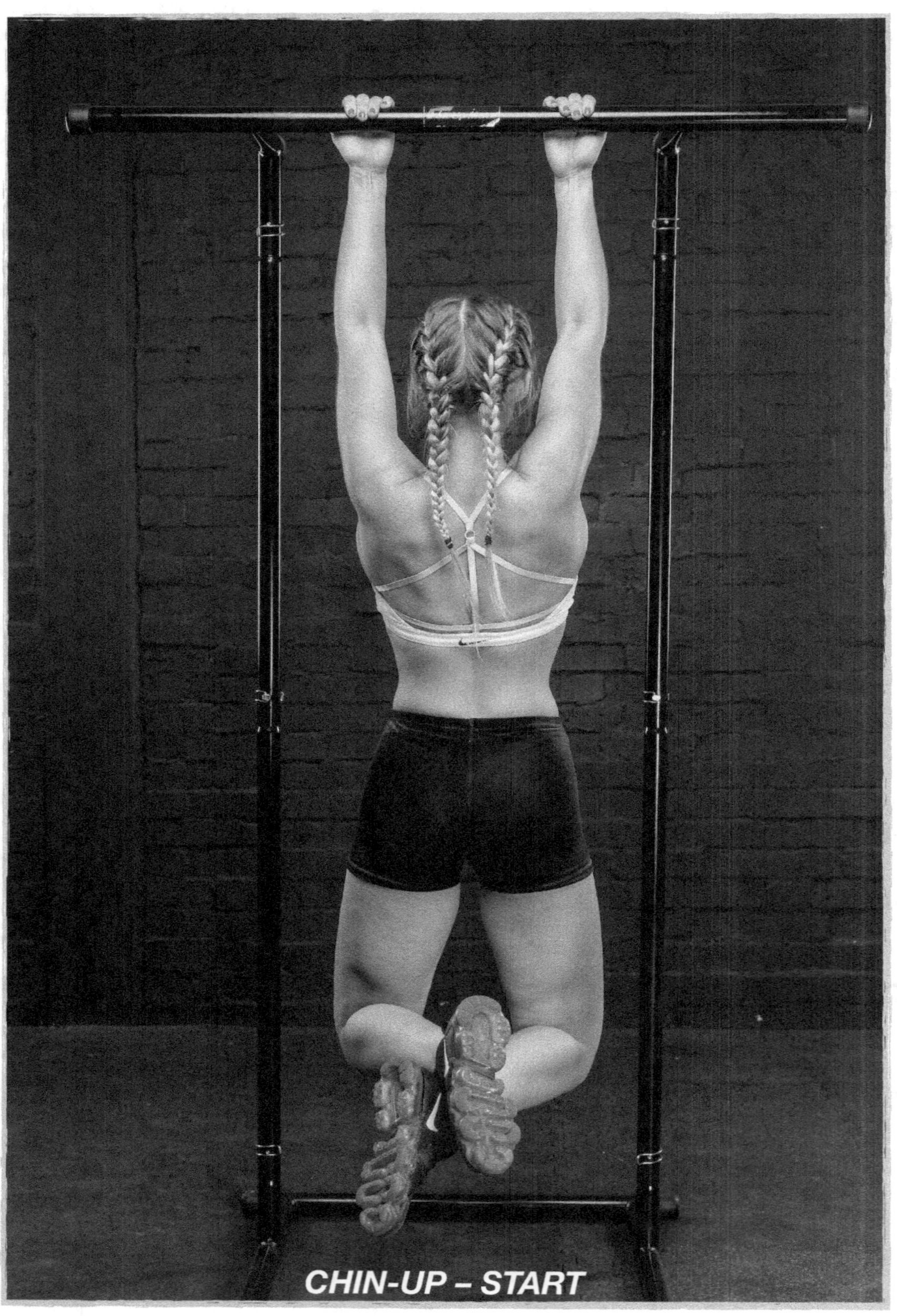

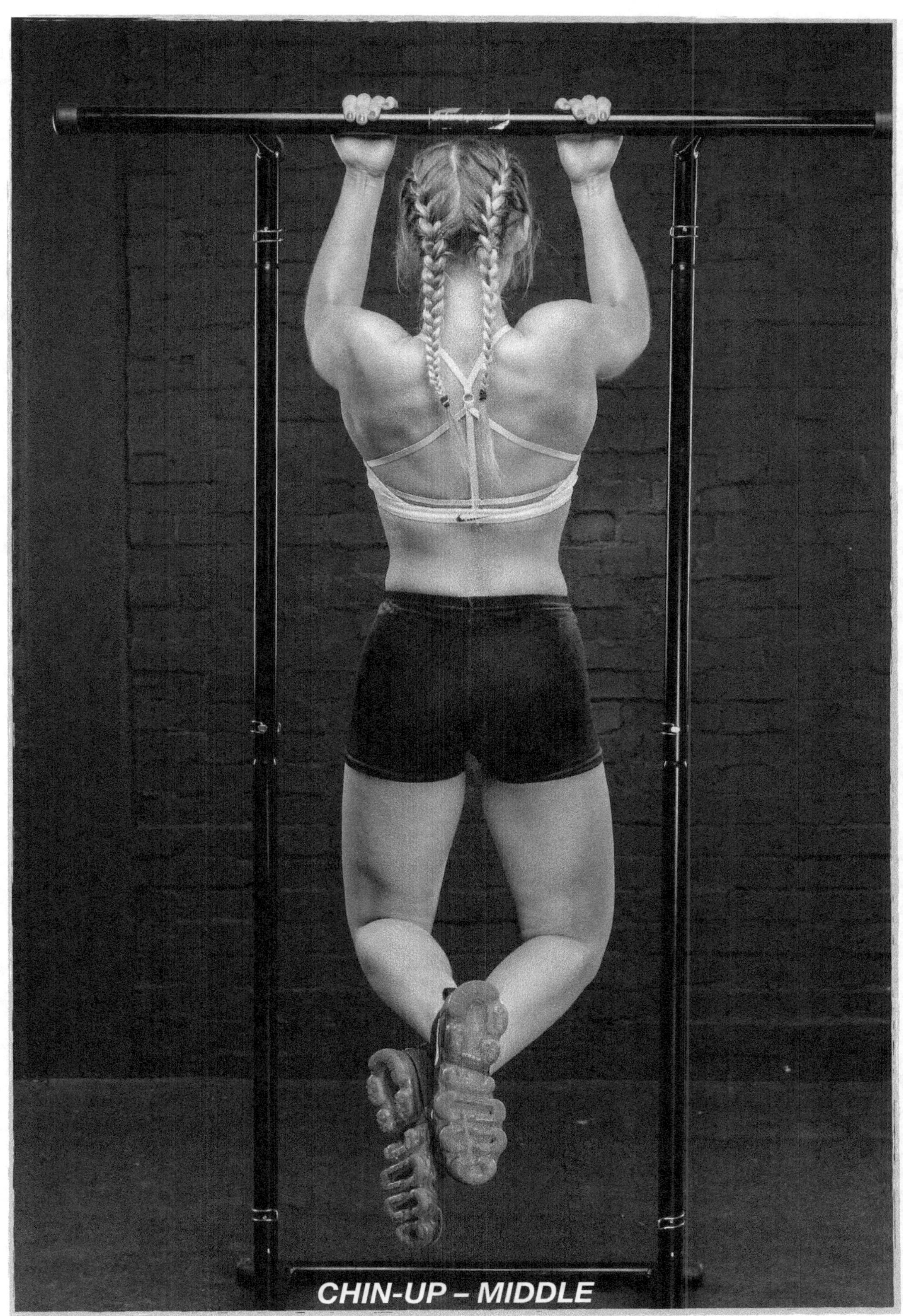

CHIN-UP – MIDDLE

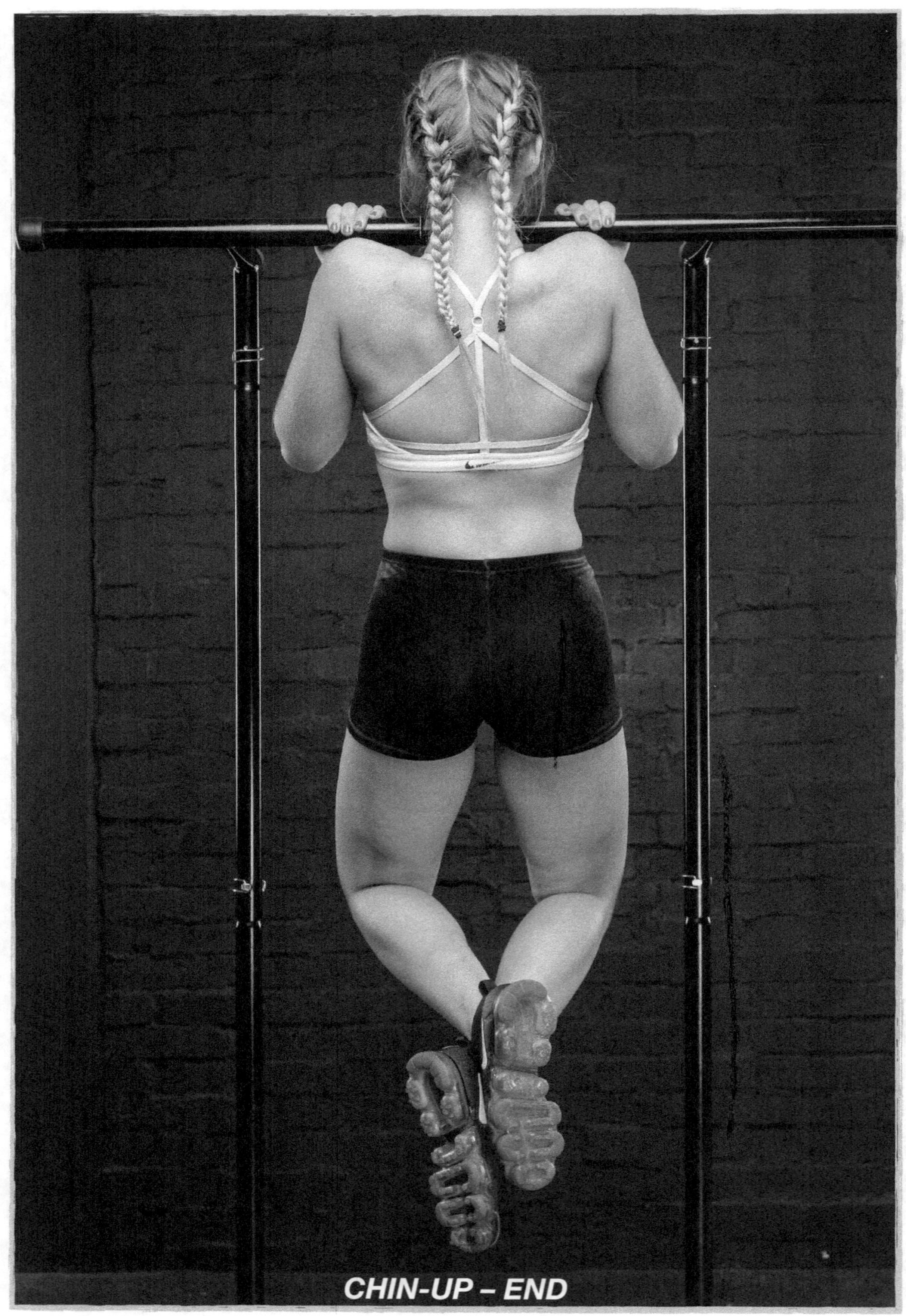

CHIN-UP – END

7.4 PULL-UP

At first glance this entire section may look very similar to the chin-up section; and that's because it is! The chin-up and pull-up are very similar in terms of the muscles that they work, but they differ enough to warrant their own sections here.

The main difference between the chin-up and pull-up is the fact that the chin-up is performed with your palms facing you (or in a supinated grip), and the pull-up is performed with the palms facing away from you (or in a pronated grip). This difference might seem small, but it actually affects the difficulty of the exercise a lot! Pull-ups are generally much harder than chin-ups, for many different reasons, but the main one being that the back is much more involved in the pull-up, and the body position is a little more awkward.

STAGE 1: ROW (PRONATED)

The first stage to learning the pull-up is the pronated row, a movement identical to the row in the previous section, but with the palms facing away from you, or in a "pronated" position.

HOW DO I SET THE EQUIPMENT UP?

For the pronated row you will need a bar that is set at shoulder height, and that can be adjusted up or down in small increments. A squat rack, smith machine, and even a suspension trainer are suitable for this.

HOW DO I DO IT?

1. To perform the pronated row stand in front of the bar and grab it with both hands. Your grip should be shoulder width apart, and your palms should be facing forwards.

2. Position your feet under the bar to start with (the same as with the standing row) then move them forward by a few inches.

3. From here pull on the bar until your chest touches it, or you cannot pull any further. Keep your body straight and head in a neutral position.

4. Pause for a second, and then return to the starting position. This counts as one rep.

HOW MANY SETS AND REPS?

You should be looking to perform 3 to 5 sets of 8 to 12 reps.

HOW DO I ADJUST THE DIFFICULTY?

To make the row easier raise the height of the bar and make your body position more vertical. This will move more weight off the arms and onto the legs. To make the row harder lower the height of the bar and move you feet forwards. This will move more weight onto the upper body.

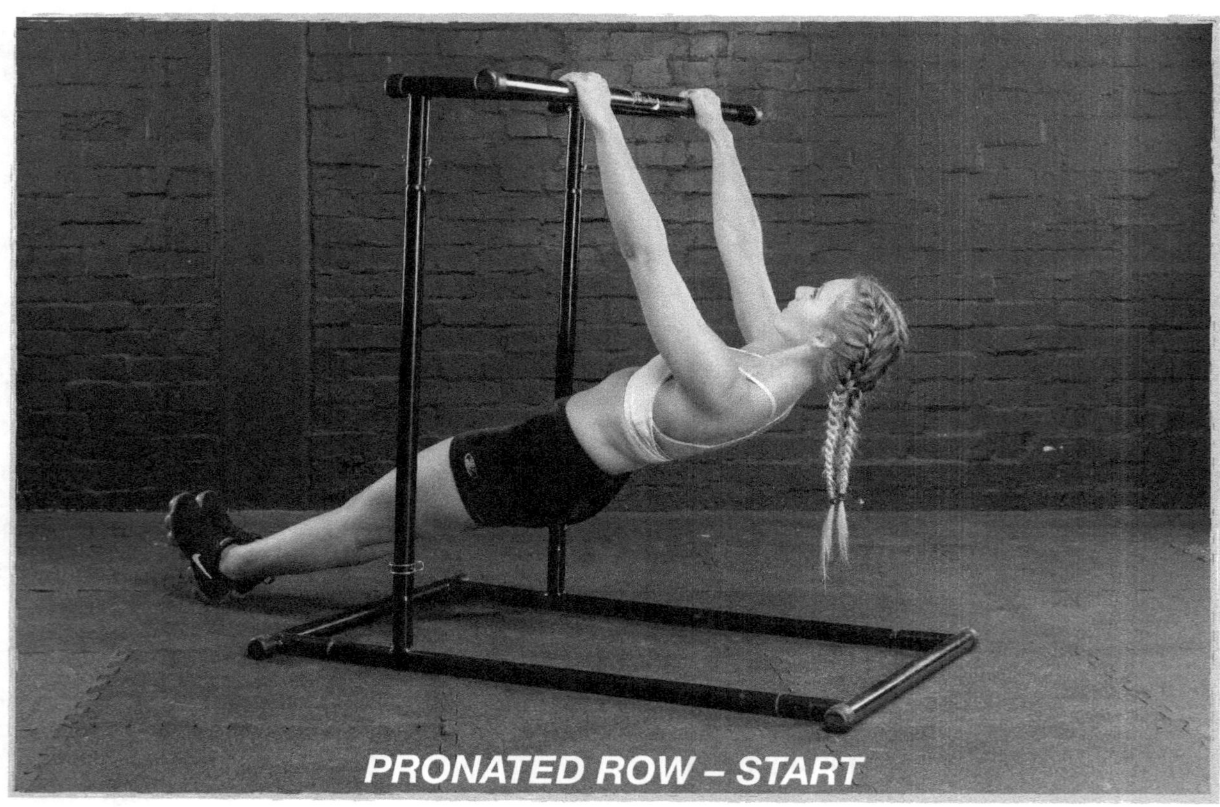

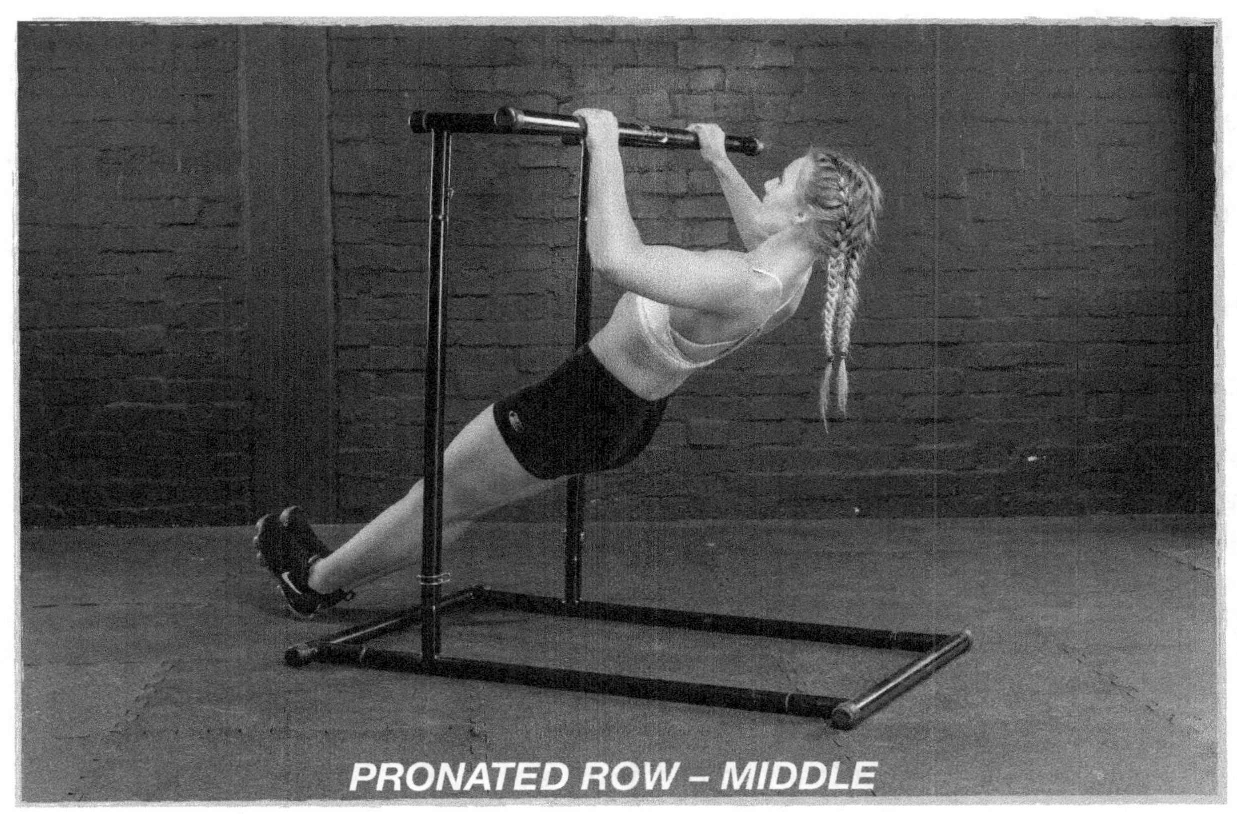

PRONATED ROW – MIDDLE

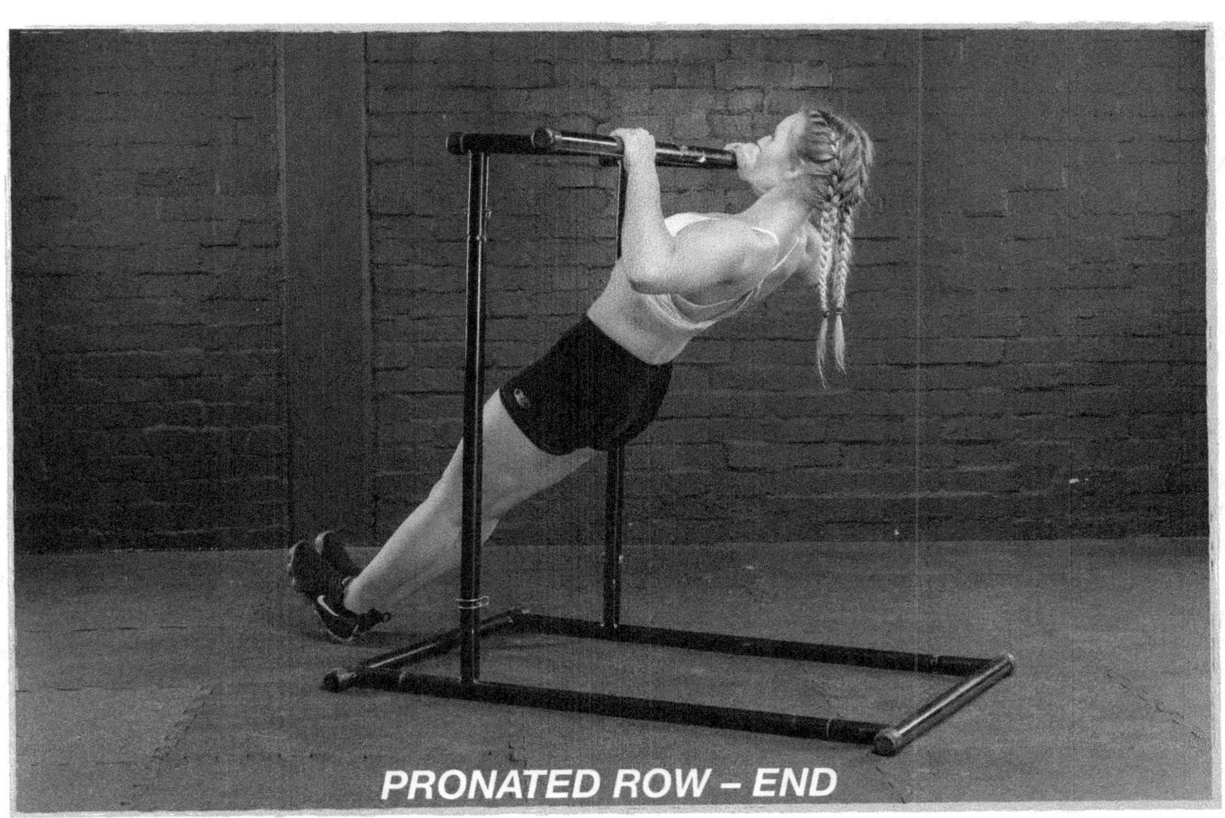

PRONATED ROW – END

STAGE 2: DEAD HANG (PRONATED)

After you've got to grips (sorry, another pun), with the Pronated Row, you will want to work on your grip strength. As with the chin-up, the best way to do this is to simply hang off a bar, in an exercise called the Dead Hang. This time however, your hands will be in the pronated position, instead of the supine one.

HOW DO I SET THE EQUIPMENT UP?

Depending on what type of pull-up bar that you have access to will depend on the set-up here. If the pull-up bar is fixed, then make sure that you can grab the bar without having to jump. Use a box or other type of step to help you here, and make sure that when you let go you are not dropping too far to the ground. Again, smith machines, squat racks, and other similar pieces of equipment are good, as you can set the bar at a height that is suitable for you individually.

HOW DO I DO IT?

1. Grab the pull-up bar with an overhand or pronated grip (palms facing away). Your hands should be slightly wider than shoulder width apart.

2. Make sure that your elbows are straight and your head is in a neutral position.

3. Now lift your feet off the ground, either by bending your knees or lifting your legs up.

4. Now hang onto the bar for as long as possible! Really concentrate on squeezing the bar very tightly, using as much force from your hands and forearms as you can.

5. As soon as you start to feel your grip loosen, or feel that you are going to drop off the bar, then let go and rest. This counts as one rep.

HOW MANY SETS AND REPS?

Perform 5 reps, hanging for as long as you can on each rep, with 45 to 60 seconds rest between each set.

HOW DO I ADJUST THE DIFFICULTY?

To make the dead hang easier use a thinner bar, and to make it more difficult use a thicker bar.

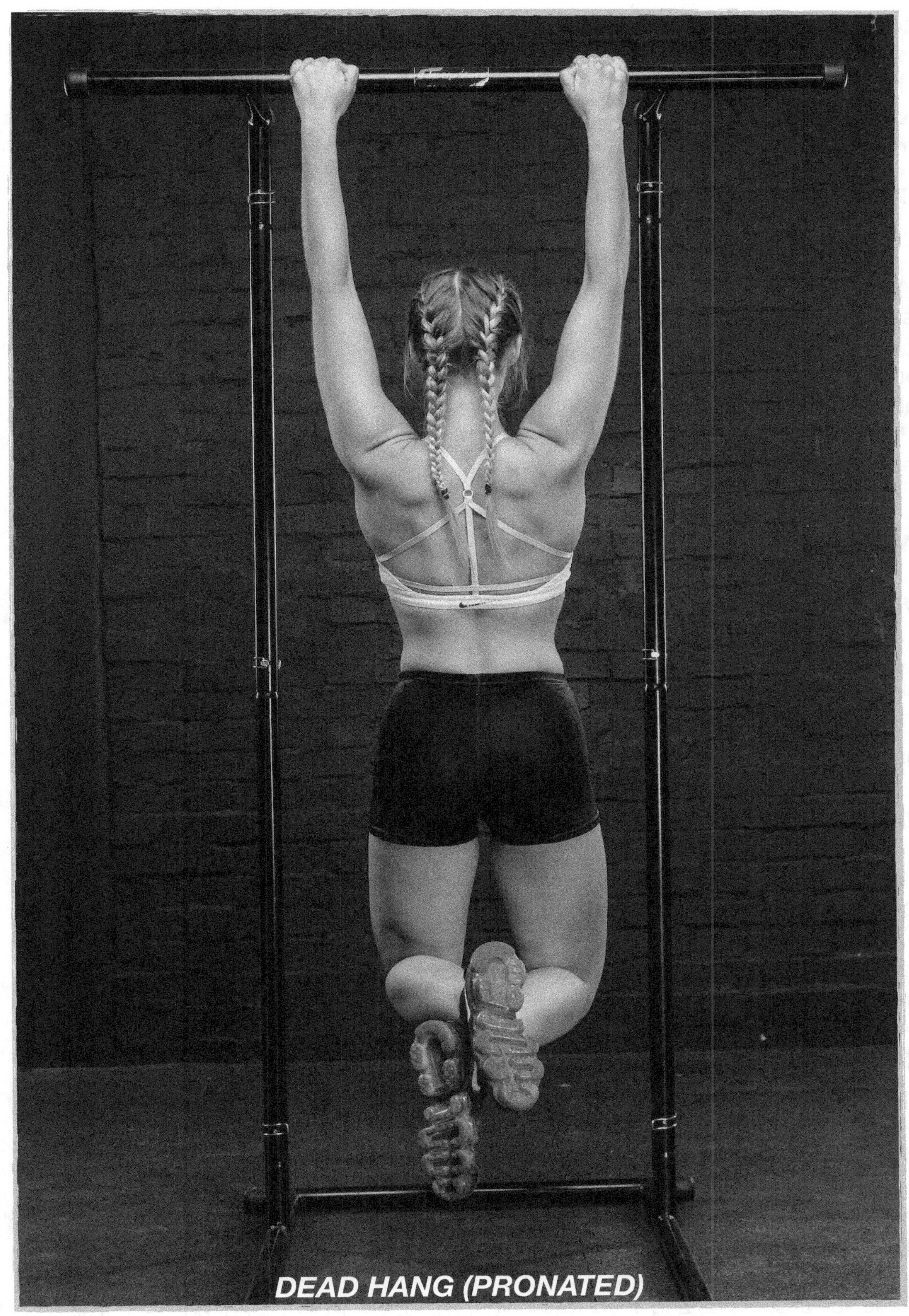

DEAD HANG (PRONATED)

STAGE 3: ASSISTED PULL-UP

The next stage in learning the pull-up is the assisted version. This is exactly the same as the assisted chin-up, except that the hands are in the pronated, or overhand grip position.

HOW DO I SET THE EQUIPMENT UP?

If you're performing the exercise with assistance bands, then choose a band that's heavy in resistance, to make the movement as easy as possible. There will be time to use lighter bands once you've got the hang of the exercise.

If you have access to an assisted machine, start with at least 75% of your body weight. For example, if you weigh 60 kilograms (130 pounds), then put 45 kilograms (100 pounds) on the machine. Remember, the more weight that is on the machine the *easier* the exercise will be!

HOW DO I DO IT?

For the exercise band version:

1. Secure the band on the pull-up bar as detailed earlier. If the pull-up bar is too high to reach without jumping, place a step or box underneath as well.

2. Place your foot or knee (depending on how long the band is), in the loop, and grab the bar with both hands in an overhand (pronated) grip. Hang with your arms straight, allowing the band to stretch and build up resistance.

3. Now pull up hard, keeping your leg straight so that the band can give assistance. Keep pulling until your chin rises above the bar.

4. Pause for a second, and then lower down to the start position. This counts as one rep.

For the assisted machine version:

1. Grip the bar with your palms facing forward, your knees or feet should be in contact with the support pad, and your torso should be vertical.

2. Make sure your arms are completely straight, and then start to pull-up slowly and strongly. Keep going until your chin goes over the bar.

3. Pause for a second, and then lower yourself down to the start position. This counts as one rep.

HOW MANY SETS AND REPS?

You should be looking to perform 3 to 5 sets of 3 to 5 reps.

HOW DO I ADJUST THE DIFFICULTY?

To make the assisted pull-up easier use a heavier band or use more weight on the machine. To make them harder use a lighter band or less weight on the machine.

WHEN DO I MOVE ON?

If you're using an exercise band, then you should move onto the next stage when you can perform 3 sets of 5 to 8 reps with a light band. Many bands are different, so it's impossible to give an exact estimate here, but you should be looking at pulling at least 50% of your body weight.

If you're using an assisted machine, you should move on to the next stage when you can perform 3 sets of 5 to 8 reps with 25% of your body weight on the machine. For example, if you weigh 60 kilograms (130 pounds), then you need to have 15 kilograms (37 pounds) on the machine.

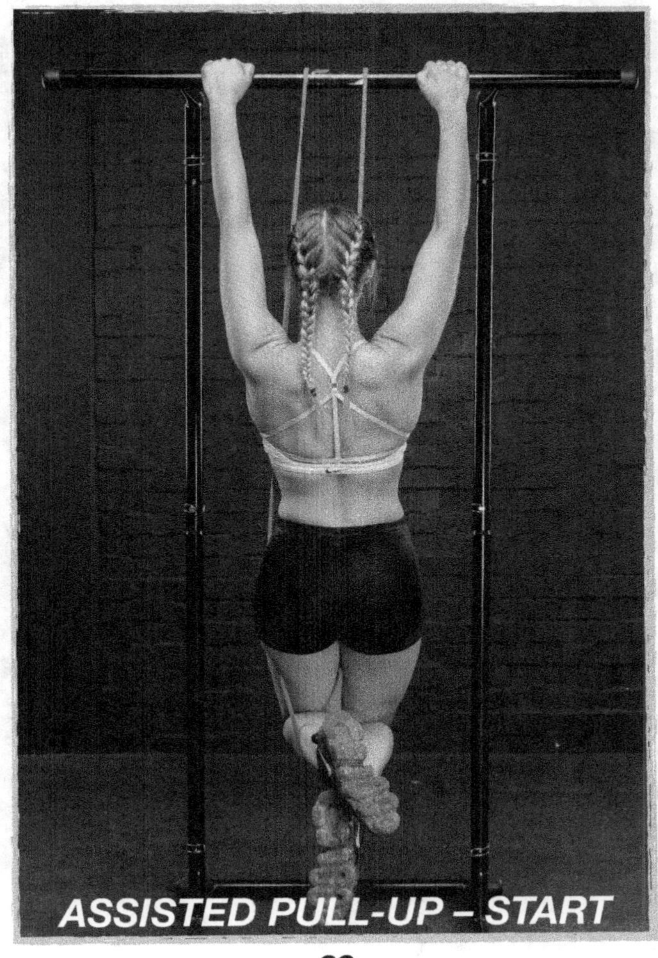

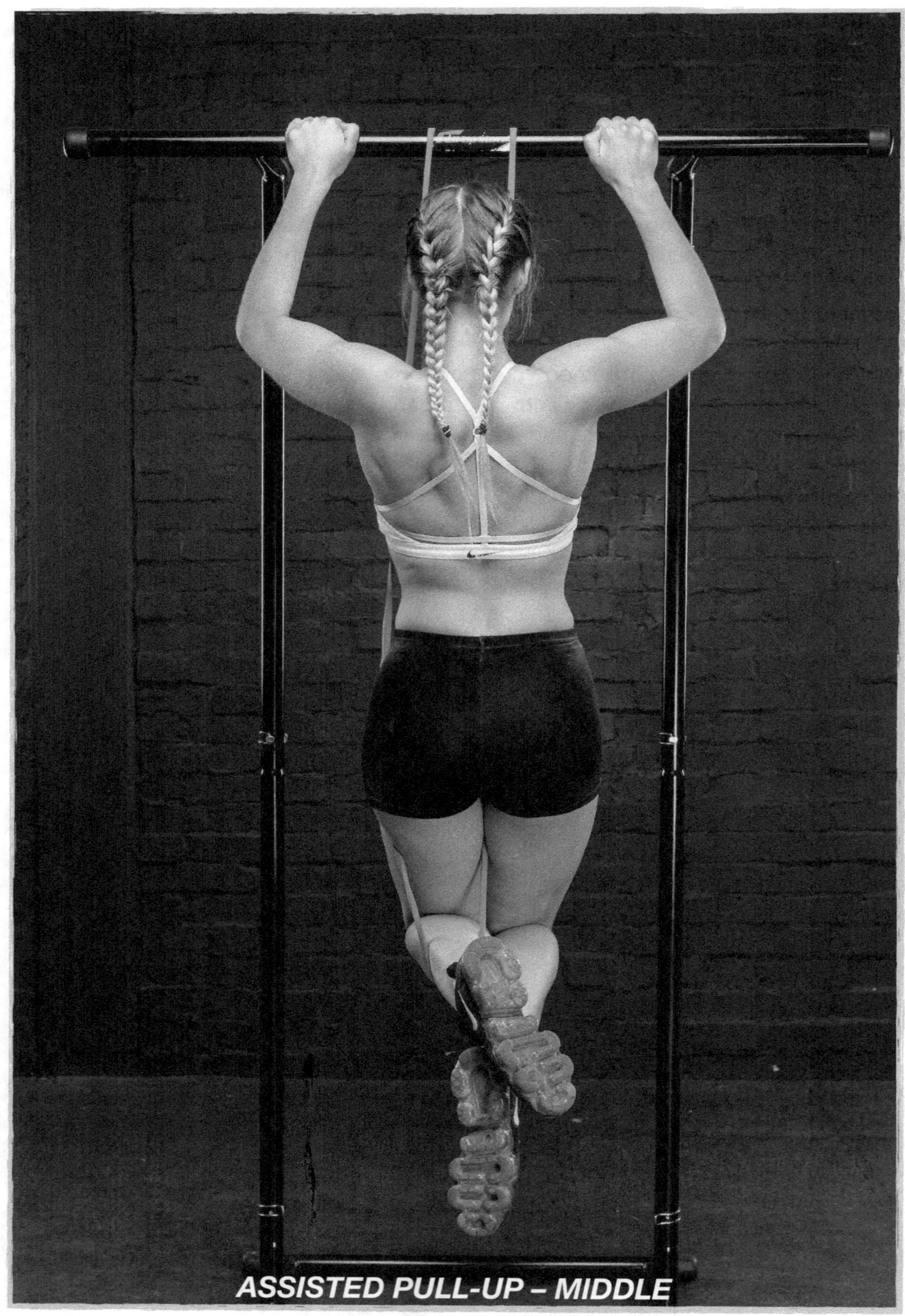

ASSISTED PULL-UP – MIDDLE

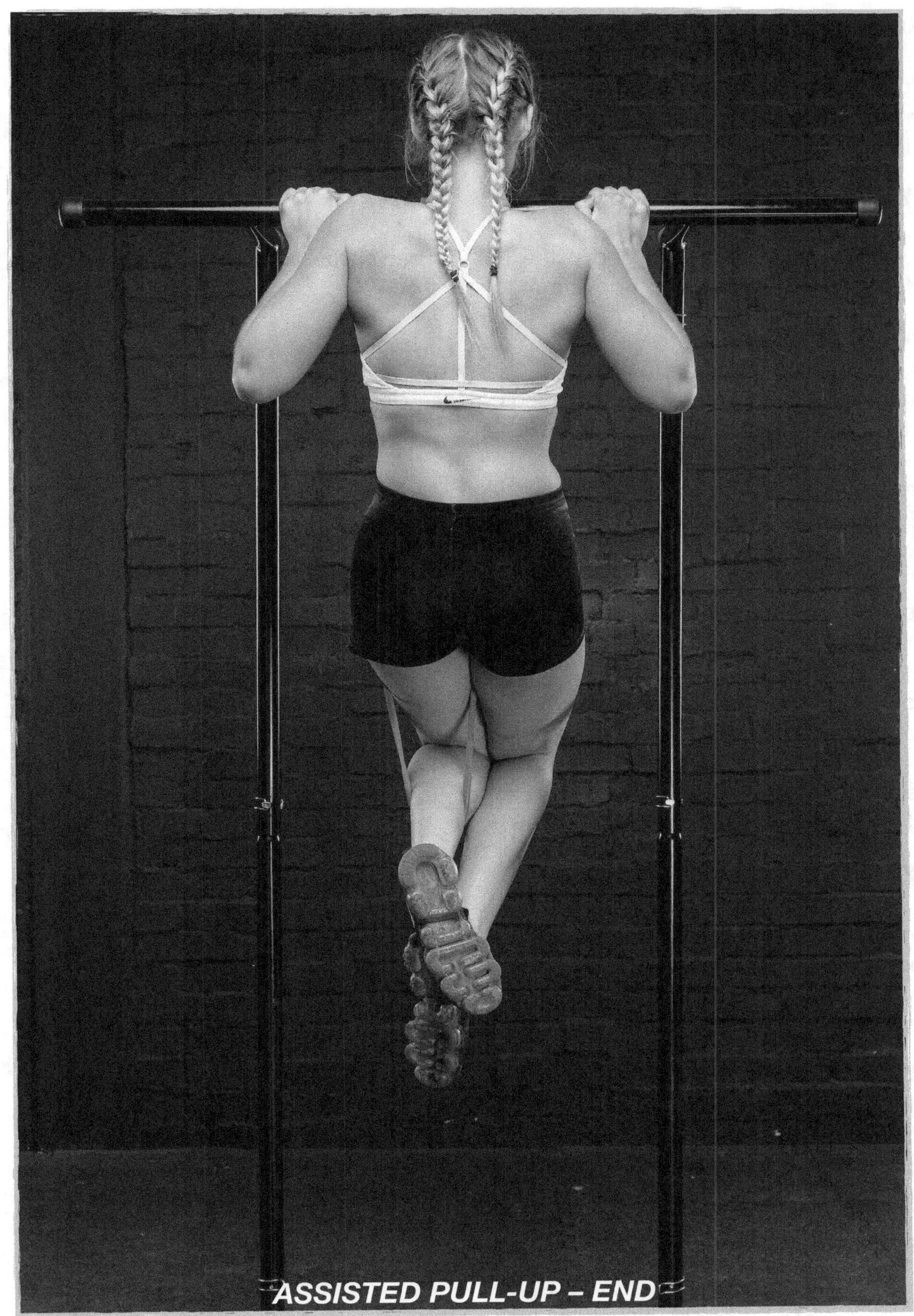
ASSISTED PULL-UP – END

STAGE 4: NEGATIVE PULL-UP

The penultimate stage to learning the pull-up is the negative version, which, like the negative version of the chin-up, really taxes the muscles in a way that builds real strength.

HOW DO I SET THE EQUIPMENT UP?

You will need a pull-up bar, and if the pull-up bar is too high for you to reach comfortably, an exercise step or platform to stand on.

HOW DO I DO IT?

1. Grab the pull-up bar with both hands in an overhand (pronated) grip, hands slightly wider than shoulder width apart.

2. Step onto the platform and stand up straight, so that your chin is either level with the bar or over it (if your bar is low then you may be able to stand on the floor and get into this position).

3. Contract your muscles hard and pull down. Now take your feet off the box (or lift them off the ground if your bar is low) and hold yourself at the top of the position.

4. Now start to lower yourself as slowly as possible. Pull on the bar very hard, but let your muscles lengthen as gravity pulls you down.

5. Keep going all the way until your arms are completely straight, then drop off or let go of the bar, and rest. This counts as one rep.

HOW MANY SETS AND REPS?

Again, as the negative exercises work differently to the other exercises, you should be looking to do 3 to 5 sets of 1. So, you would do 1 rep, taking as long as possible to lower yourself to the bottom position, then rest, and then repeat 2 to 4 more times.

HOW DO I ADJUST THE DIFFICULTY?

To make the negative pull-up more difficult simply take longer to lower yourself down to the bottom position. To make it easier take less time to lower yourself down to the bottom position.

WHEN DO I MOVE ON?

You should move on to the next stage when it takes you at least 15 to 20 seconds to do a single rep.

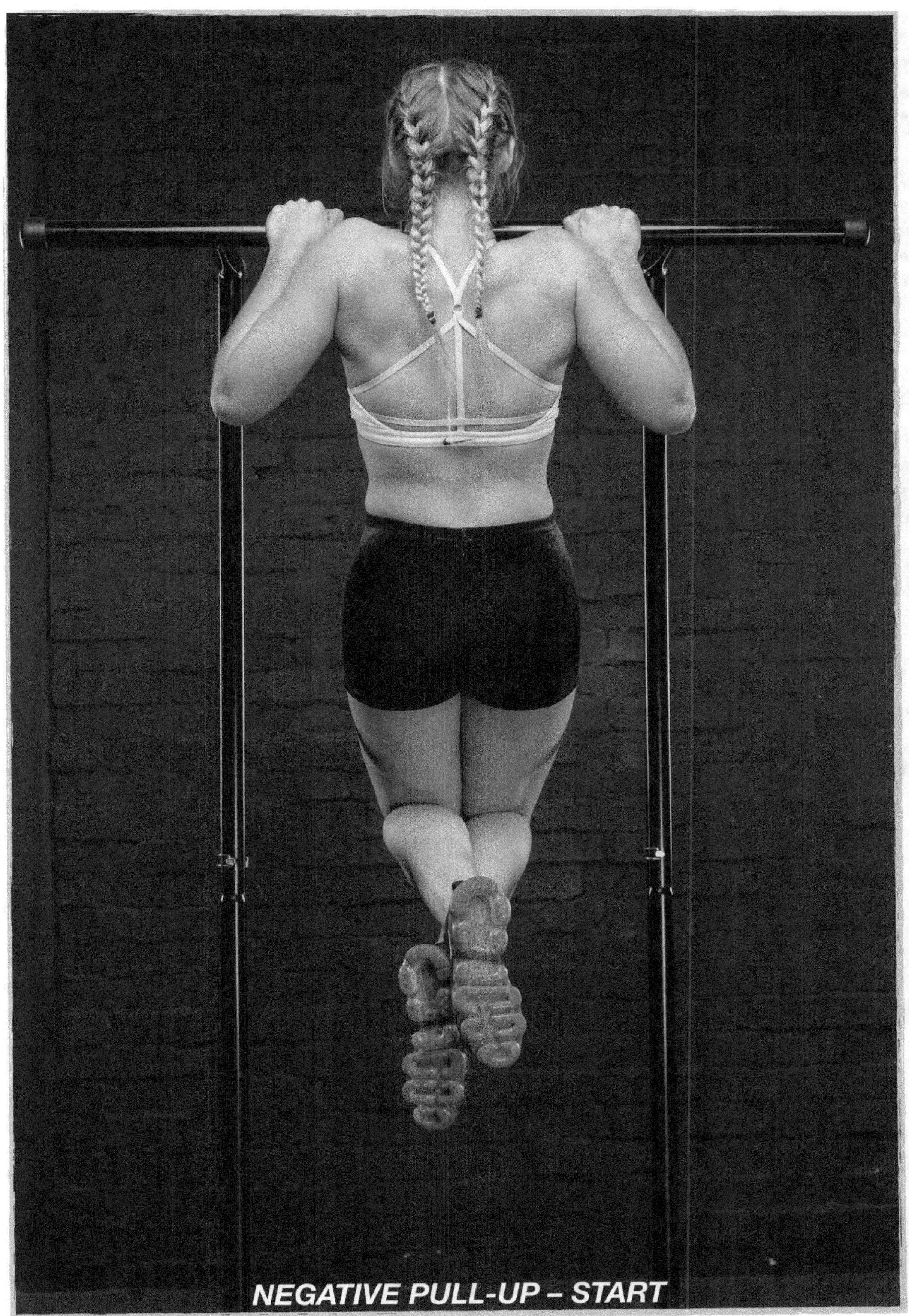

NEGATIVE PULL-UP – START

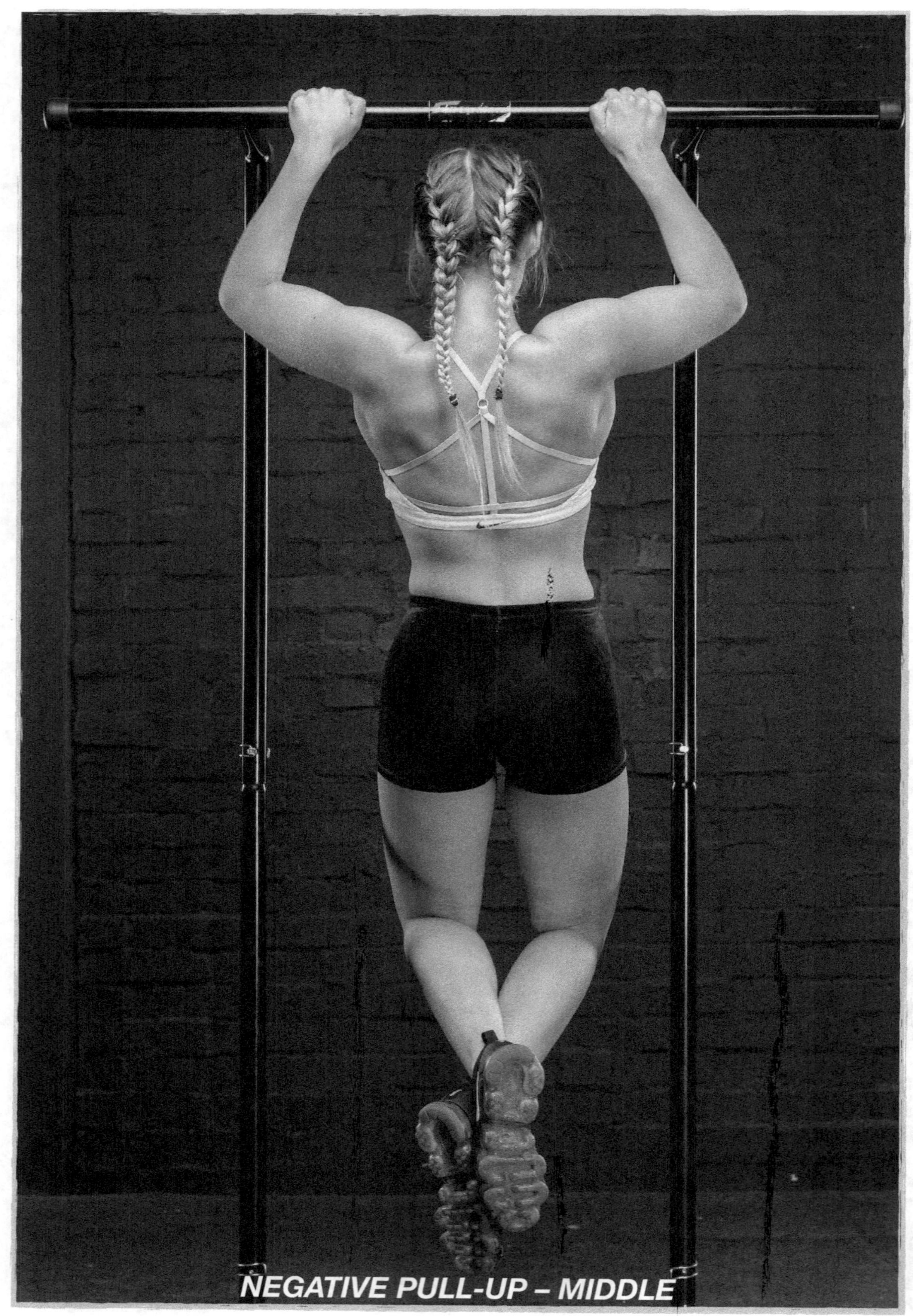

NEGATIVE PULL-UP – MIDDLE

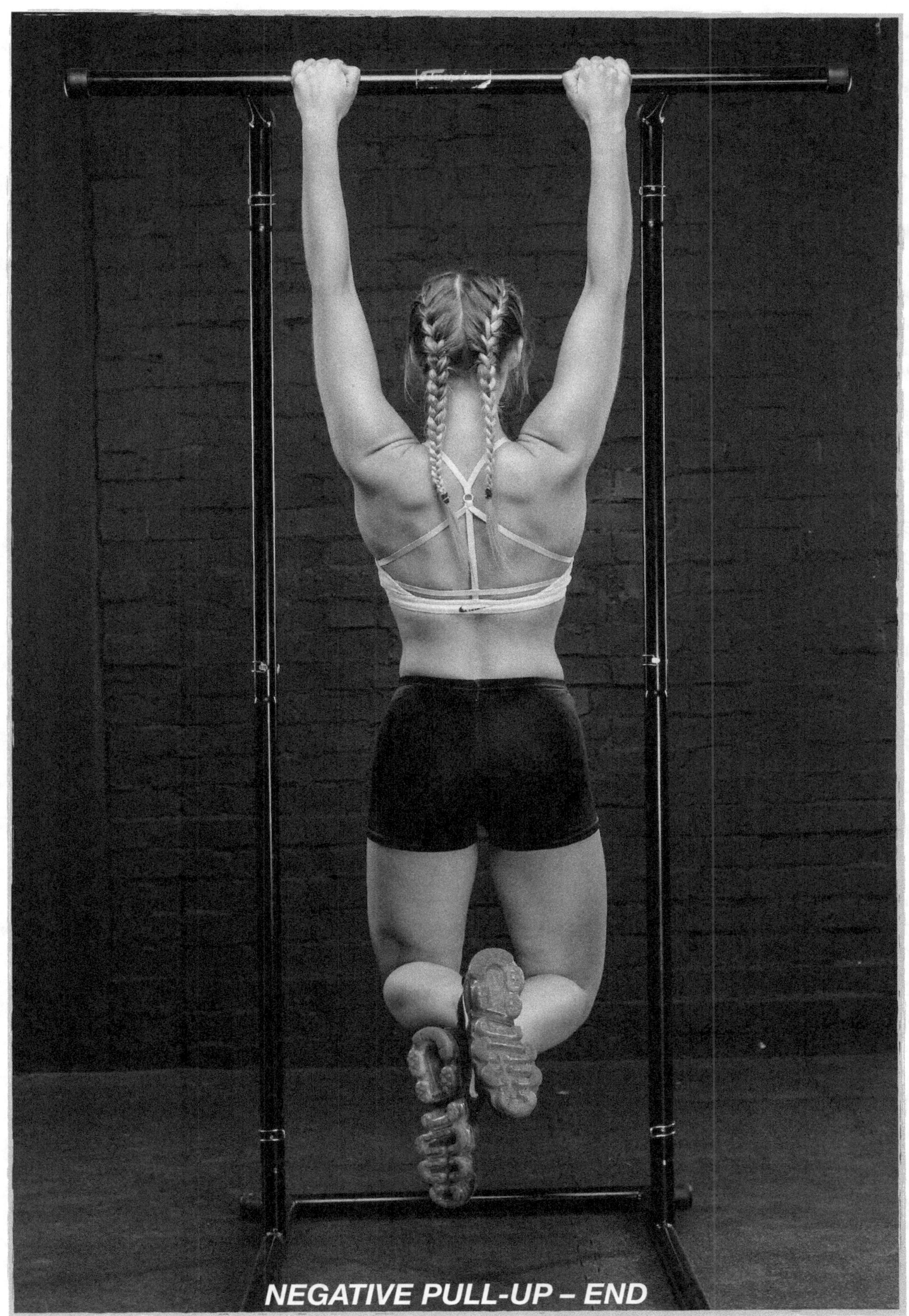

NEGATIVE PULL-UP – END

PULL-UP

OK, so nearly there! This stage is the pull-up for real, with no assistance, full range of motion, and proper form. It may take you a while to get these, so don't worry if it doesn't happen straight away. Also, feel free to go back and visit the earlier variations if these prove too tough.

HOW DO I SET THE EQUIPMENT UP?

You will need a pull-up bar, and if it's too high to reach comfortably, an exercise step or platform to stand on.

HOW DO I DO IT?

1. Grab the pull-up bar with an overhand (pronated) grip, with your hands slightly wider than shoulder width apart.

2. Hang from the bar, making sure your arms are completely straight, and then start to pull-up slowly and strongly. Keep going until your chin goes over the bar.

3. Pause for a second, and then lower yourself down to the start position. This counts as one rep.

HOW MANY SETS AND REPS?

Ideally you should be aiming for 3 to 5 sets of 3 to 5 reps. It may be a while until you can do this, so start by doing 3 to 5 sets of 1 rep, and build up from there.

HOW DO I ADJUST THE DIFFICULTY?

To make the pull-up easier you can reduce the range of motion, and keep a slight bend in the arms at the bottom of the movement. To make them harder (are you mad?!) you can remain in the dead hang position for longer, hold yourself in the top position for longer, slow the movement down, and increase the range of motion as much as possible.

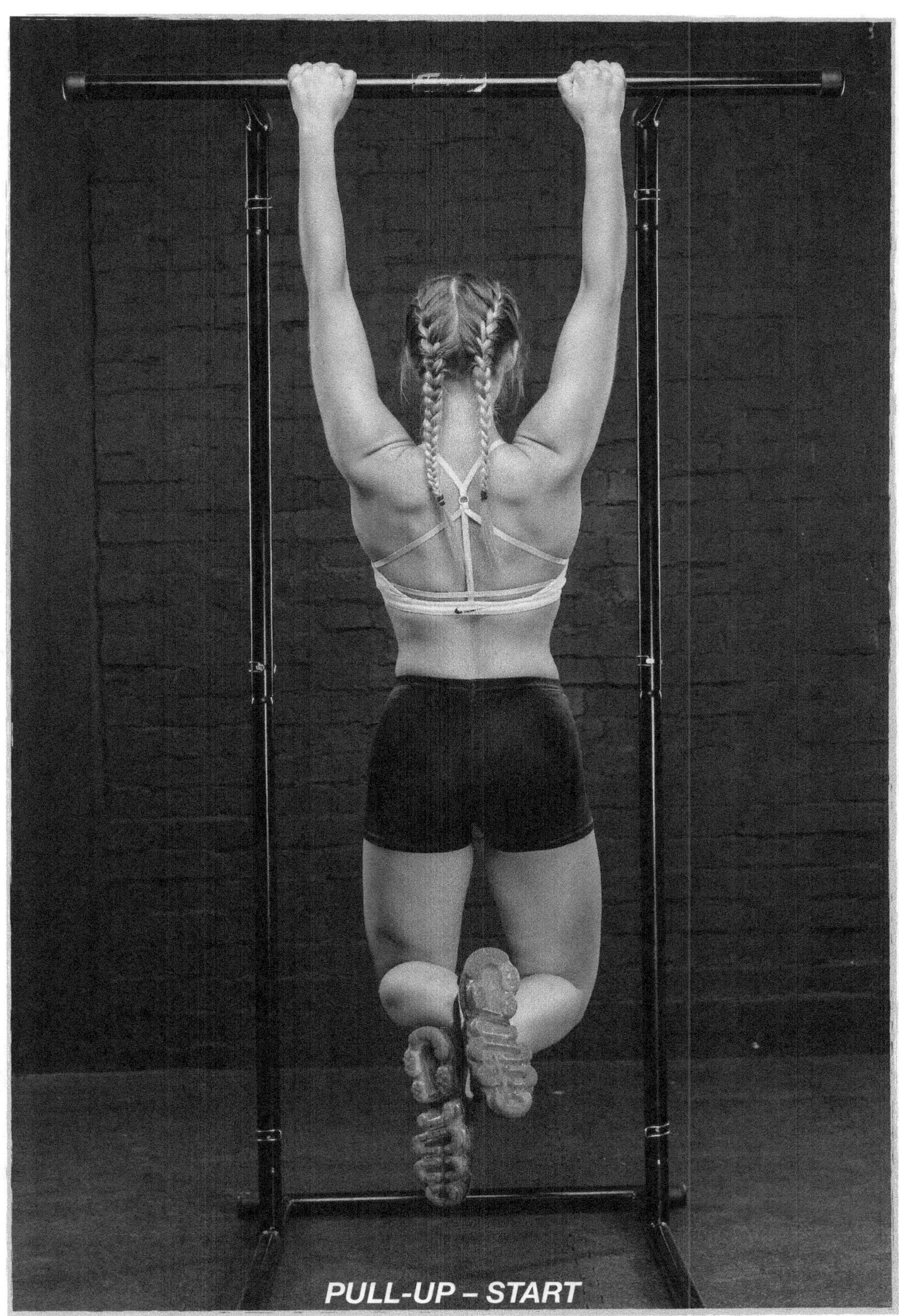

PULL-UP – START

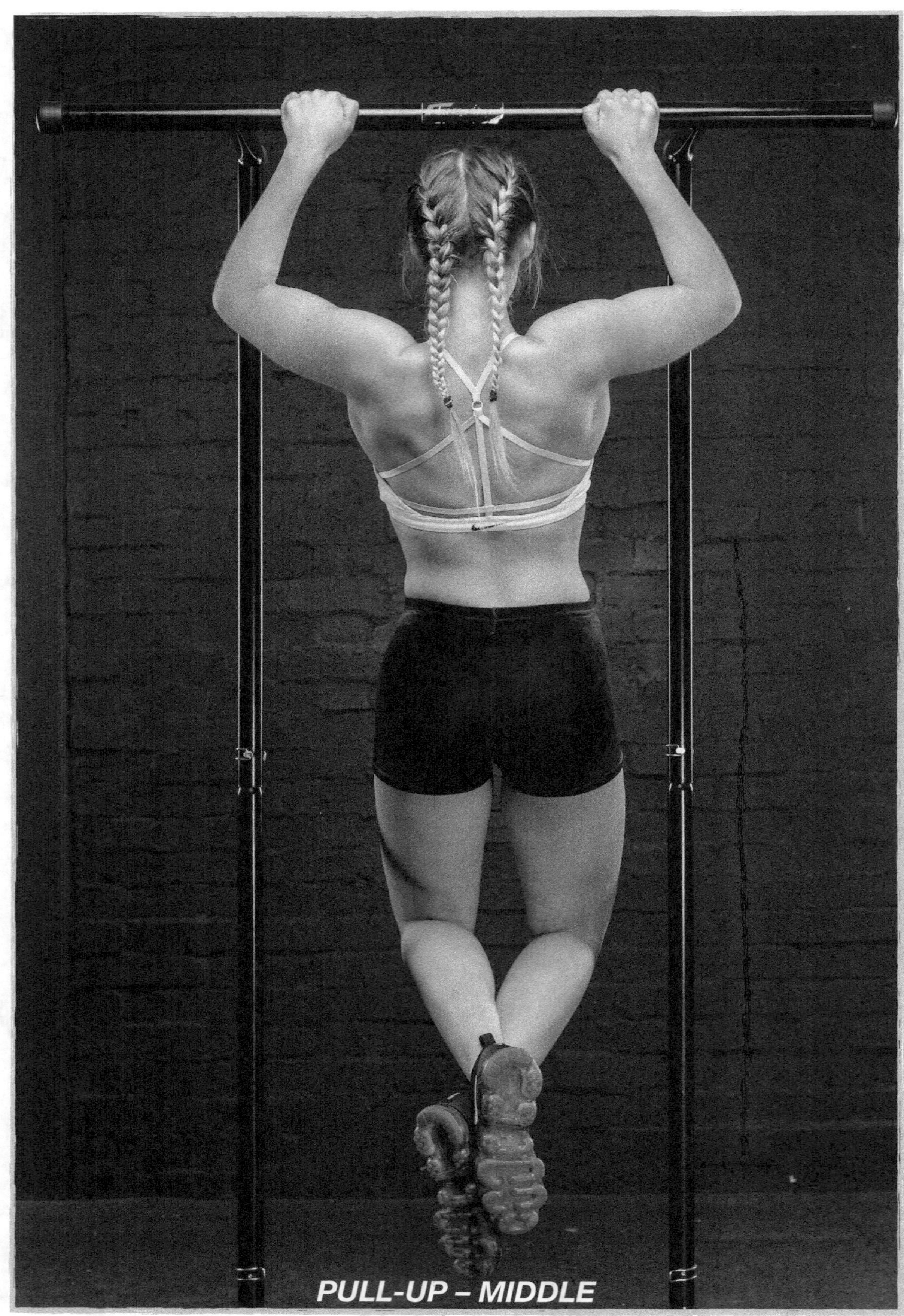

PULL-UP – MIDDLE

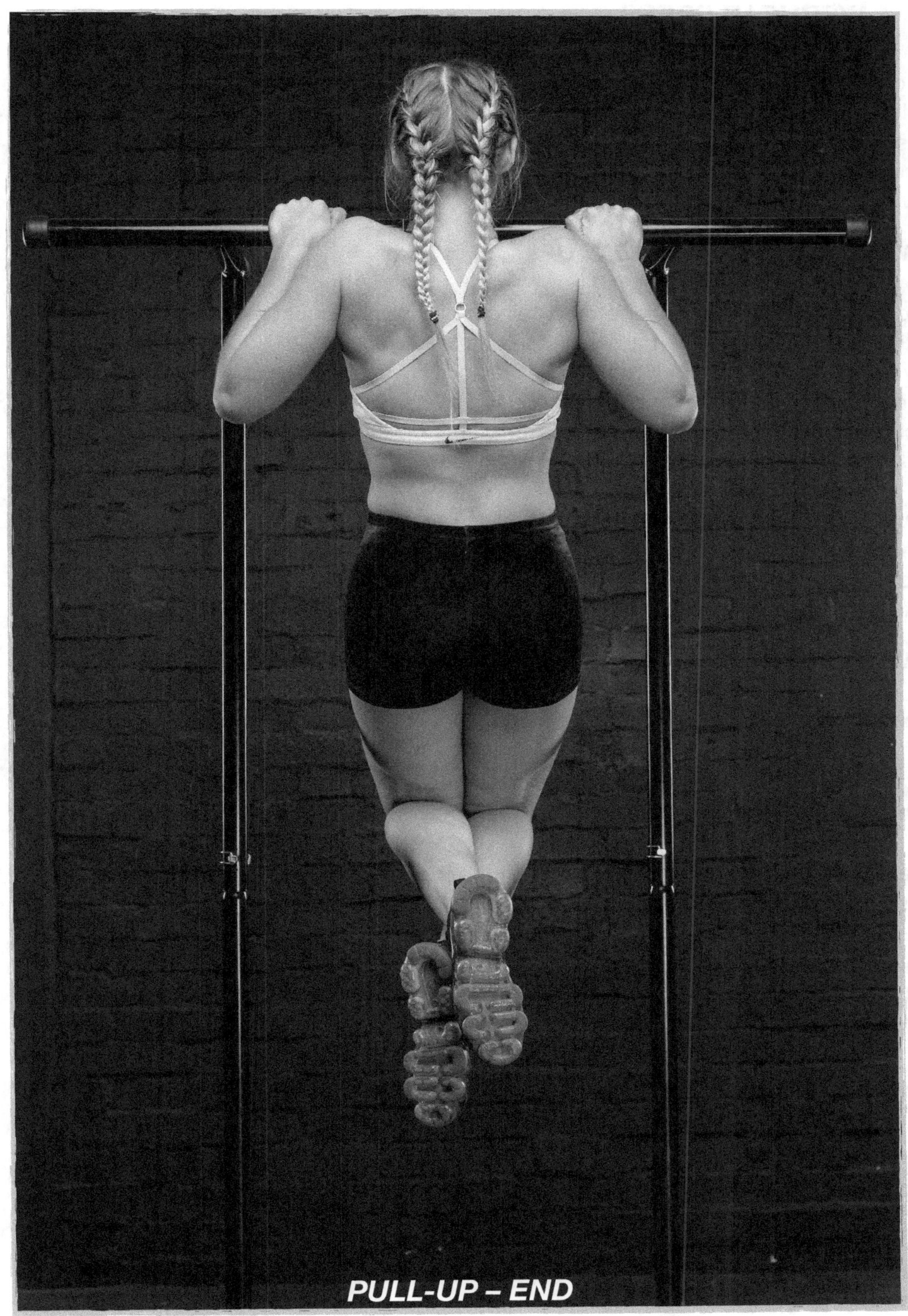

PULL-UP – END

7.5 Overhead Press

The overhead press is a very popular strongman event, but before you run away, stop! It's also great for building strength throughout the entire body, and will sculpt and shape the shoulders and arms like nothing else. It's scalable for a wide range of abilities, and using a squat rack will enable safe performance of the exercise every time.

HOW DO I SET THE EQUIPMENT UP?

The overhead press is best performed using a barbell and squat rack.
Starting with Olympic style barbells (the ones that are 15 to 20 kg / 30 to 45 lbs) is likely to be too difficult for most people, so it is best to use an exercise class barbell, or one that is light enough for you to lift easily. If you are using weight plates check that you have the same number of plates on each end of the bar. It's also a good idea to use clips to secure the plates in place.

If you are using the squat rack to support the bar make sure that the hooks are the correct level. You should be able to grab the bar with knees slightly bent, and then stand up wit the bar safely. This way you can also replace the bar back on the hooks without bending down, which is safer.

HOW DO I DO IT?

1. Load the bar with the correct weight, and place it on the hooks of the squat rack.

2. Stand directly underneath the bar, and grip it with you hands. Your hands should be about shoulder width apart, with your thumb wrapped around the bar.

3. Make sure that the bar is in contact with the top of your chest, and then stand up fully so that you take control of the bar.

4. Take a small step backwards so that the bar will clear any obstacle above your head. Make sure that your feet are planted, and slightly wider than shoulder width apart.

5. Now press the bar overhead strongly and smoothly, moving your head and shoulders as they need to. Keep your eyes looking forward.

6. Keep pressing until your arms become straight. At this point the bar should be directly overhead, and your head should be directly between your arms.

7. Pause for a second, and then lower the bar back to the starting position. This counts as one rep.

8. To replace the bar, simply take a step forward and lower the bar on to the hooks.

HOW MANY SETS AND REPS?

You should be looking to perform 3 to 5 sets of 8 to 12 reps.

HOW DO I ADJUST THE DIFFICULTY?

The difficulty of the overhead press can be adjusted in a number of ways. To make the movement easier reduce the weight, reduce the range of motion, use your legs to drive the bar into the air, do fewer reps, or do fewer sets. To make the exercise harder increase the weight, increase the range of motion, don't allow the legs to help out, do more reps, and do more sets.

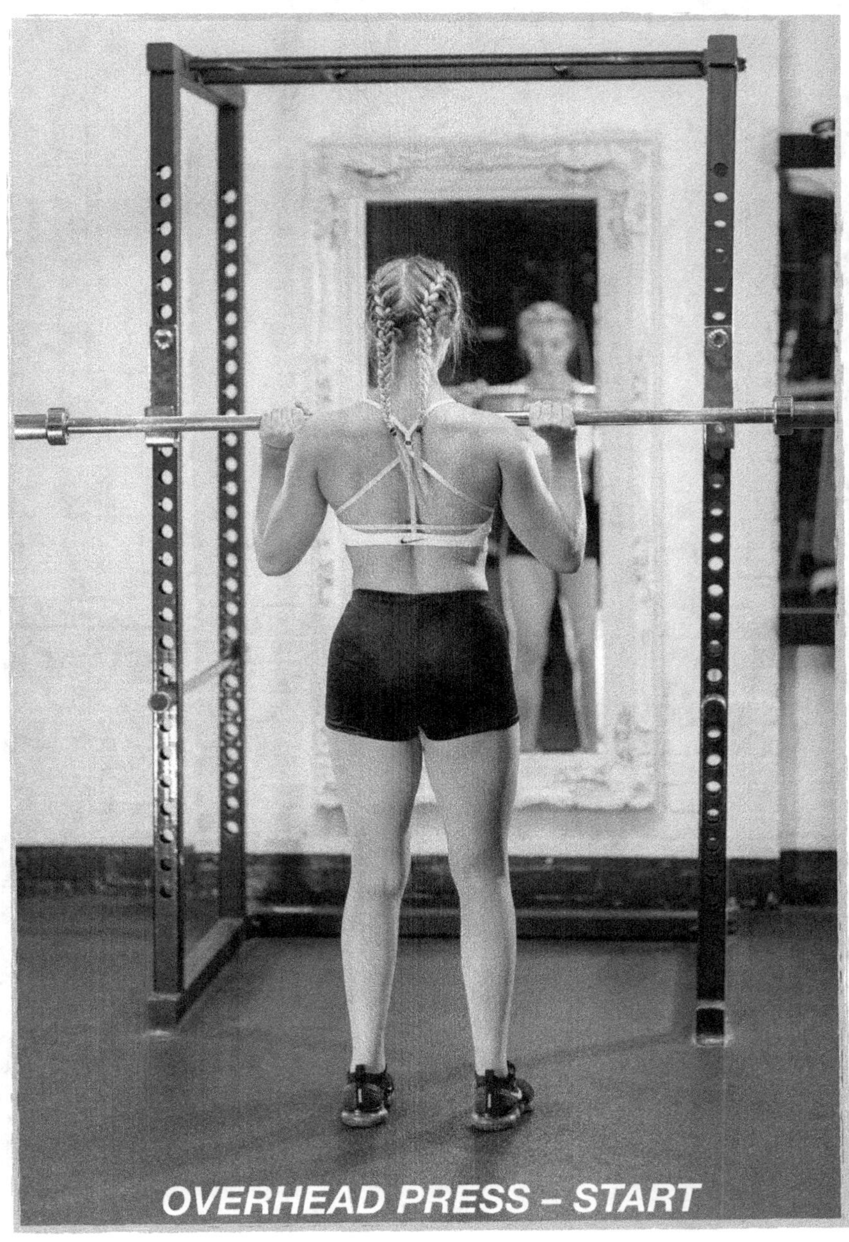

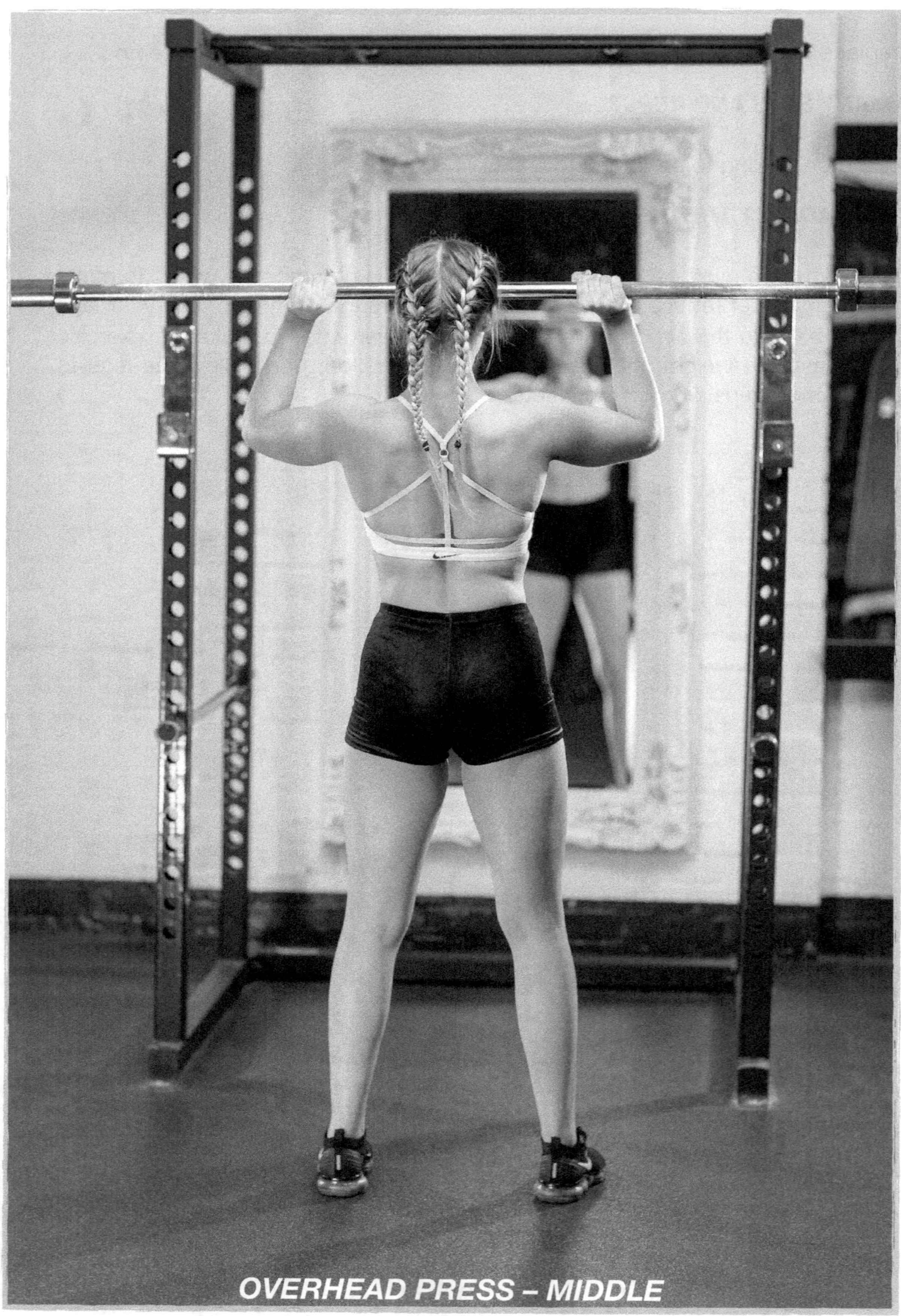

OVERHEAD PRESS – MIDDLE

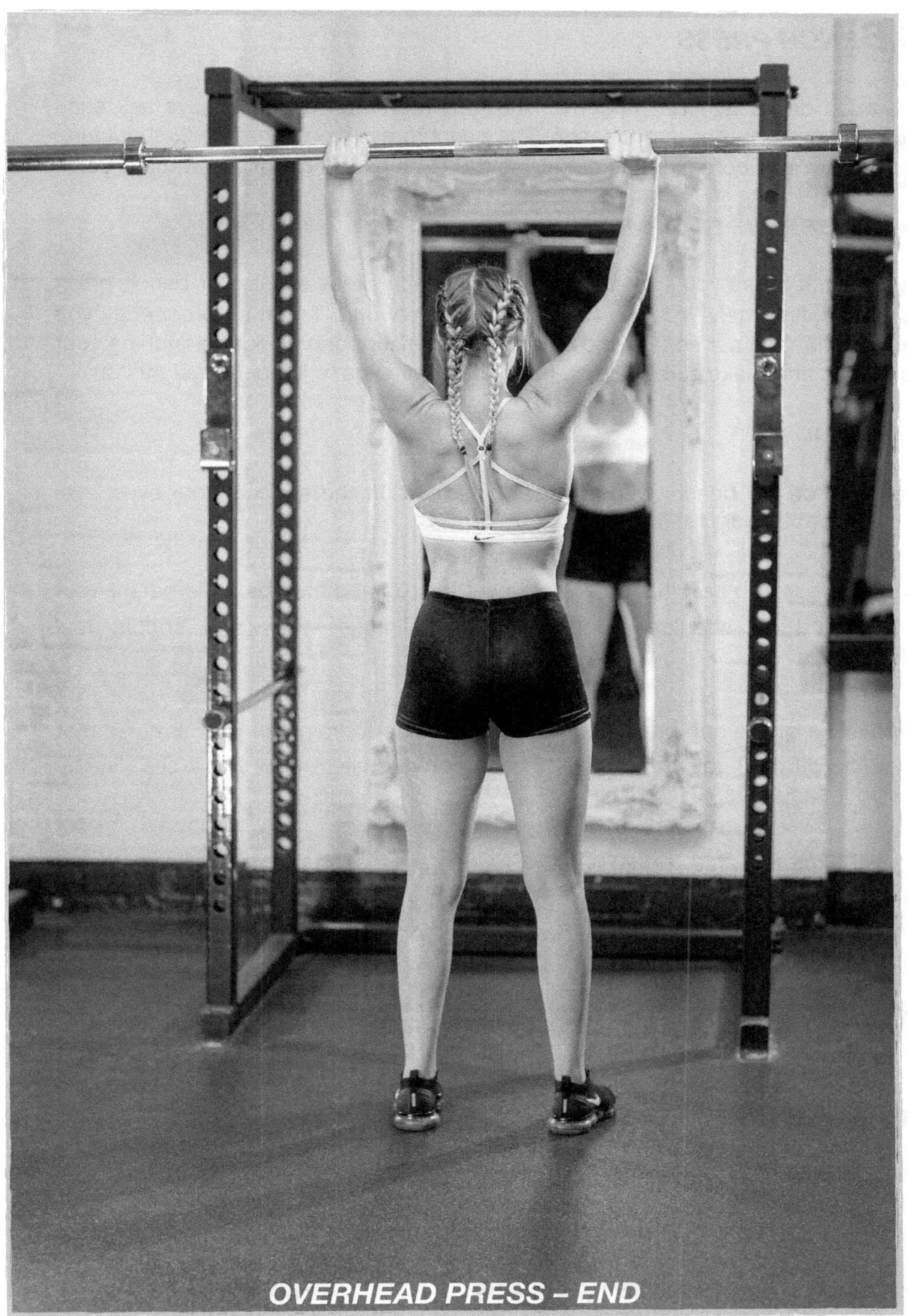

OVERHEAD PRESS – END

7.6 BENCH PRESS

"How much do ya bench?" might be the most common question guys ask each other in the gym, but for good reason! The bench press works the chest, shoulders, backs of the arms, core, and the glutes, so this is an exercise that you want to do!

HOW DO I SET THE EQUIPMENT UP?

For the bench press you'll need access to a bench press station, or bench press bench. You'll find these in almost every gym in the world. To set it up correctly you should position the bar so that you can lift it off the supports without stretching your arms too far, and make sure that you have collars or clips to keep the weights on.

HOW DO I DO IT?

1. Lie down on the bench, with your back flat against the surface, your eyes level with the bar, and your feet flat on the floor.

2. Grab the bar with both hands, fingers over the top and thumbs underneath. Your hands should be shoulder width apart, or slightly wider, and should feel comfortable.

3. Tense your glutes and press your feet into the floor. Straighten your arms so that the bar lifts off the hooks, and move the bar forward slightly so that it sits directly above your shoulders.

4. Making sure you core is tight, start to bend your elbows and lower the bar down towards your chest. Keep lowering the bar until it touches your chest. Make sure that the bar doesn't wander towards your head or feet; it should stay above your shoulders at all times.

5. Pause for a second, and then press upwards, straightening the elbows until your arms are straight. This counts as one rep.

HOW MANY SETS AND REPS?

You should be looking to perform 3 to 5 sets of 8 to 12 reps.

HOW DO I ADJUST THE DIFFICULTY?

There are a few ways the difficulty of the bench press can be adjusted. To make it easier you can reduce the weight, reduce the range of motion, and do fewer reps and sets. To increase the difficulty you can increase the weight, increase the range of motion, and do more sets and reps.

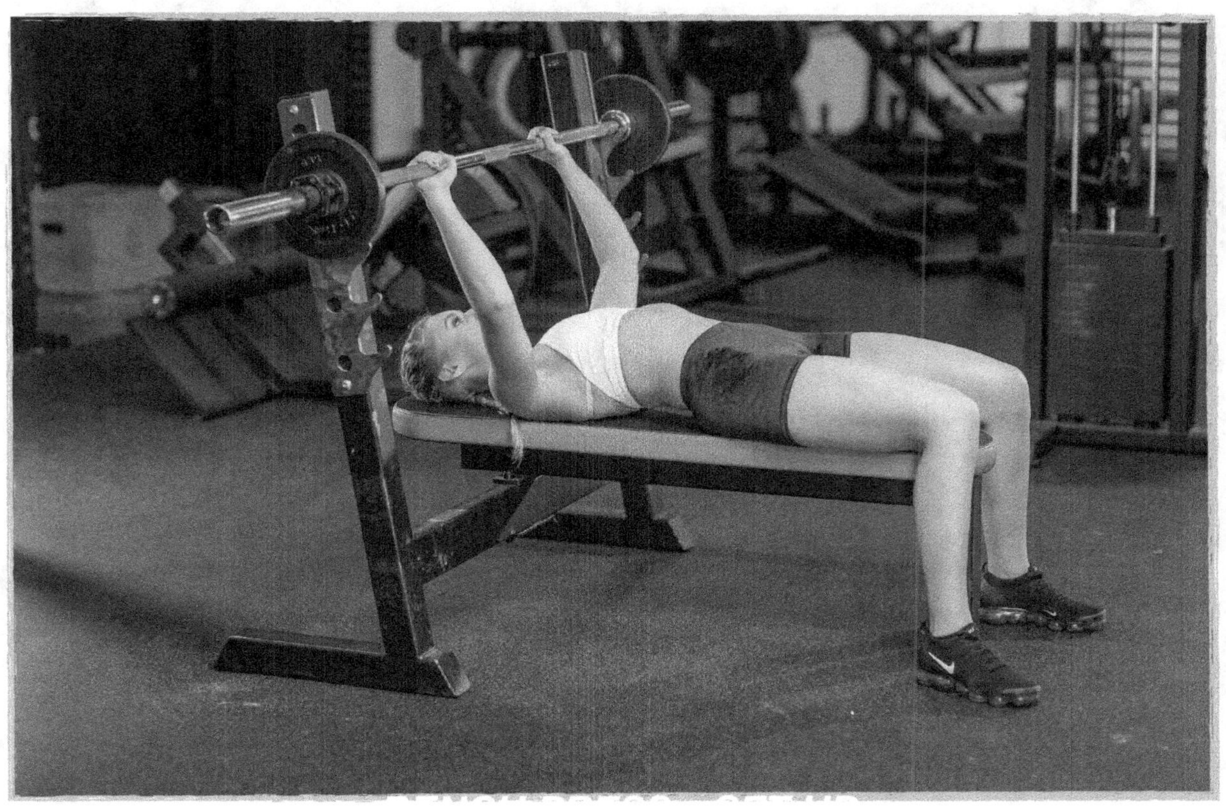

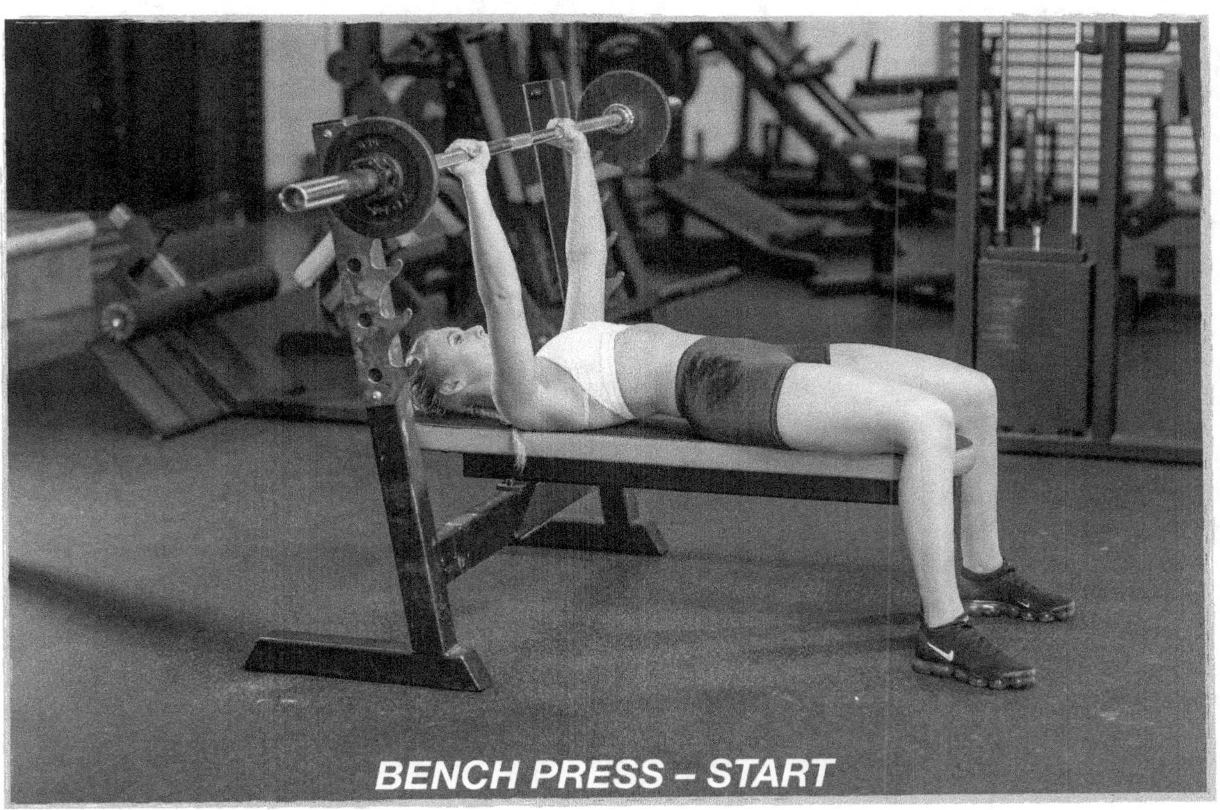

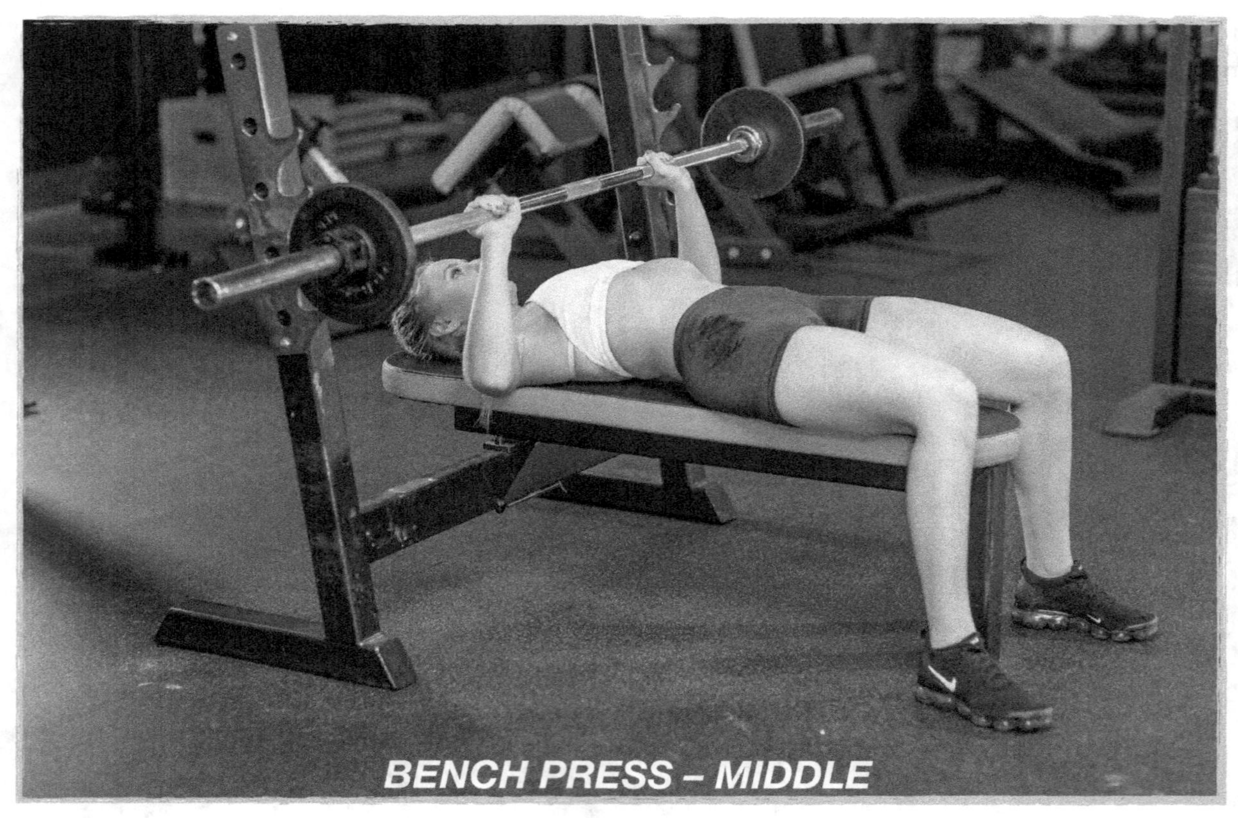

BENCH PRESS – MIDDLE

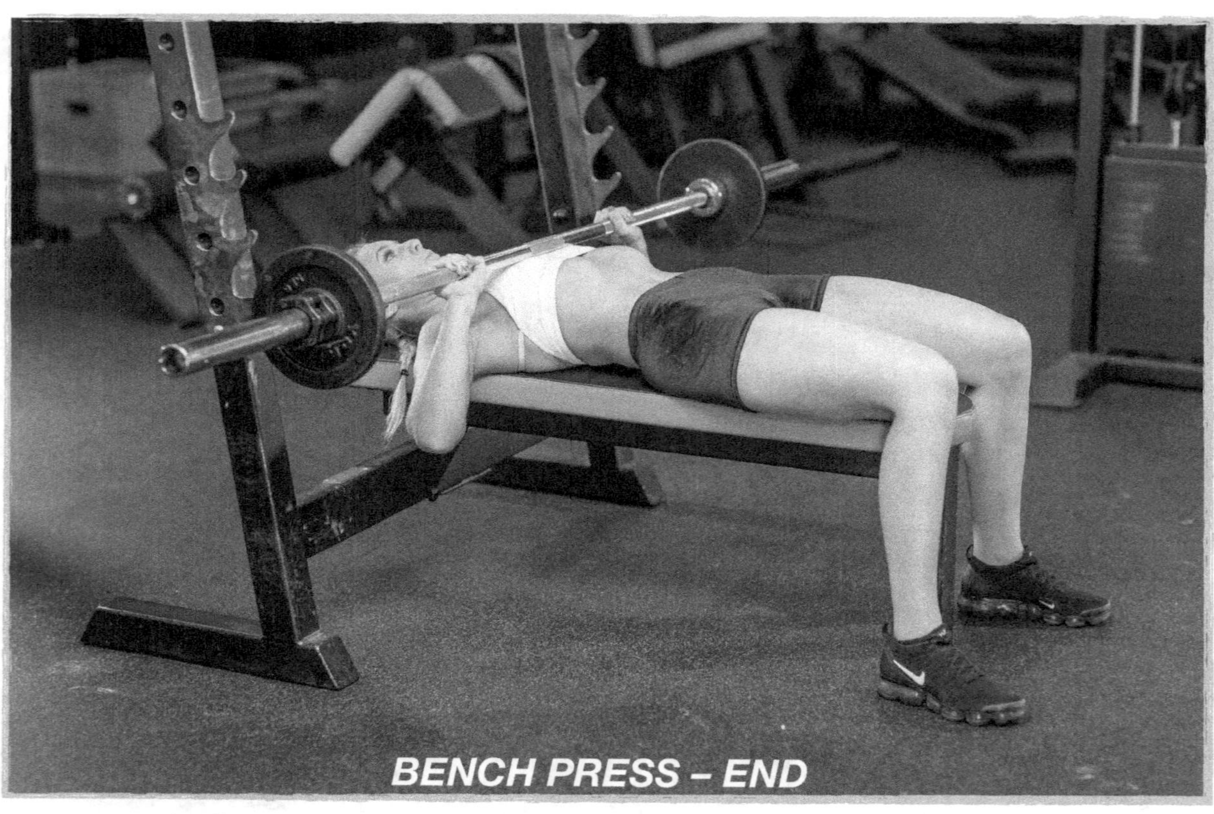

BENCH PRESS – END

7.7 *Shoulder Press*

The shoulder press is the seated, dumbbell version of the overhead press. It is a little easier to set-up and do, as it allows the bench to provide support for the torso.

HOW DO I SET THE EQUIPMENT UP?

You will need a pair of dumbbells that are suitable for your level. Try 5 kg (10 lbs) to start with, and then work up gradually from there. Don't be a heroine and try and do the fifties; your arms will fall off!

The bench should be raised so that the back of it is just shy of vertical. Double check the locking mechanism to make sure that everything is secure.

HOW DO I DO IT?

1. Place the dumbbells down on the floor, one each side of the bench, where they can be reached comfortably.

2. Sit on the bench with your bum against the back, legs spread out so that your feet are flat on the floor and give you plenty of support.

3. Reach down and pick the dumbbells off the ground. Lift them up so that they rise above your shoulder, using your biceps muscles to curl them. Your arms should be flared out to the sides, a 90 degree bend in the elbows.

4. The starting position should have the dumbbells above your shoulders, back flat against the bench, feet spread wide and flat against the floor, and head and neck neutral.

5. From here start to press the dumbbells into the air, allowing them to come closer together as they rise. Keep going until both arms are completely straight.

6. Pause for a second, and then reverse the movement, allowing the dumbbells to move apart as they get lower, and stop when the elbows reach 90 degrees again. This counts as one rep.

HOW MANY SETS AND REPS?

You should be looking to perform 3 to 5 sets of 8 to 12 reps. If you can't perform this number then lower the amount of weight that you are using. If you can perform this number easily then add more weight until it starts to test your ability.

There are a few ways to adjust the difficulty of the shoulder press. To make the exercise easier you can use less weight, use a reduced range of motion (not straightening the arms fully, only bending the elbow to 90 degrees at the bottom), and doing fewer reps and sets. To make the exercise harder you can use more weight, use an increased range of motion (lowering the dumbbells as far as your flexibility allows), and doing more sets and reps.

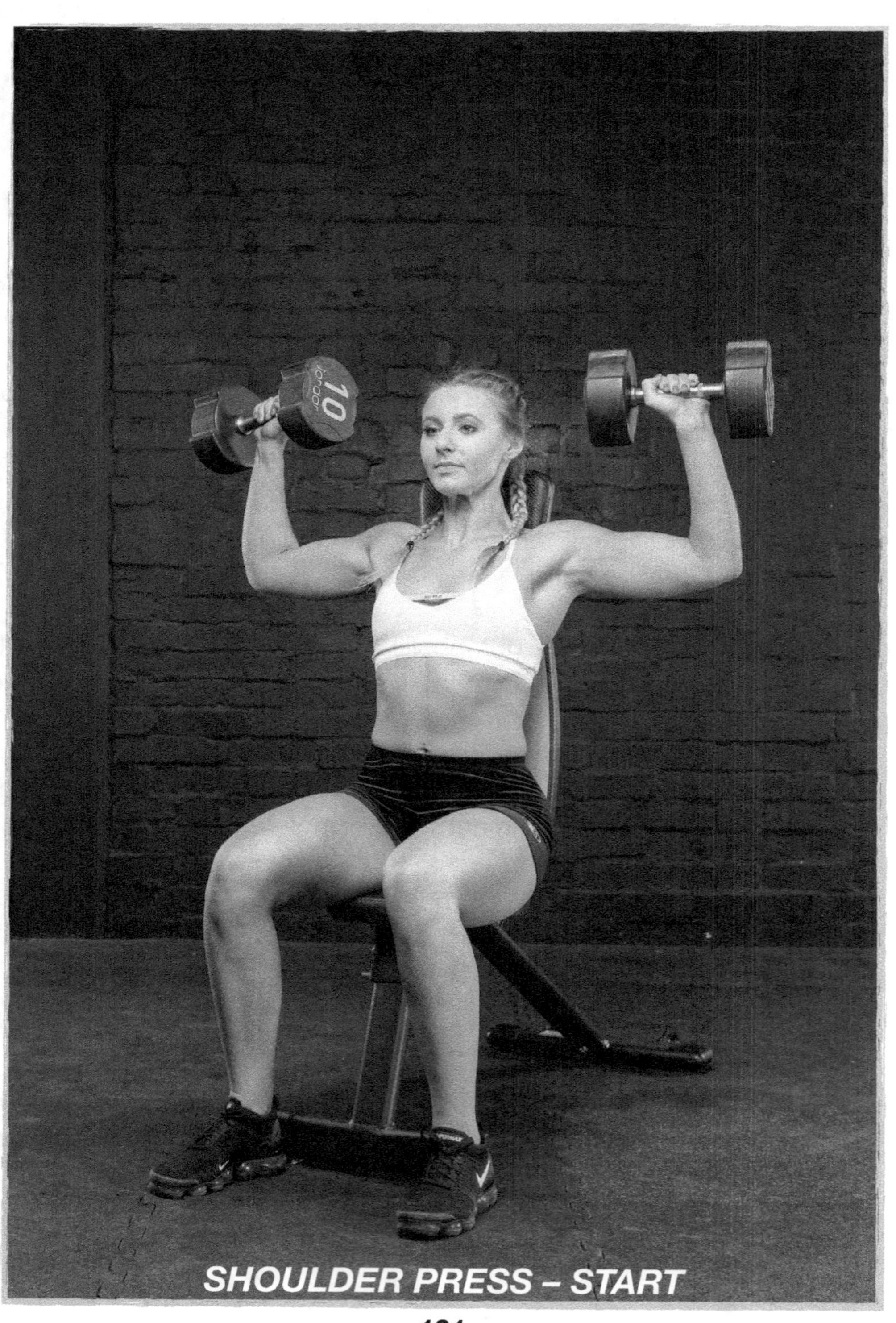

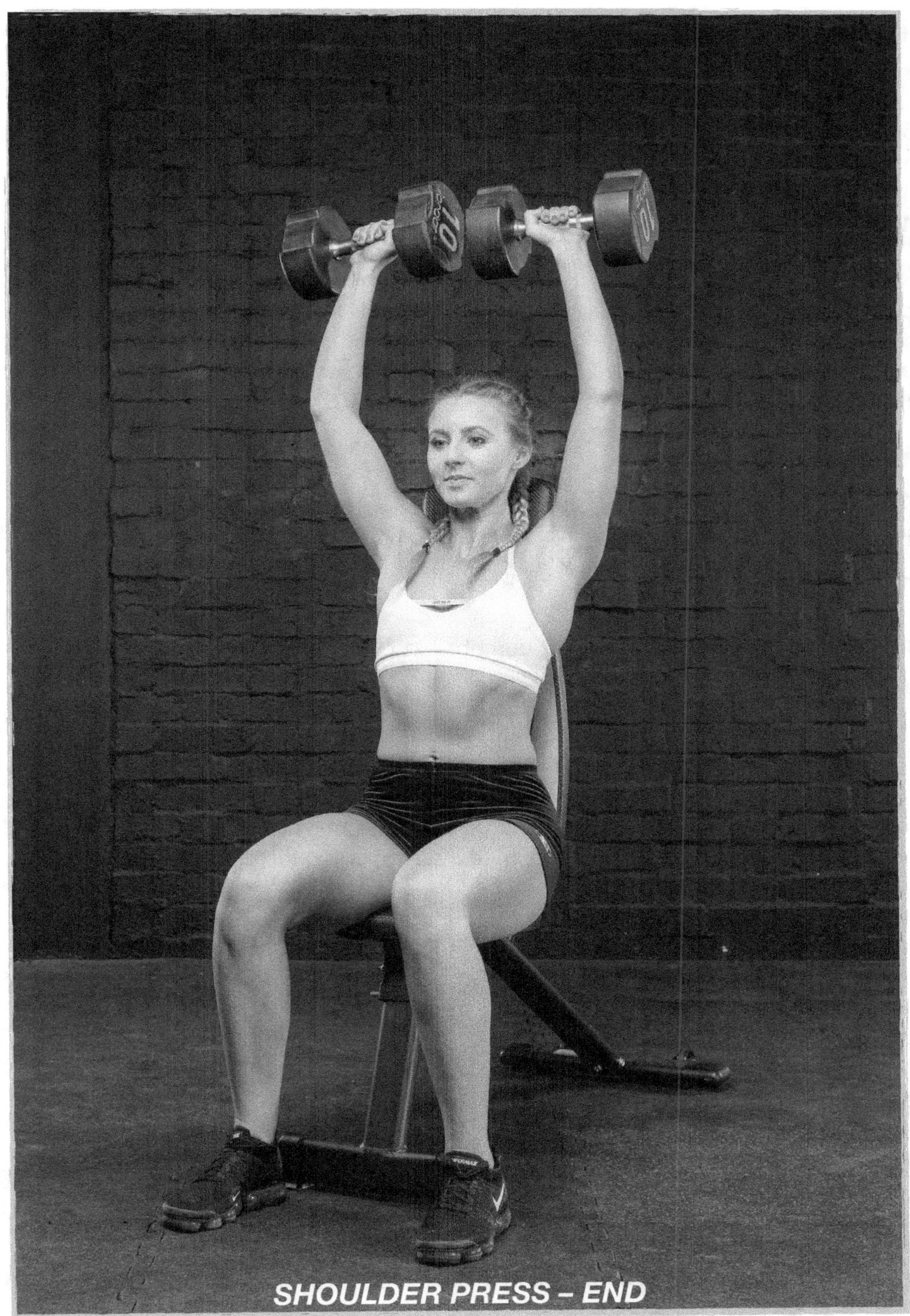

SHOULDER PRESS – END

7.8 BICEPS CURL

The biceps are the front of the upper arm, and should be trained to get toned, shapely looking arms. Making them stronger will also help with pulling exercises, such as the chin-up.

HOW DO I SET THE EQUIPMENT UP?

Dumbbells and barbells can both be used for biceps curls, and they can also be performed seated or standing. We recommend the seated version using dumbbells. This helps keep the lower body from helping out, and also allows the hands to be in a more comfortable position. Try 2.5 to 5 kg (5 to 10 lbs) to start with, and work up from there.

HOW DO I DO IT?

1. Set up the equipment as detailed above, and place a dumbbell on each side of the bench.

2. Sit down on the bench and grab a dumbbell in each hand. Allow your arms to hang loosely.

3. Plant your feet flat on the floor, wide apart, to form a solid base.

4. Now start to curl the dumbbells up by contracting your biceps muscles. Keep your butt and back pressed into the bench, and do not swing the dumbbells up!

5. Keep curling the dumbbells until your forearms are vertical. Pause for a second, and then lower the weights under control to the start position. This counts as one rep.

HOW MANY SETS AND REPS?

You should be looking to perform 3 to 5 sets of 8 to 12 reps.

HOW DO I ADJUST THE DIFFICULTY?

Adjusting the difficulty of the biceps curl is easy. Simply reduce the amount of weight, or reduce the range of motion to make the exercise easier, and increase the weight and increase the range of motion to make the exercise harder.

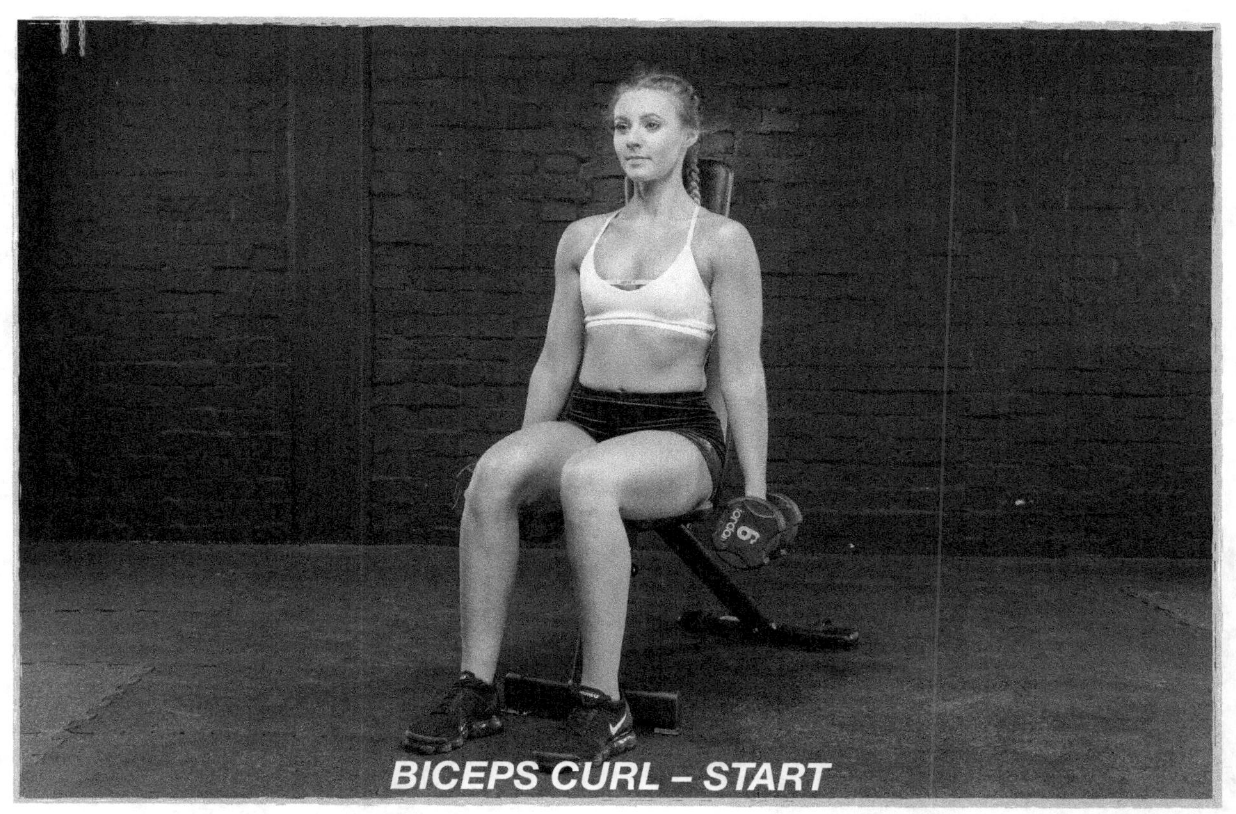

BICEPS CURL – START

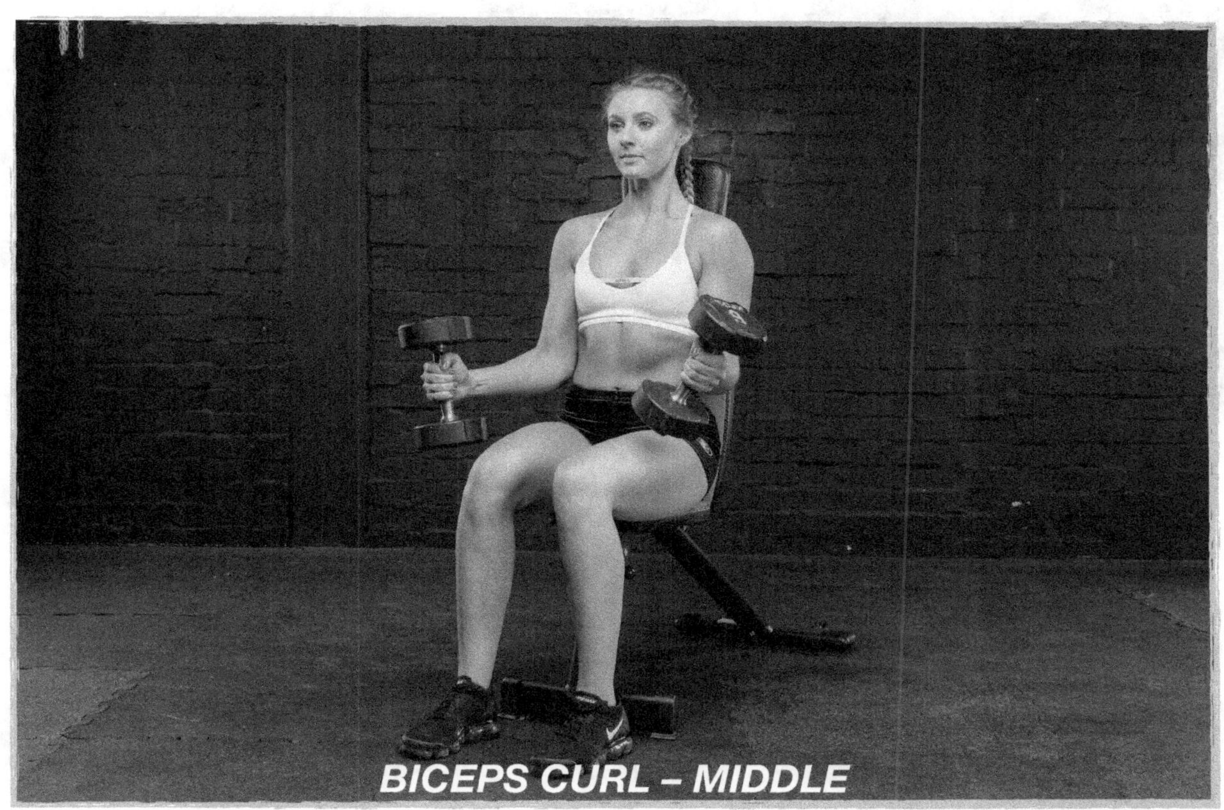

BICEPS CURL – MIDDLE

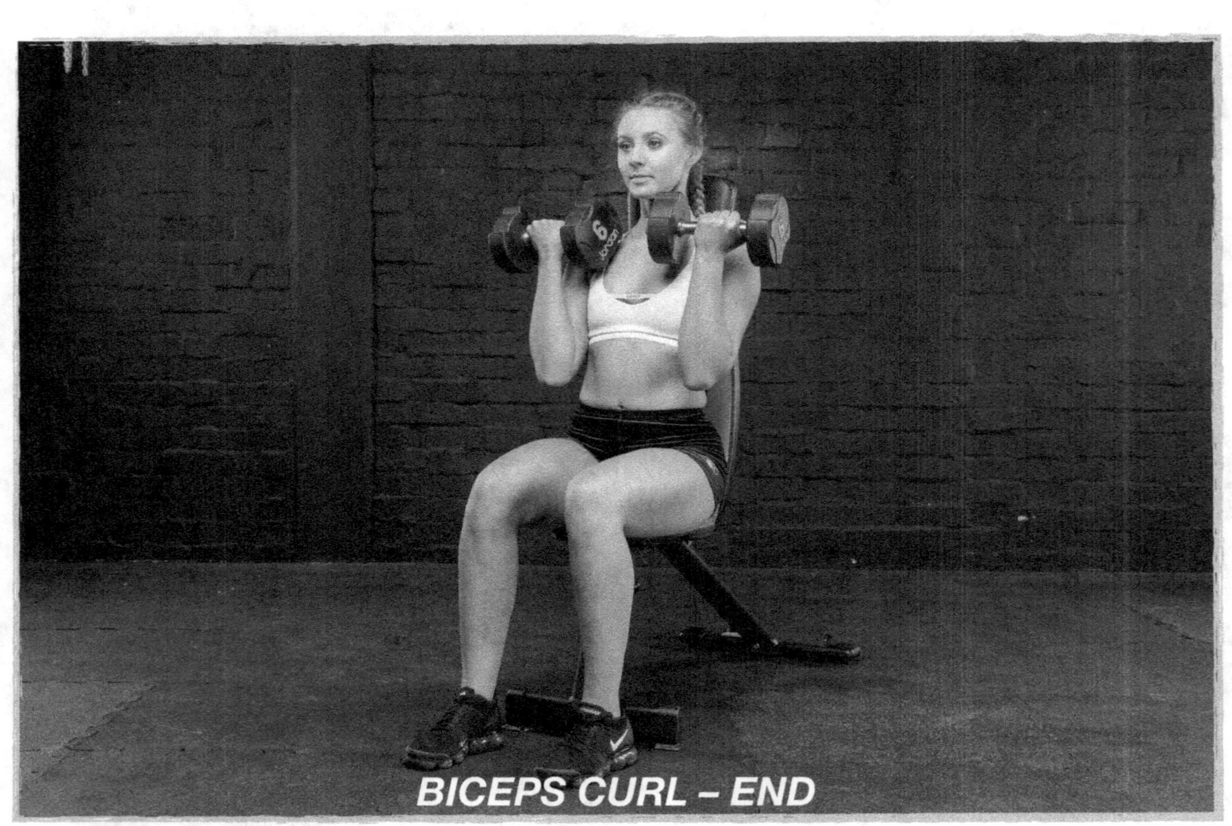

BICEPS CURL – END

7.9 Triceps extension

Although the body weight exercises for the triceps (push-up, triceps dip) are great, as you progress you may want to add weight to challenge yourself in a different way. The triceps extension is a good way of doing this, and is another exercise that is perfect for tackling the muscles at the back of the arms, and strengthening and toning them.

HOW DO I SET THE EQUIPMENT UP?

For the triceps extension you will need an upright bench and a dumbbell. Set up the bench so that it is just shy of vertical, and place the dumbbell in front of the bench.

In terms of weight start out light, and work your way up to a suitable weight for you. We suggest starting with 2.5 kilograms (5 pounds) just so you can learn the technique, before moving on to heavier weights.

HOW DO I DO IT?

1. Sit down on the bench and make sure that your lower back is pressed firmly into the rest. Spread your feet wide to aid in support.

2. Lean forward and grab the dumbbell in both hands, with your fists touching each other.

3. Sit up straight and raise the dumbbell over your head, straightening your arms.

4. Get comfortable, and make sure that you feel stable and secure.

5. Keeping your upper arms still, bend you elbows and allow the dumbbell to drop slowly behind your head.

6. Keep going until you reach the limit of your range of motion, or the dumbbell touches the bench.

7. Reverse the movement and press the dumbbell overhead again until your arms become straight. This counts as one rep.

HOW MANY SETS AND REPS?

You should be looking to perform 3 to 5 sets of 8 to 12 reps.

HOW DO I ADJUST THE DIFFICULTY?

As with other barbell and dumbbell movements, adjusting the difficulty can be done in two main ways: altering the range of motion, or altering the weight. Increasing the range of motion and the weight will make the exercise more difficult, and decreasing the range of motion and the weight will make it easier.

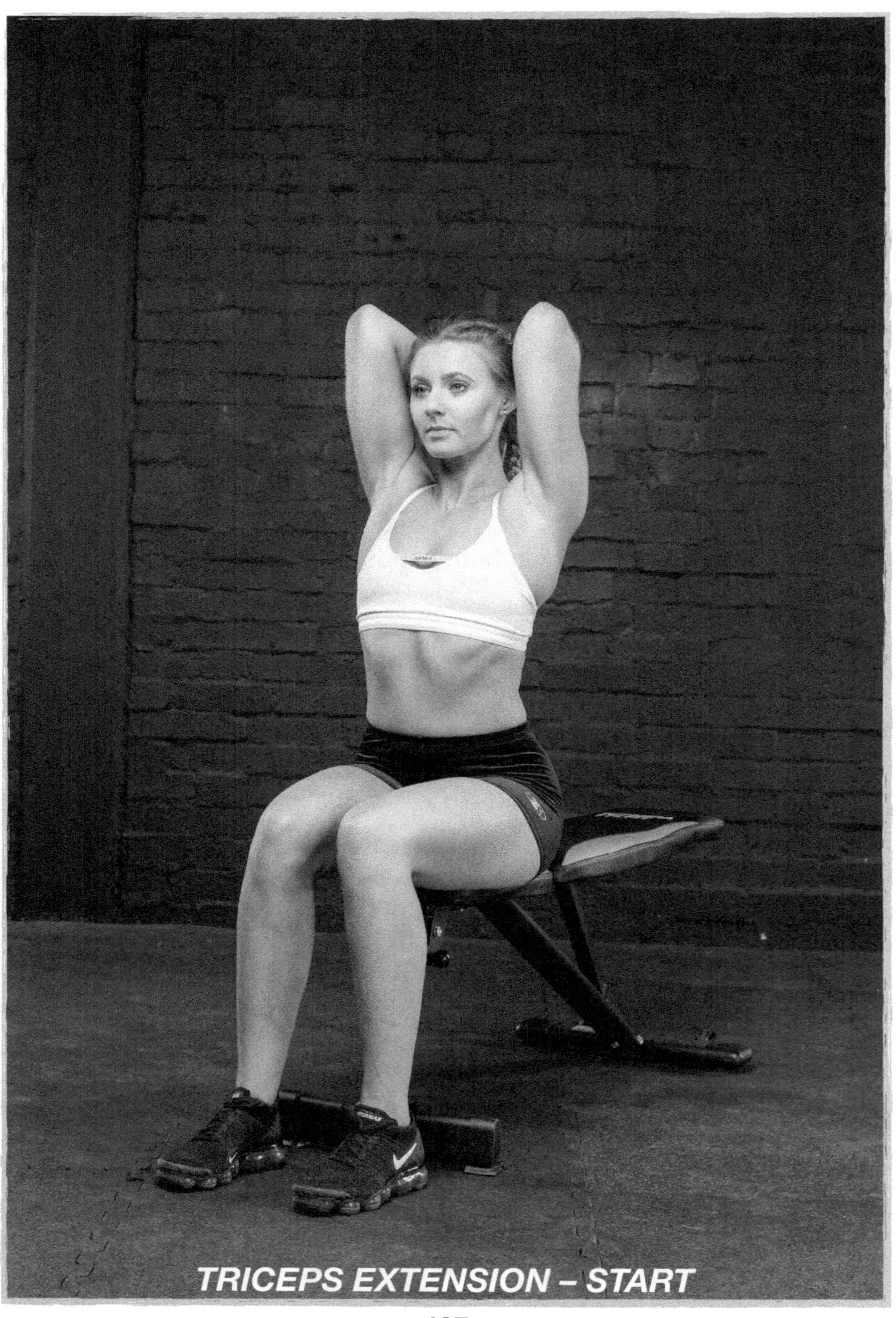

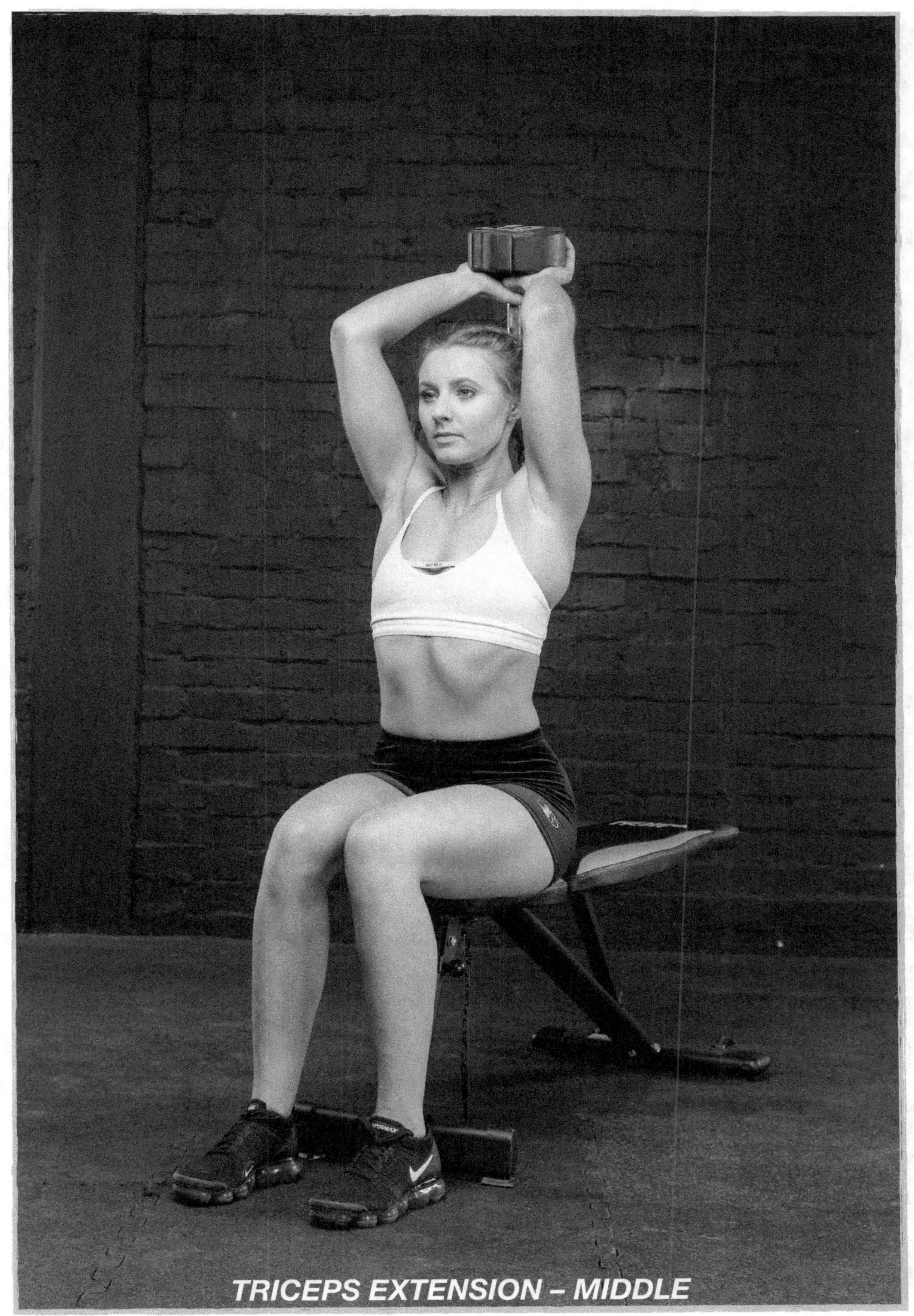

TRICEPS EXTENSION – MIDDLE

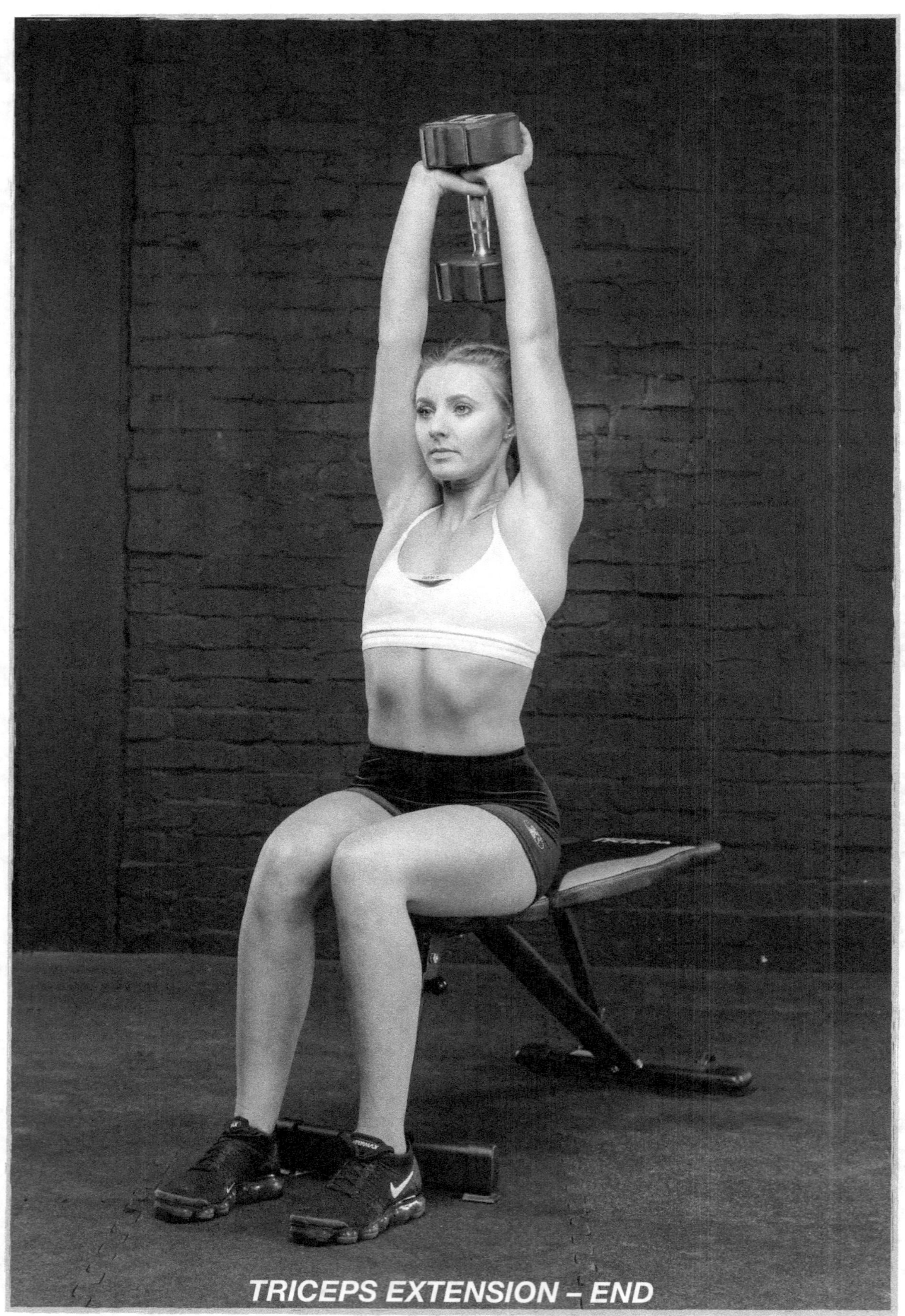

TRICEPS EXTENSION – END

7.10 Barbell row

The barbell row is kind of the weighted version of a pull-up, which works the muscles from a different angle. The upper back, lower back, shoulders, biceps, and core are all worked here, making it an awesome exercise for shaping the upper body.

HOW DO I SET THE EQUIPMENT UP?

You will need a barbell, preferably an Olympic style one, either 15 kg (30 lbs) or 20 kg (45 lbs) depending on your strength, ability, and what's available in your gym. If this is too heavy for you, then try an exercise class barbell. These are usually much lighter and shorter, and will still allow enough weight to be used.

HOW DO I DO IT?

1. Set the bar up with weight. This should be low enough so that you are confident that you can perform the exercise immediately. If you are unsure, go very light to start, or use the bar only.

2. Crouch down and grab the bar with both hands in an overhand grip, shoulder width apart. Your feet should also be shoulder width apart with a slight bend in the knee.

3. At this point you should be in the deadlift starting position (see page **177** for more information on the deadlift)!.

4. Now stand up with the bar, but only go halfway, so that your back is angled at about 45 degrees, and your knees are bent. The bar should be hanging straight down and your arms should be relaxed.

5. From here contract you're biceps, back, and shoulders, so that the bar begins to rise. Keep your body position the same, and don't change the angle of your back!

6. Keep pulling the bar until it touches your chest, or until you reach the limit of your range of motion.

7. Pause for a second, and then lower the bar to the starting position again. This counts as one rep.

HOW MANY SETS AND REPS?

You should be looking to perform 3 to 5 sets of 8 to 12 reps.

HOW DO I ADJUST THE DIFFICULTY?

To adjust the difficulty of the barbell row is easy. If you need to make it less difficult then use a reduced range of motion or use less weight, and if you need to make it more difficult then increase the range of motion or use more weight.

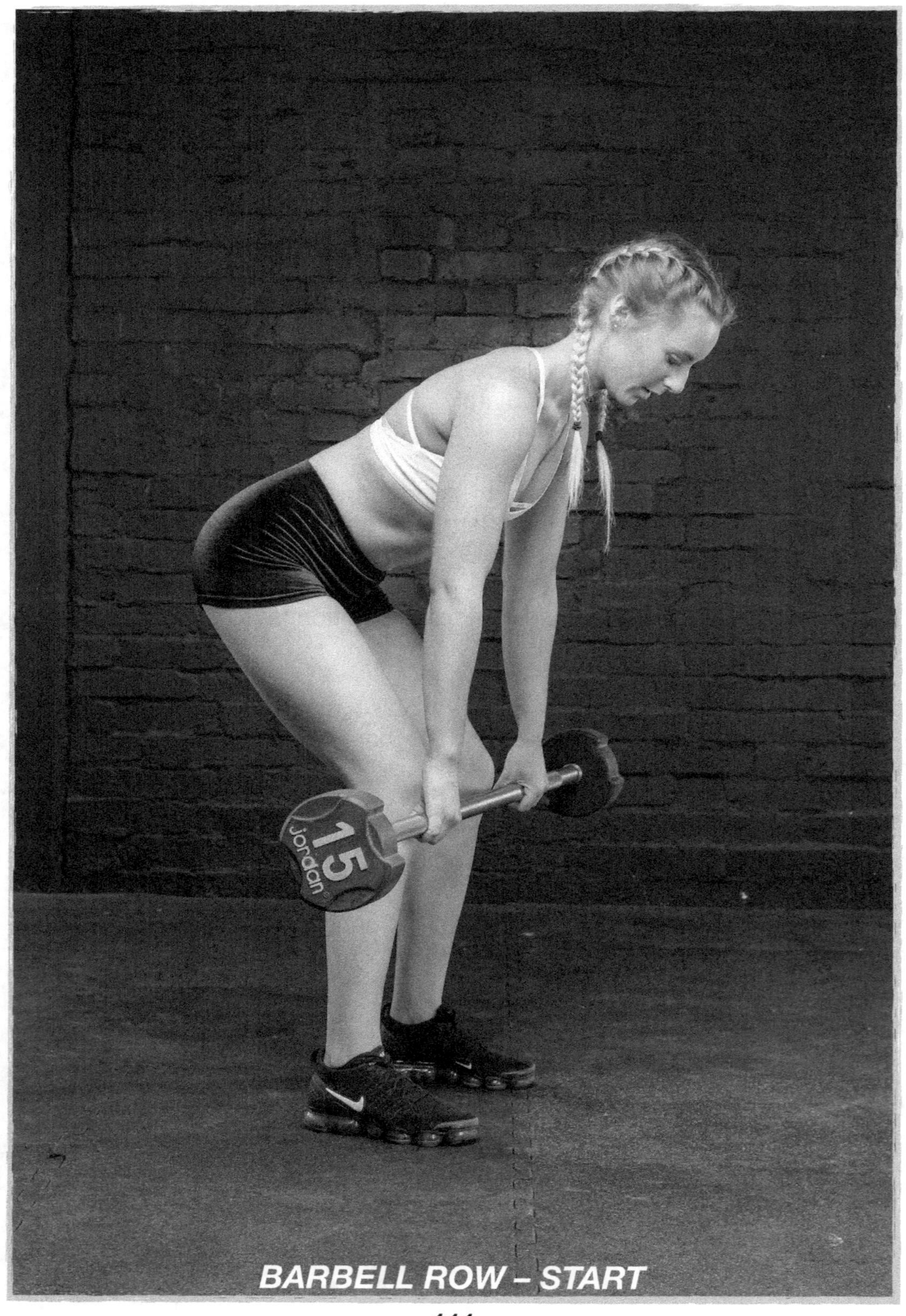

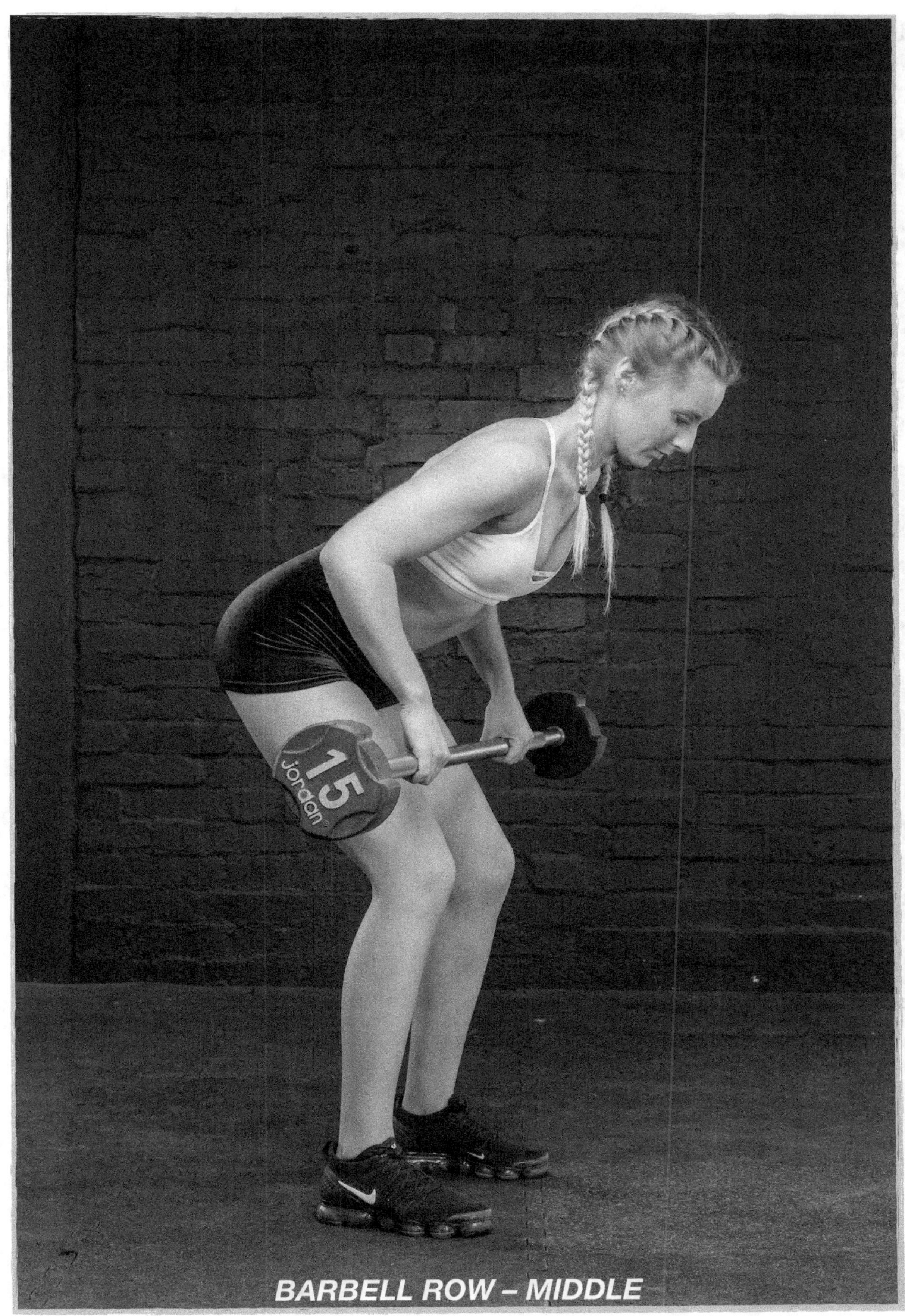

BARBELL ROW – MIDDLE

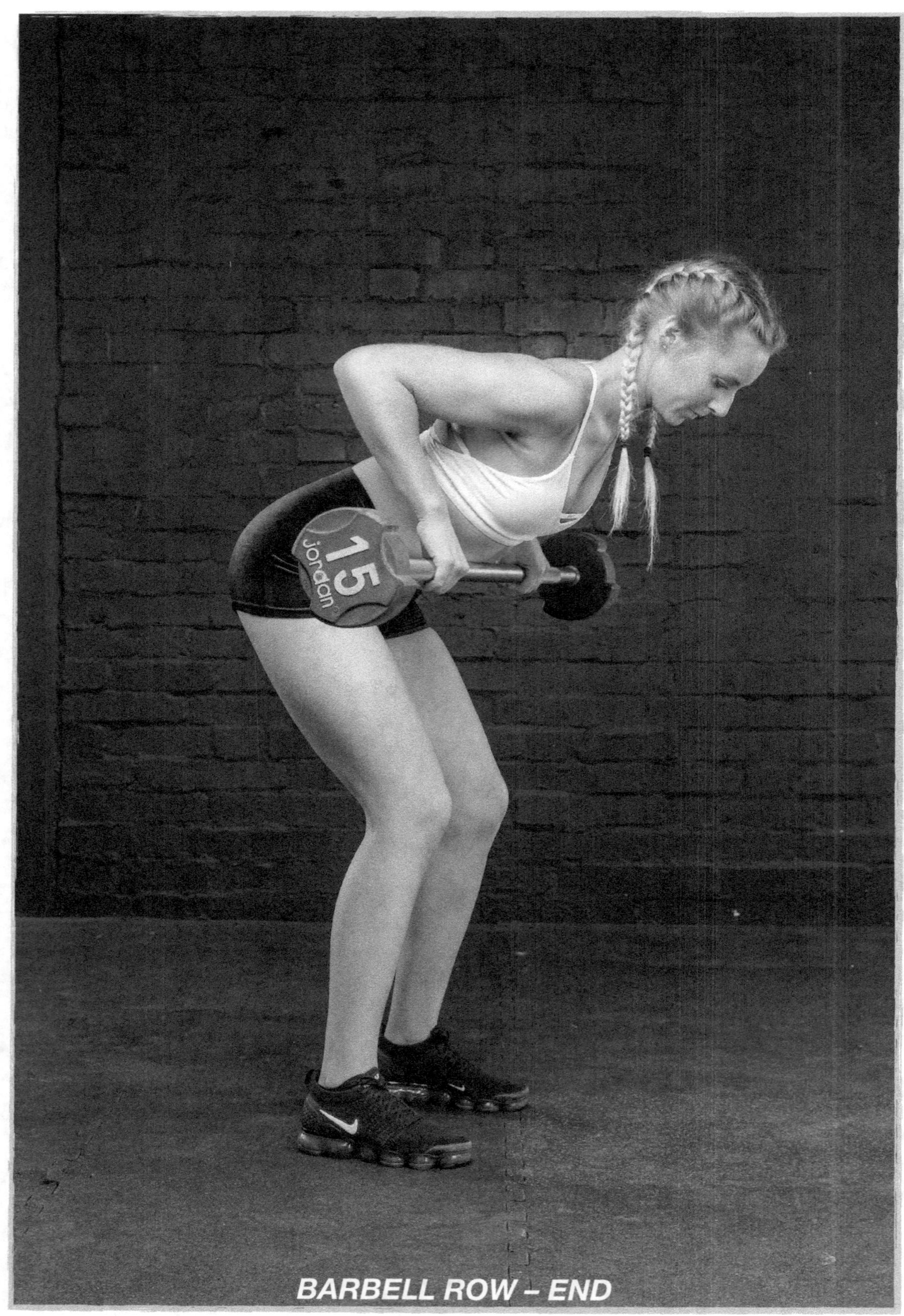

BARBELL ROW – END

Section Two: Abs and Core

This section will be a popular one, as many women seek to tighten their abs and make their core stronger. It's important to remember that this book won't have you doing millions of reps; this isn't how you get strong abs or how you lose body fat and get a toned stomach!

What we will focus on instead are core exercises that work the entire core, build strength from the inside out, and which are suitable for lots of different abilities.

It's also worth mentioning that although in the other exercise sections we cover both body weight and weighted exercises, for the core there are plenty of very difficult exercises using just body weight, so adding weight really is unnecessary.

8.1 Plank

The plank sure looks like a simple exercise, but try holding it for 2 minutes and you'll change your mind! It can also be regressed (made easier) and progressed (made harder) very easily, to suit a wide range of abilities. There are loads of more complicated and more fancy core exercises, but the plank is a great starting point, and will give you a good base of strength to build on.

HOW DO I SET THE EQUIPMENT UP?

All you need for the plank is some floor space and maybe a mat to cushion your hands. Stretching areas or functional training areas in gyms are great for this!

HOW DO I DO IT?

1. Place your forearms on the ground and stretch your legs out behind you, balancing on your toes.

2. Make sure that your forearms are parallel, positioned shoulder width apart.

3. Push your hips up into the air, so that a straight line can be drawn through the shoulders, hips, and feet.

4. Now hold this position as long as possible.

HOW MANY SETS AND REPS?

You should be looking to hold the plank for at least 3 sets of 30 seconds.

HOW DO I ADJUST THE DIFFICULTY?

Adjusting the difficulty of the plank is pretty easy, and can be done in a few ways. First, you can perform the exercise with your knees on the ground instead of your toes. This makes the distance between your upper and lower body smaller, which makes the exercise easier!

To make the plank harder you can increase the distance between your arms and feet, even moving up into a push-up position if needed. If you do this then you can keep moving your hands further and further forward to increase the challenge by a large amount, meaning that you can continue to use the plank for a long time!

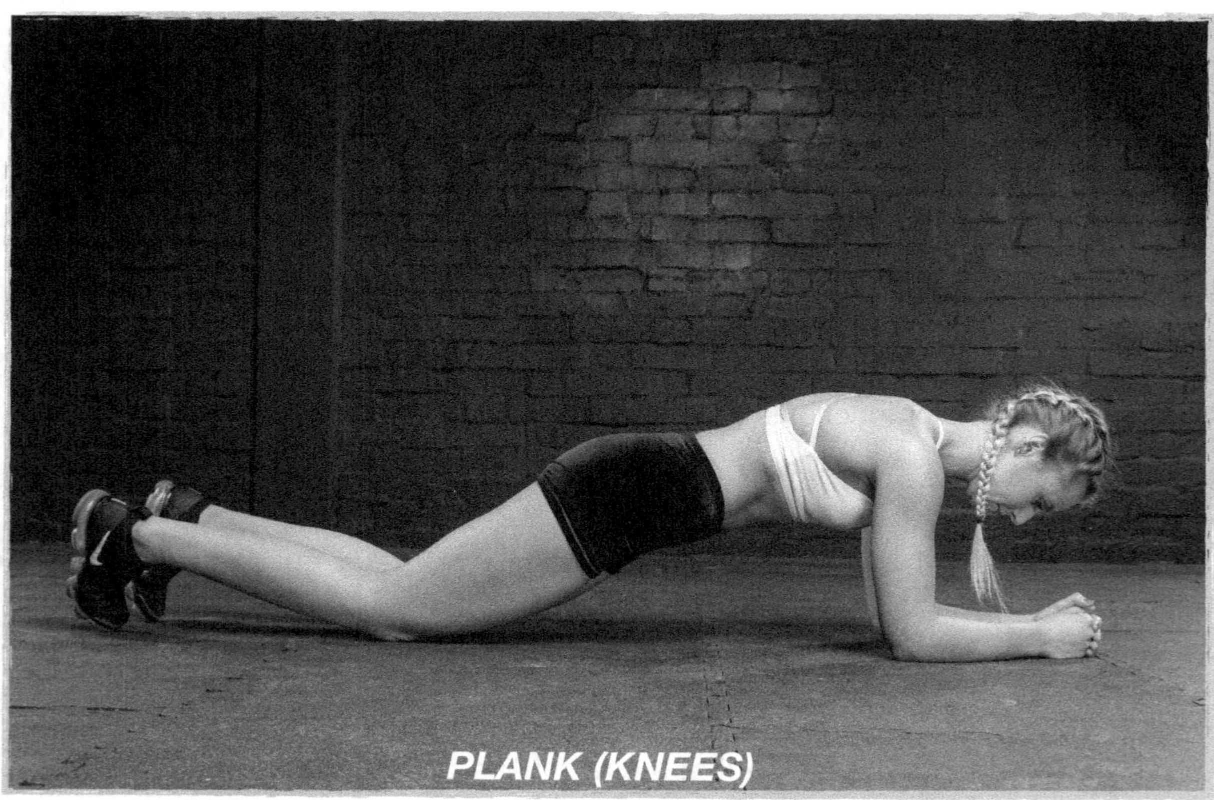

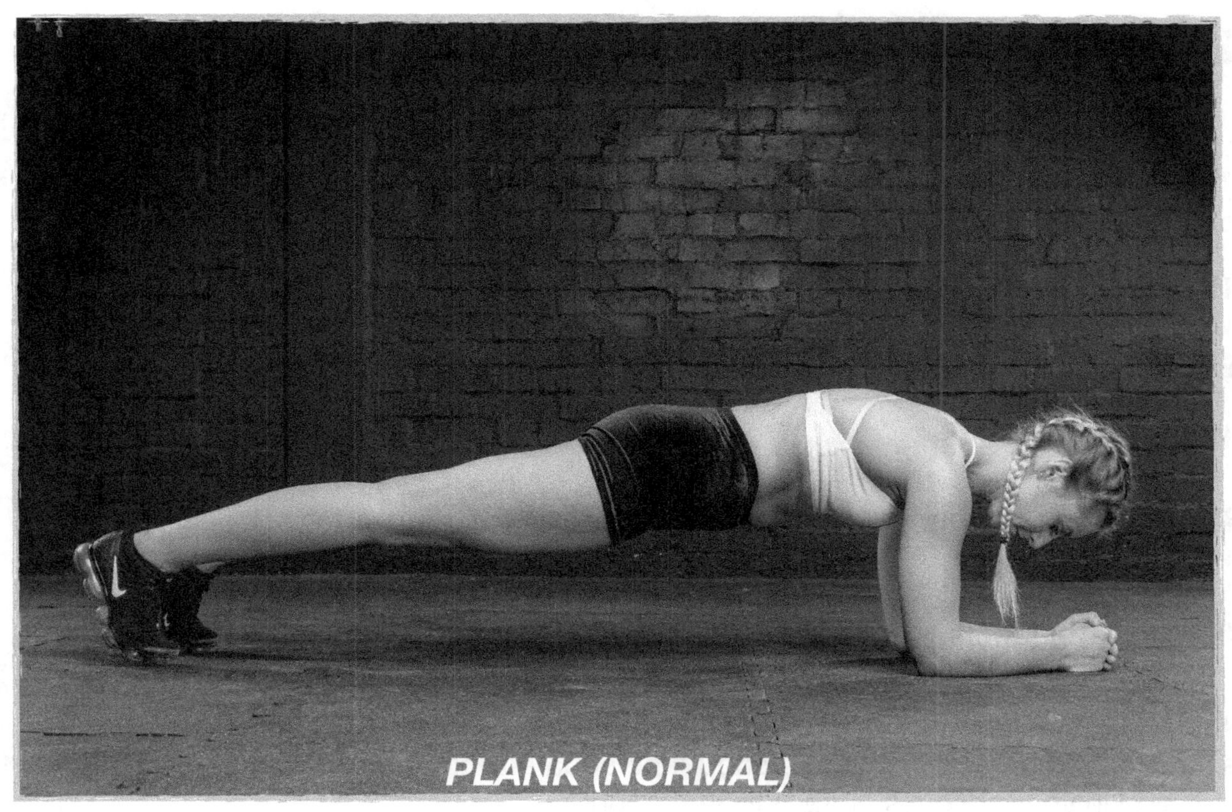

PLANK (NORMAL)

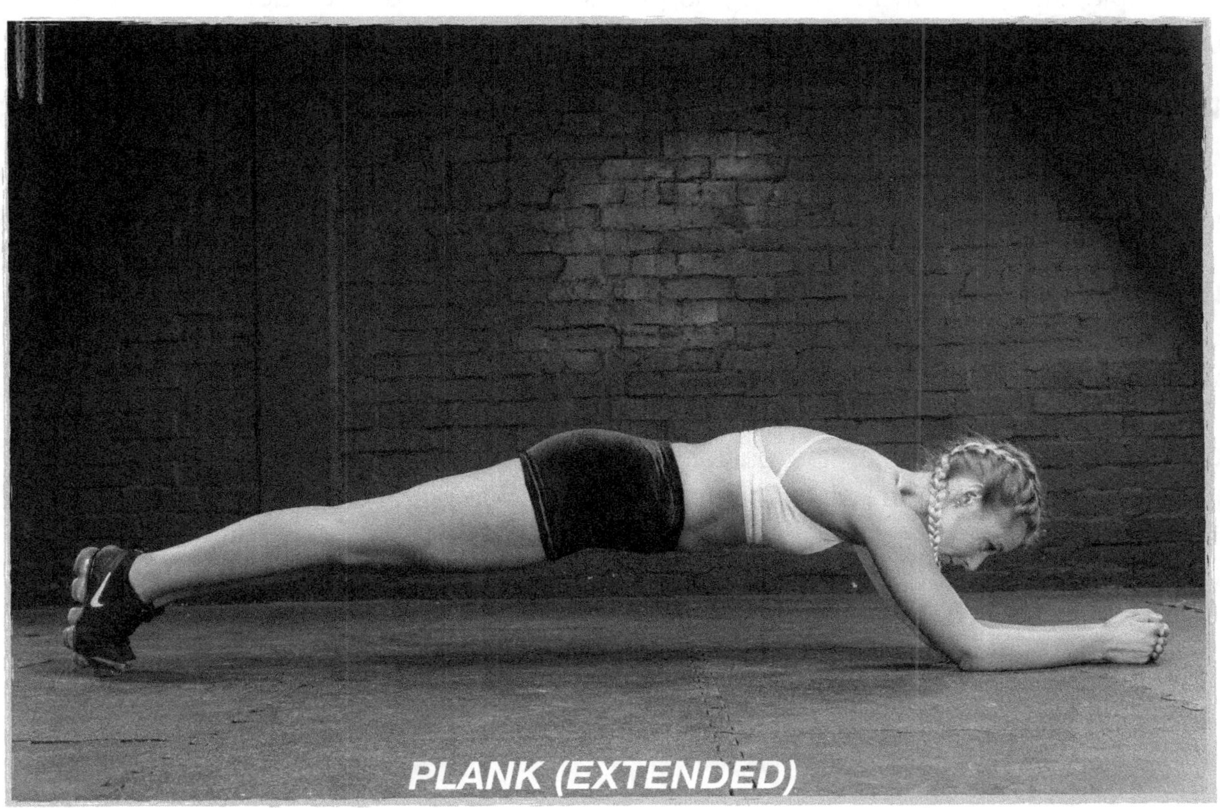

PLANK (EXTENDED)

8.2 SIDE PLANK

The side plank is a great core exercise that works the sides of the stomach (or the obliques), and can help to bring in and tighten that area of your stomach. It's pretty much the same method as the normal plank, but with your body turned on its side.

HOW DO I SET THE EQUIPMENT UP?

You'll need some floor space, and an exercise mat to cushion the arms.

HOW DO I DO IT?

1. Place one forearm on the ground and stretch out your legs at ninety degrees to this arm.

2. Place your bottom foot on its side, and then place your other foot on top of this.

3. Now raise your hips up until a straight line can be drawn through your shoulders, hips, knees, and ankles. Your torso should be square to the ground and you should feel tension in your obliques closest to the ground.

4. Now hold this position for as long as possible. Once you have done your reps and sets on one side, switch over and repeat for the other side of your body.

HOW MANY SETS AND REPS?

You should be looking to perform 3 sets of 30 second holds, on both sides of the body.

HOW DO I ADJUST THE DIFFICULTY?

As with the normal plank, the side plank can be made easier by moving from the feet to the knees, as this decreases the distance between the upper body and the lower body, making the exercise easier. You can make the side plank harder by raising your free arm into the air, or even performing side plank crunches, where you raise and lower the hips for reps.

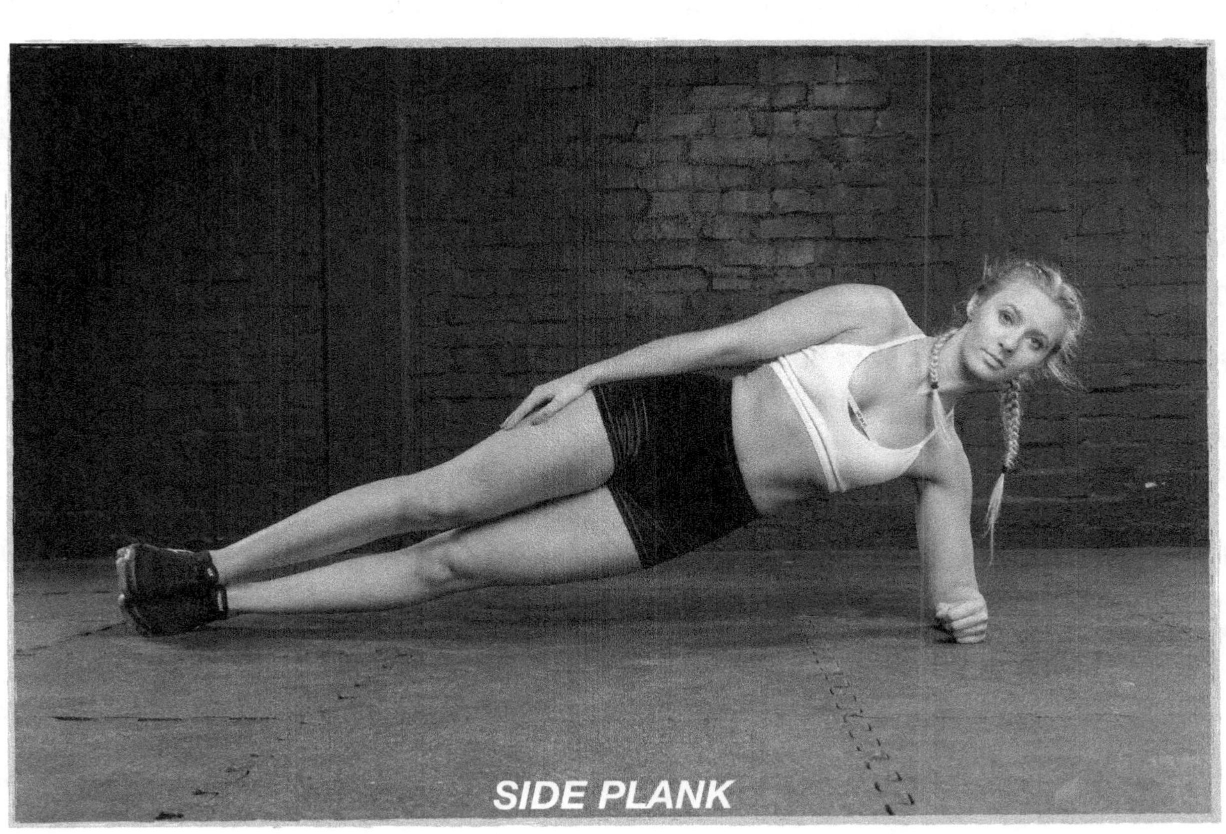

SIDE PLANK

8.3 CRUNCH

Ah, the crunch! A classic staple exercise in aerobics classes and infomercials, the crunch has a bit of a bad rep when it comes to core training. However, this is mostly because people think you have to perform hundreds of them to get any benefit. We're here to tell you that there is no benefit to doing hundreds of crunches. It will not build lots of strength, it will not burn fat off your stomach, and you will likely just get a bad back and sore neck from curling forwards all day long.

HOW DO I SET THE EQUIPMENT UP?

For the crunch you will need some floor space and exercise mat.

HOW DO I DO IT?

1. Lie down on your back with your knees bent at 45 degrees or slightly less.

2. Fold your arms across your chest, OR, place your arms by your sides.

3. Keeping your lower and middle back pressed firmly into the floor, use your ab muscles to curl up, raising your shoulders off the ground.

4. Keep curling up until your shoulders cannot rise any further. Keep your head and neck neutral, and don't strain the muscles at the front of the neck.

5. Hold for a second, and then reverse the movement to arrive at the start position again. This counts as one rep.

HOW MANY SETS AND REPS?

You should be looking to perform 3 to 5 sets of 8 to 12 reps.

HOW DO I ADJUST THE DIFFICULTY?

To make the crunch easier you can bend the legs more, or secure the feet and ankles underneath an object. This will give you more leverage and allow you to complete the exercise more easily. To make the crunch harder you can stretch the legs out completely, and hold at the top for a longer period of time.

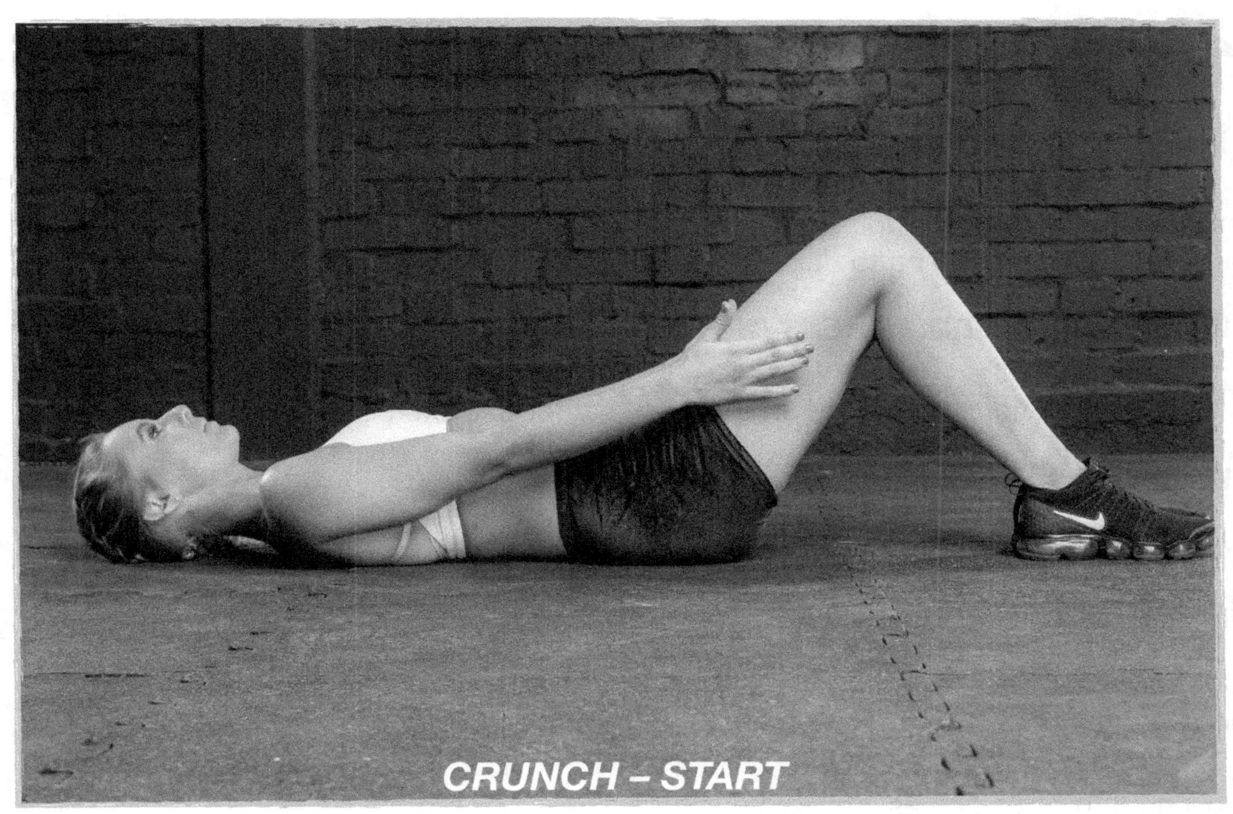

CRUNCH – START

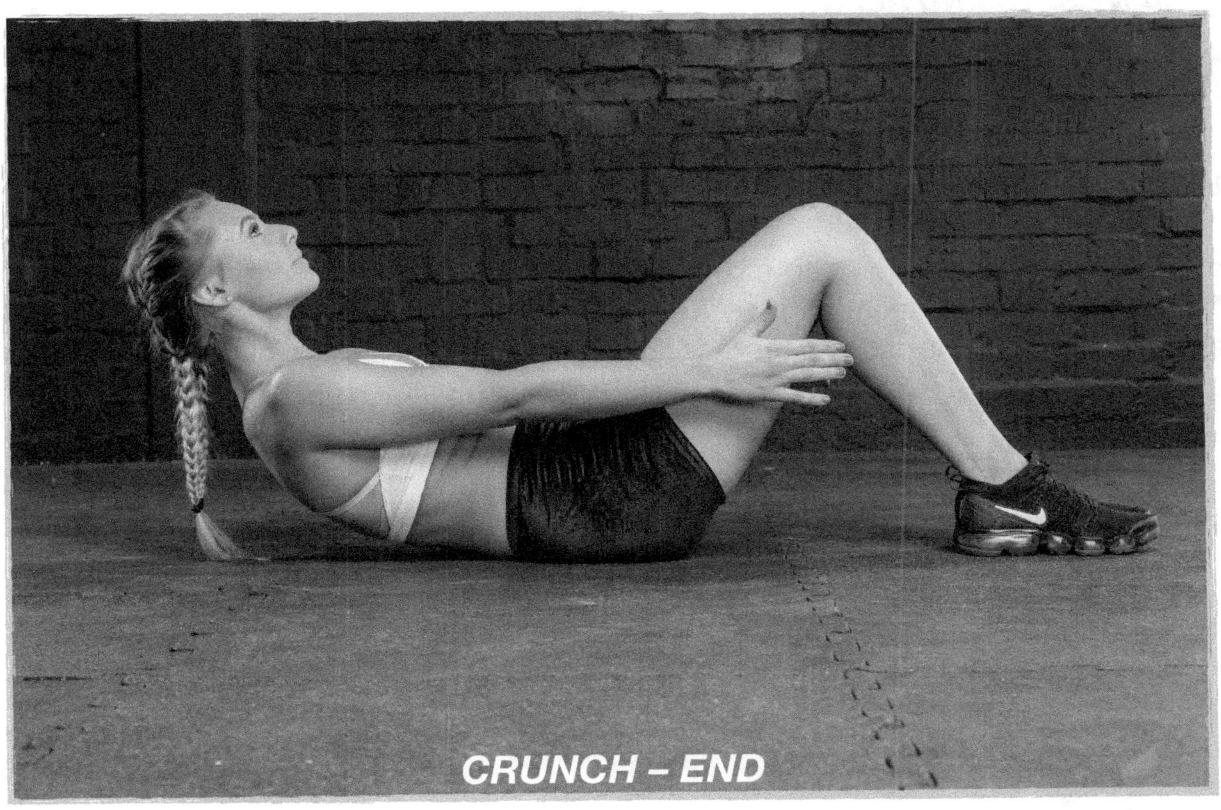

CRUNCH – END

8.4 ARCH

As important as the abs are, you shouldn't forget the lower back! Although this exercise is not really for aesthetics, the lower back is a common area of injury or niggling pain for many people, and strengthening the lower back with an exercise like the arch is a great thing to do.

HOW DO I SET THE EQUIPMENT UP?

You'll need some floor space and an exercise mat for this exercise.

HOW DO I DO IT?

1. To perform the arch, lie face down on the ground with your arms out in front of you.

2. Contract your back, bum, and leg muscles, and raise your torso and legs off the floor as far as possible.

3. Now hold this position as long as you can.

HOW MANY SETS AND REPS?

For the arch you should be looking to hold it for similar amounts of time as the plank. Try 3 sets of 30 second holds, with 60 seconds for rest.

HOW DO I ADJUST THE DIFFICULTY?

To make the arch easier you can move up and down into the arch from the lying position, doing the movement for reps. You can make it harder by keeping your legs touching throughout the movement, and also stretching your arms out in front of you.

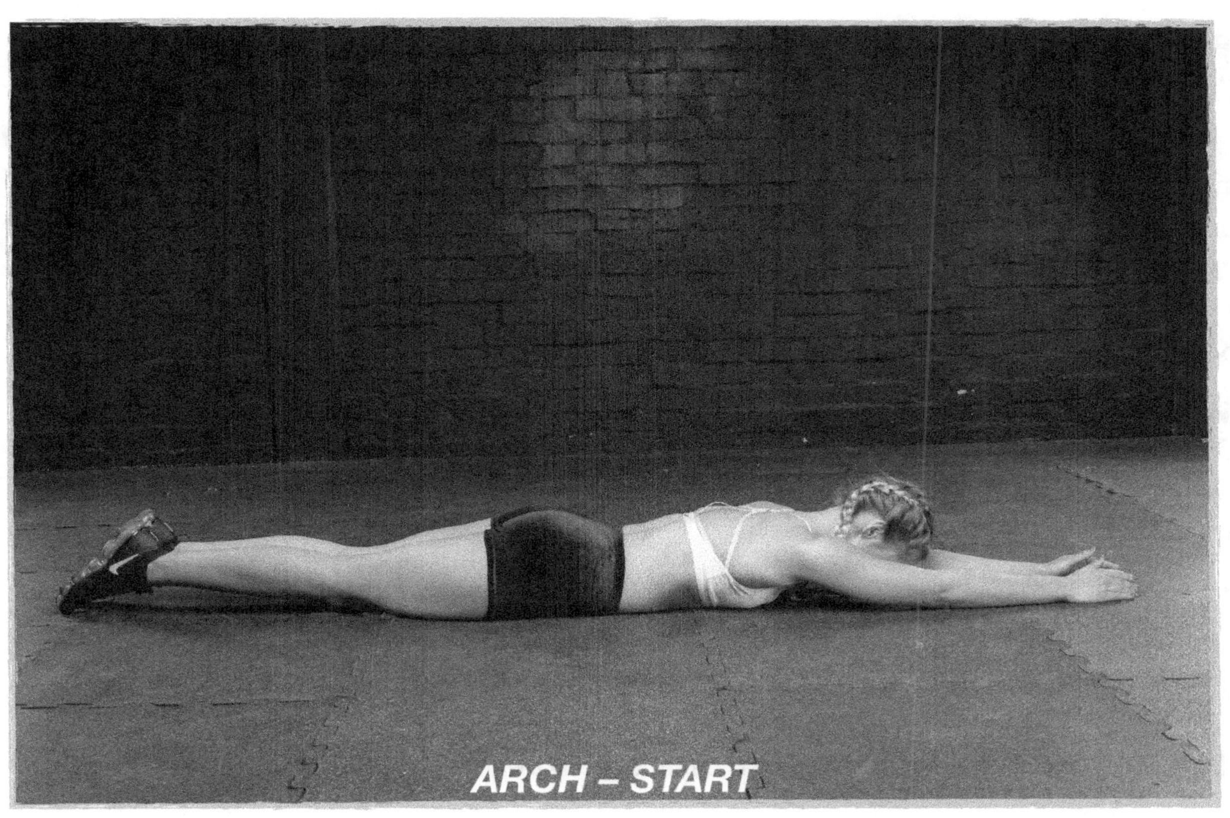

ARCH – START

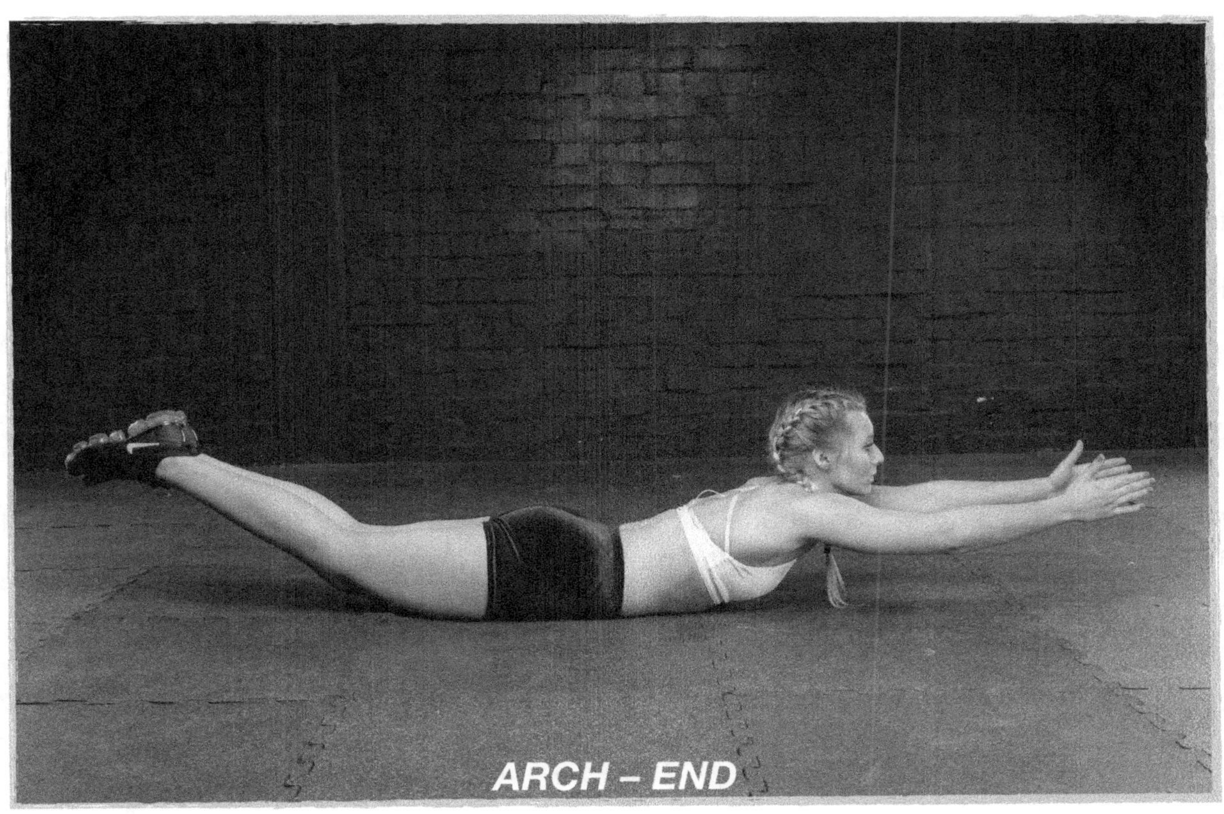

ARCH – END

8.5 Sɪᴛ-ᴜᴘ

Ah, the good old sit-up! Lots of you may have horrible memories of these, either from school, exercise classes, or infomercials that claim to give you abs of steel in 4 weeks. But, even though the humble sit-up has been relegated to the bottom of the pile when it comes to core training, this doesn't mean that it's not effective, or that you shouldn't do them. The key, as with any exercise, is the way you do them, and making sure your technique is spot on.

HOW DO I SET THE EQUIPMENT UP?

For sit-ups it is recommended that you have some floor space, and also a mat to pad your bum.

HOW DO I DO IT?

1. Lie down with your feet flat on the floor and your knees bent slightly.

2. Place your hands across your chest, behind your head, or on your temples.

3. Now tense your abs and start to sit up. Don't curl your back; keep it straight and try and pivot from the hips.

4. Keep sitting up, maintaining a neutral head and neck position, until your torso reaches a vertical position.

5. Pause for a second, and then reverse the movement until you are lying down again. This counts as one rep.

HOW MANY SETS AND REPS?

You should be looking to perform 3 to 5 sets of 8 to 12 reps.

HOW DO I ADJUST THE DIFFICULTY?

To make sit-ups easier you can reduce the range of motion, so only raise your torso up a little way. You can also curl the spine more, so the movement is more similar to the crunch.

To make it more difficult, keep your back completely straight, and slow the movement down.

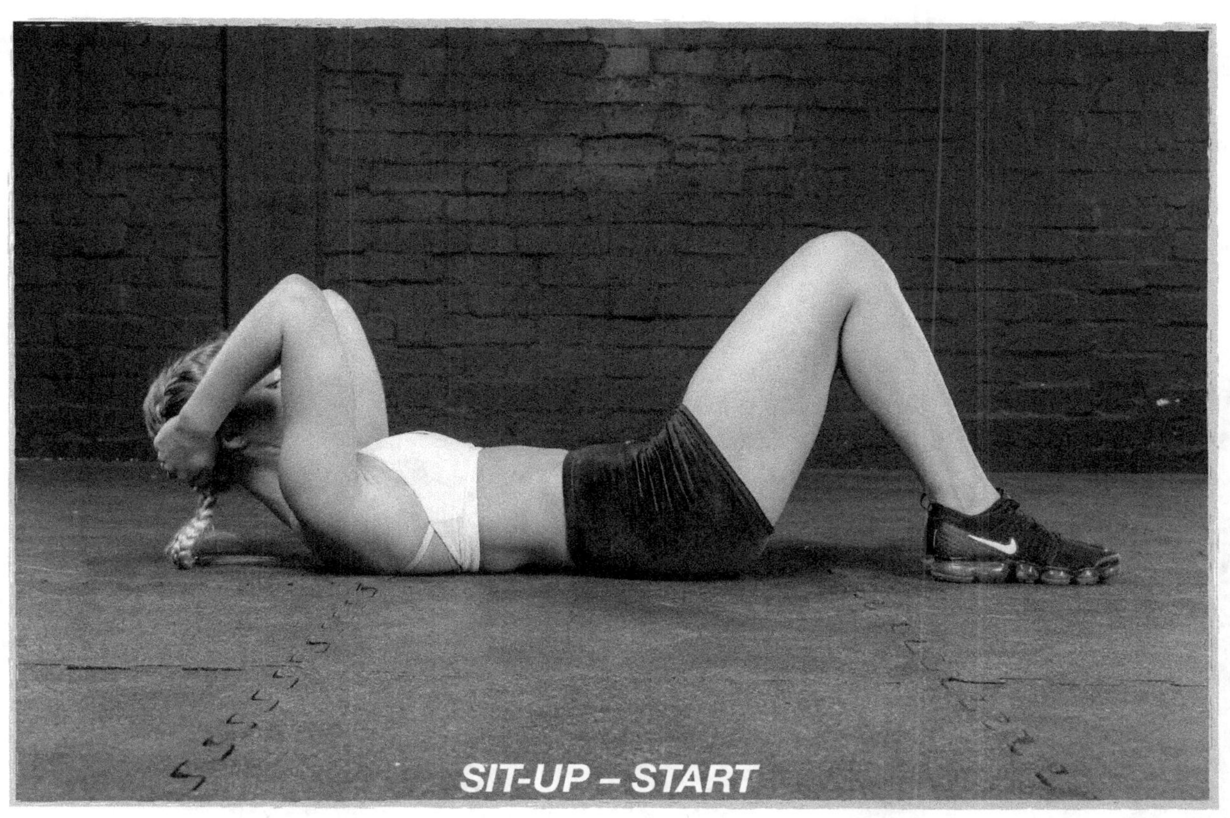

SIT-UP – START

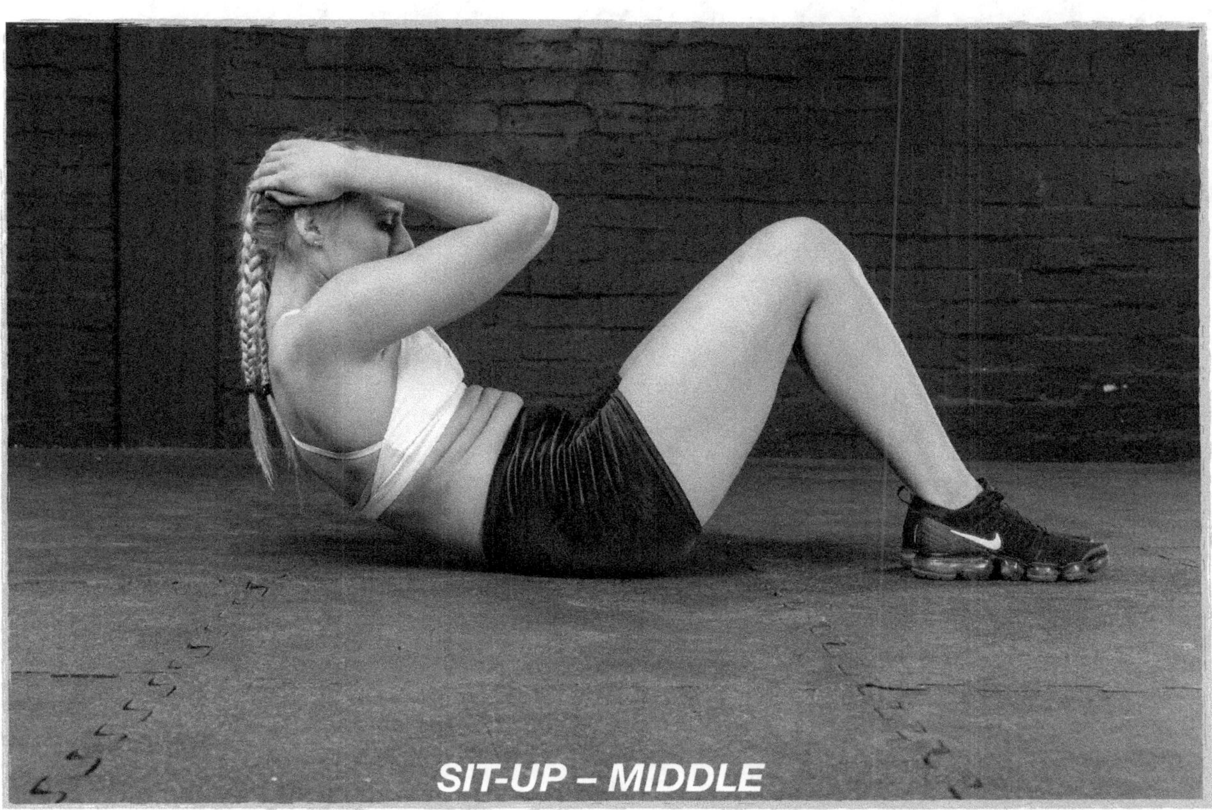

SIT-UP – MIDDLE

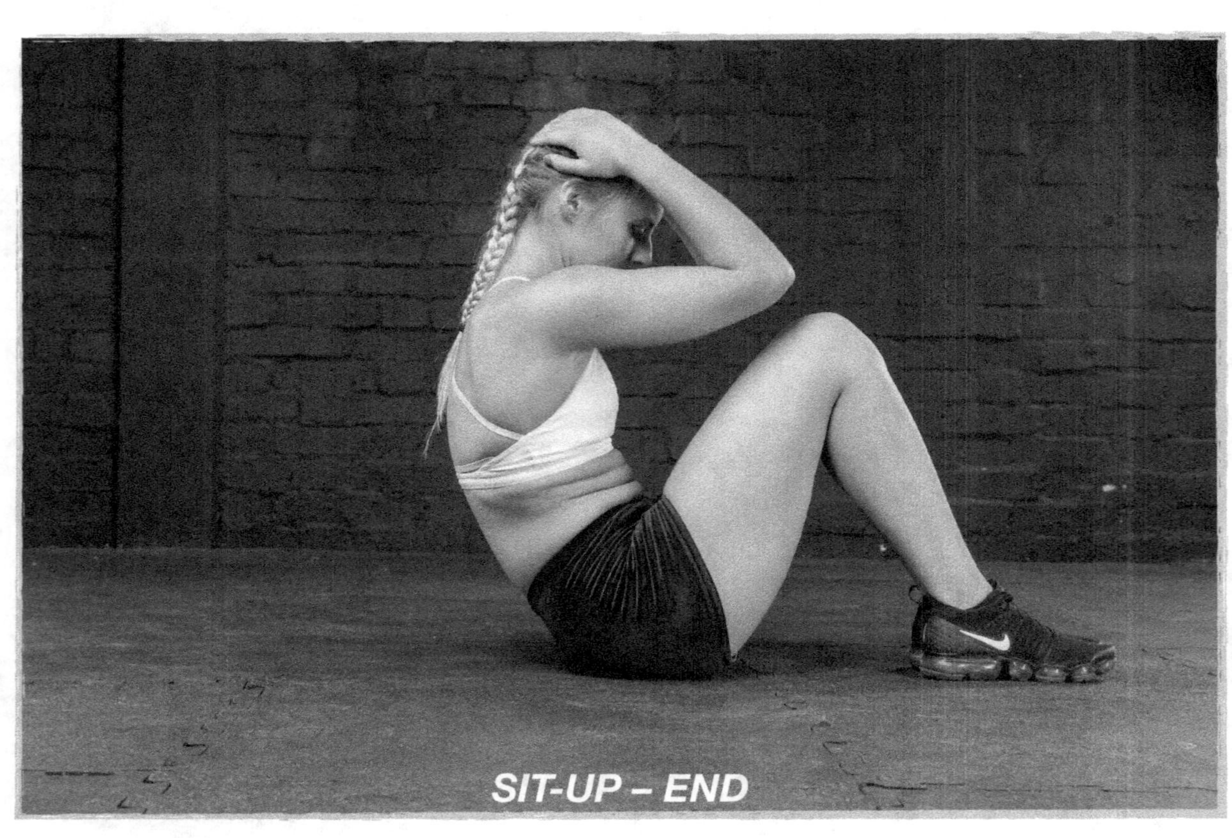
SIT-UP – END

8.6 RUSSIAN TWIST

The Russian twist isn't some dance fad, but rather a good core strengthening exercise that also targets the obliques, which are those muscles on the sides of the core. The Russian twist is great for tightening these areas up, and is a good change from the stabilisation and up and down movements of the other core exercises.

HOW DO I SET THE EQUIPMENT UP?

For the Russian twist you will need some floor space, a mat if you need to cushion the floor, and a weight of some kind. The weight can be anything that you can hold in two hands, such as a dumbbell, weight plate, kettlebell, medicine ball, or anything else of a suitable size and weight. For starters, we recommend a light weight; 2.5 to 5 kg (5 to 10 lbs), and then move up from there.

HOW DO I DO IT?

1. Sit on the floor, with your feet raised and your knees bent. Grab the weight you are using with both hands, and hold it in front of your stomach.

2. Lean back slightly so that your core goes tight; your back should be straight, but angled slightly: 45 degrees is a good starting point.

3. Now twist to one side, keeping the weight held in front of your stomach. It is important that the twisting motion comes from your core and not your arms.

4. Twist until you cannot go any further, and then twist the other way, moving past the central point to the opposite other side. This counts as one rep.

HOW MANY SETS AND REPS?

You should be looking to perform 3 to 5 sets of 8 to 12 reps.

HOW DO I ADJUST THE DIFFICULTY?

The Russian twist is tough, but mainly because the back must be angled and the core kept tense throughout. To make the exercise easier you can sit more upright, or use a lighter weight if you're struggling.

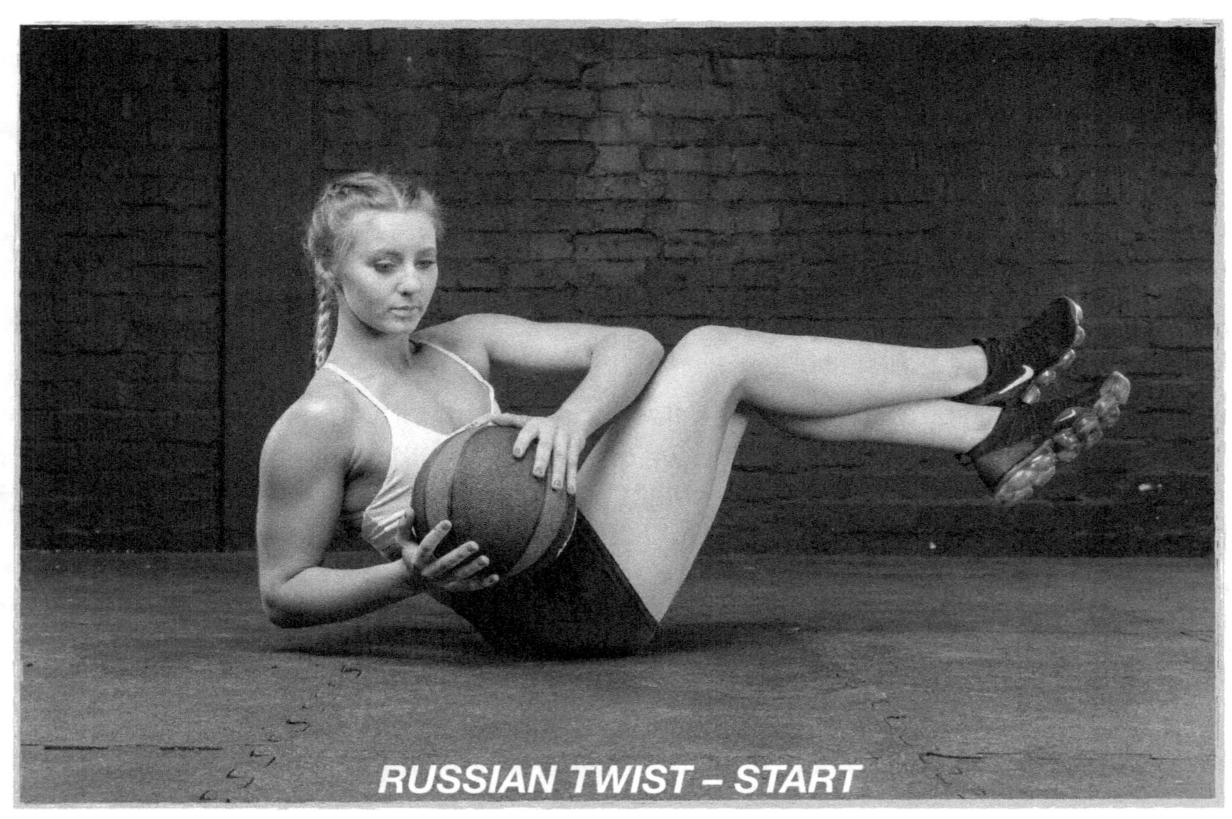

RUSSIAN TWIST – START

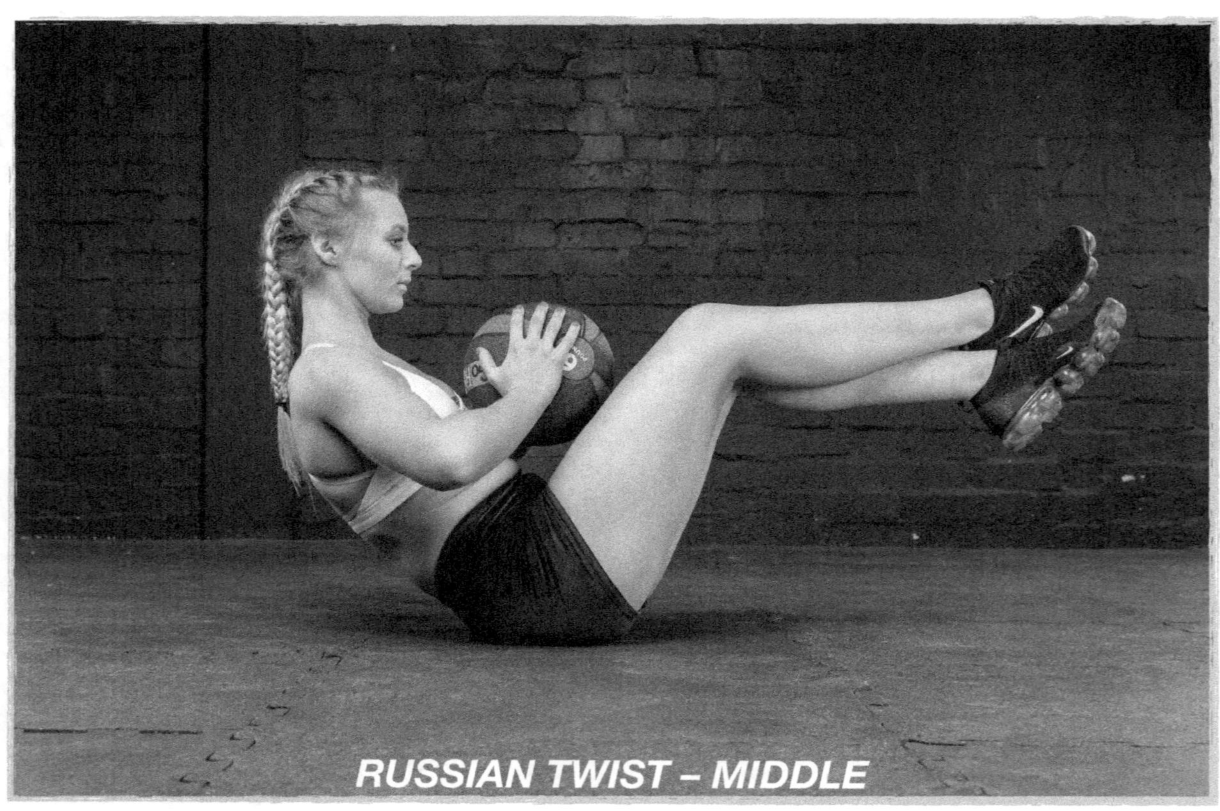

RUSSIAN TWIST – MIDDLE

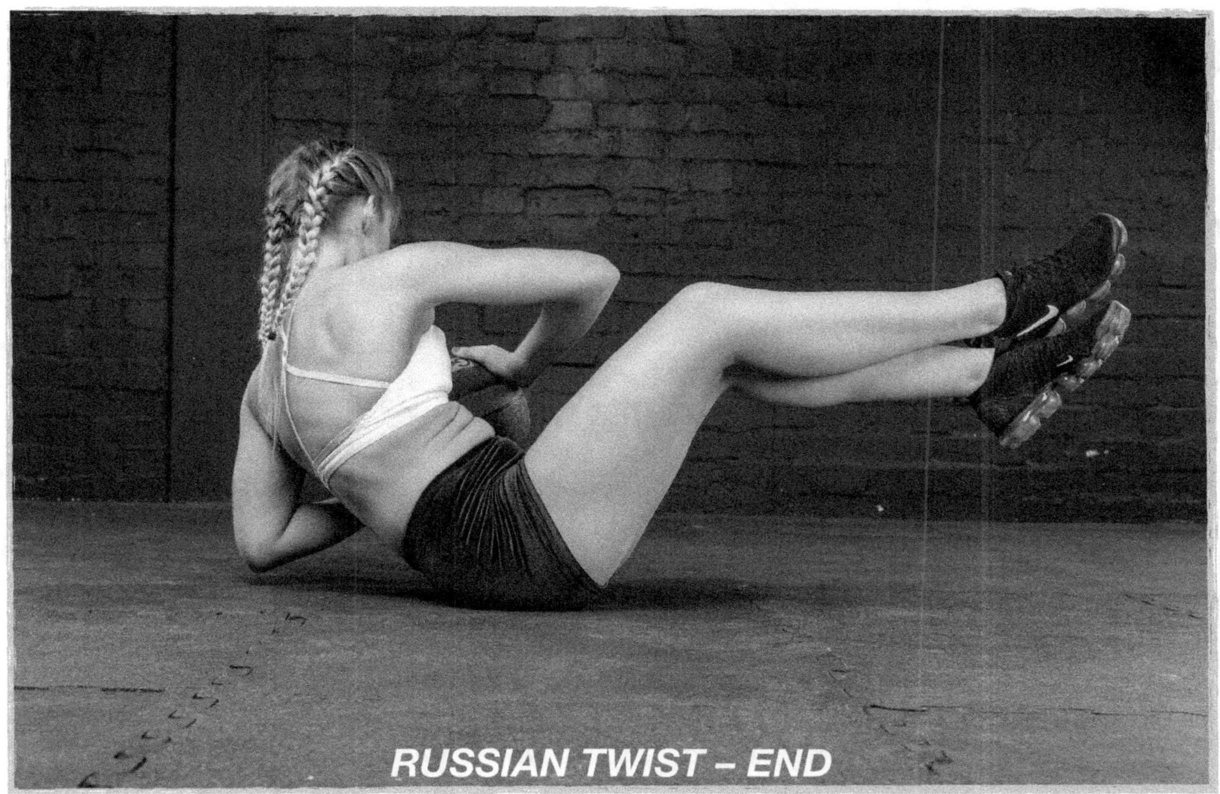

8.7 LEG EXTENSIONS

If there is one rule that rings true for core training it's that any exercise that stretches out the core works very well for building strength and muscle tone. The leg extension is one of those exercises, which lengthens the core out as far as possible and forces the muscles to contract.

HOW DO I SET THE EQUIPMENT UP?

For leg extensions you will need some floor space, and a mat to cushion your back.

HOW DO I DO IT?

1. Lie on your back and tuck your knees up to your chest. Press your lower and middle back into the ground.

2. Now extend your legs until your knees become straight, keeping your feet as close to the ground as possible. Make sure that your lower and middle back stay pressed into the ground.

3. From the extended position, bring your legs in slowly until they are tucked into your chest again. This counts as one rep.

HOW MANY SETS AND REPS?

You should be looking to perform 3 to 5 sets of 8 to 12 reps.

HOW DO I ADJUST THE DIFFICULTY?

Adjusting the difficulty of leg extensions is done with range of motion. As the exercise is hardest when the legs are fully extended, simply reduce the distance you extend the legs to make the exercise easier. Extending the legs further, and holding them outstretched for longer, will make the exercise more challenging.

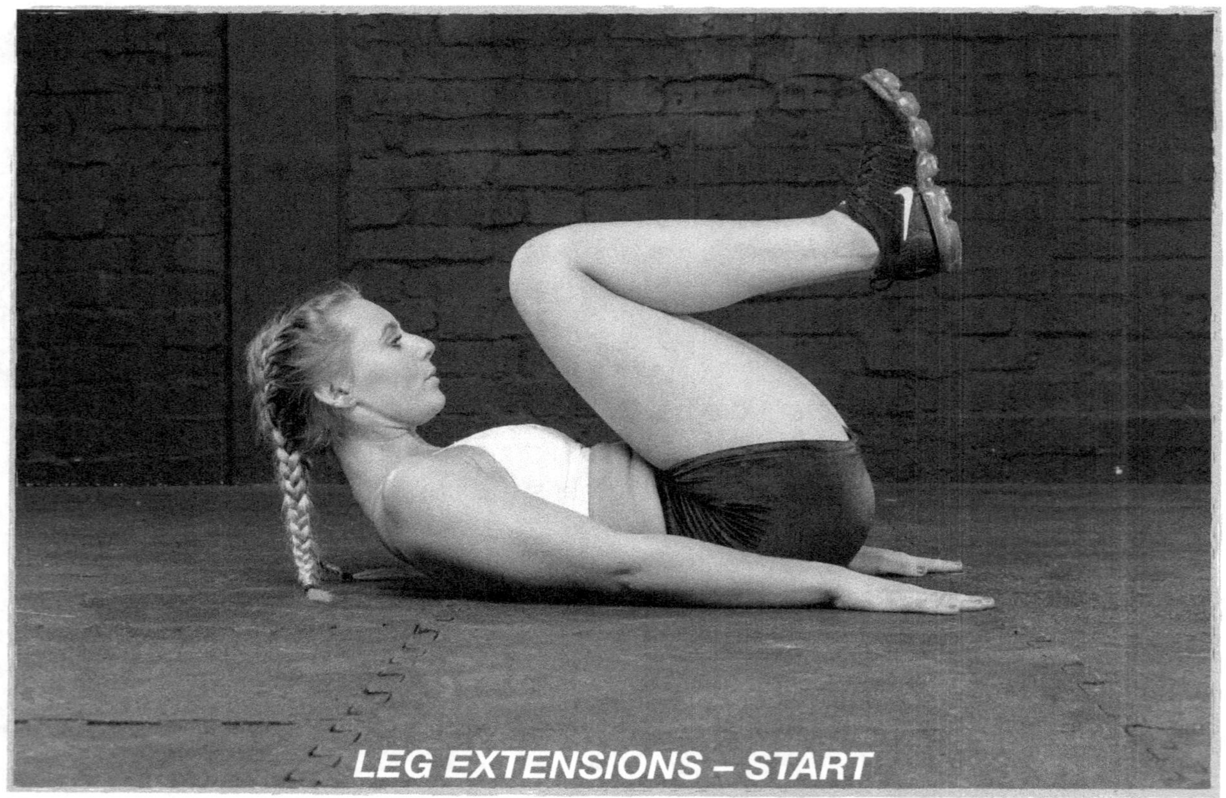

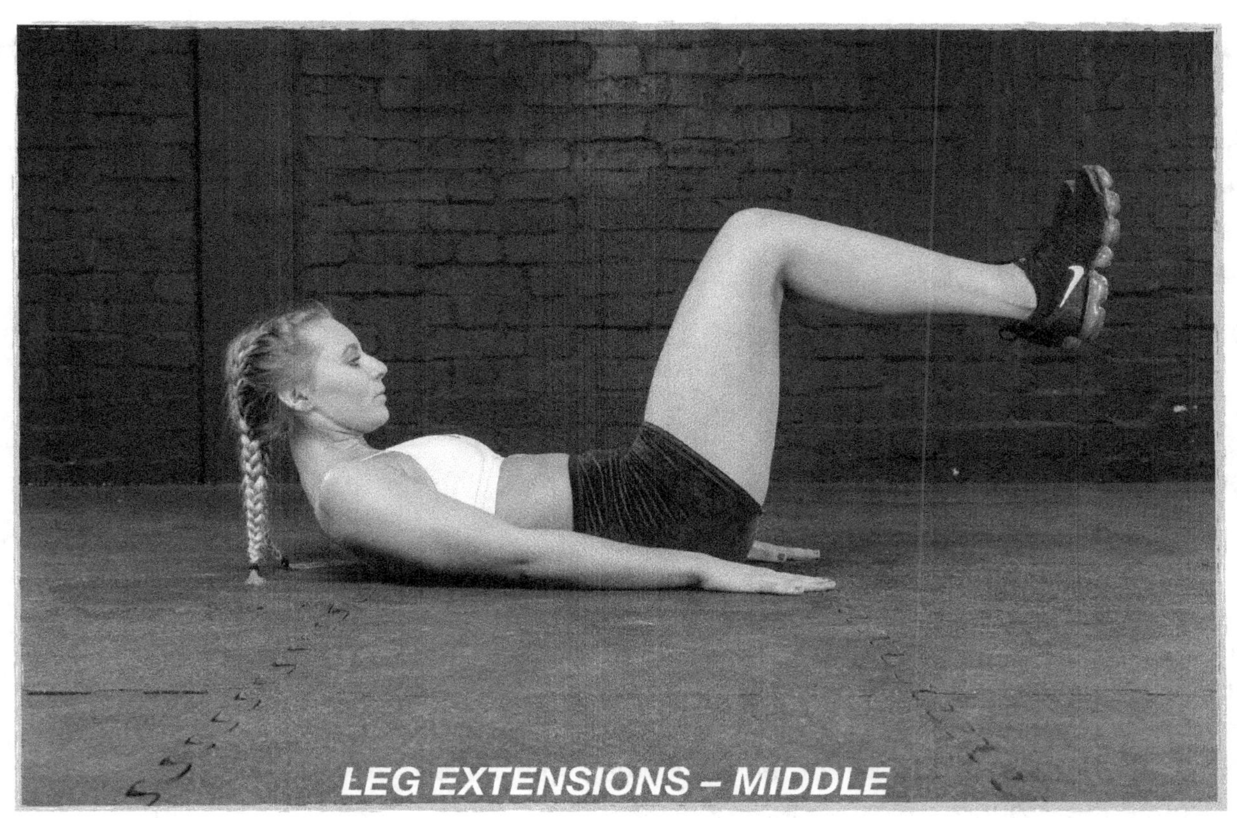

LEG EXTENSIONS – MIDDLE

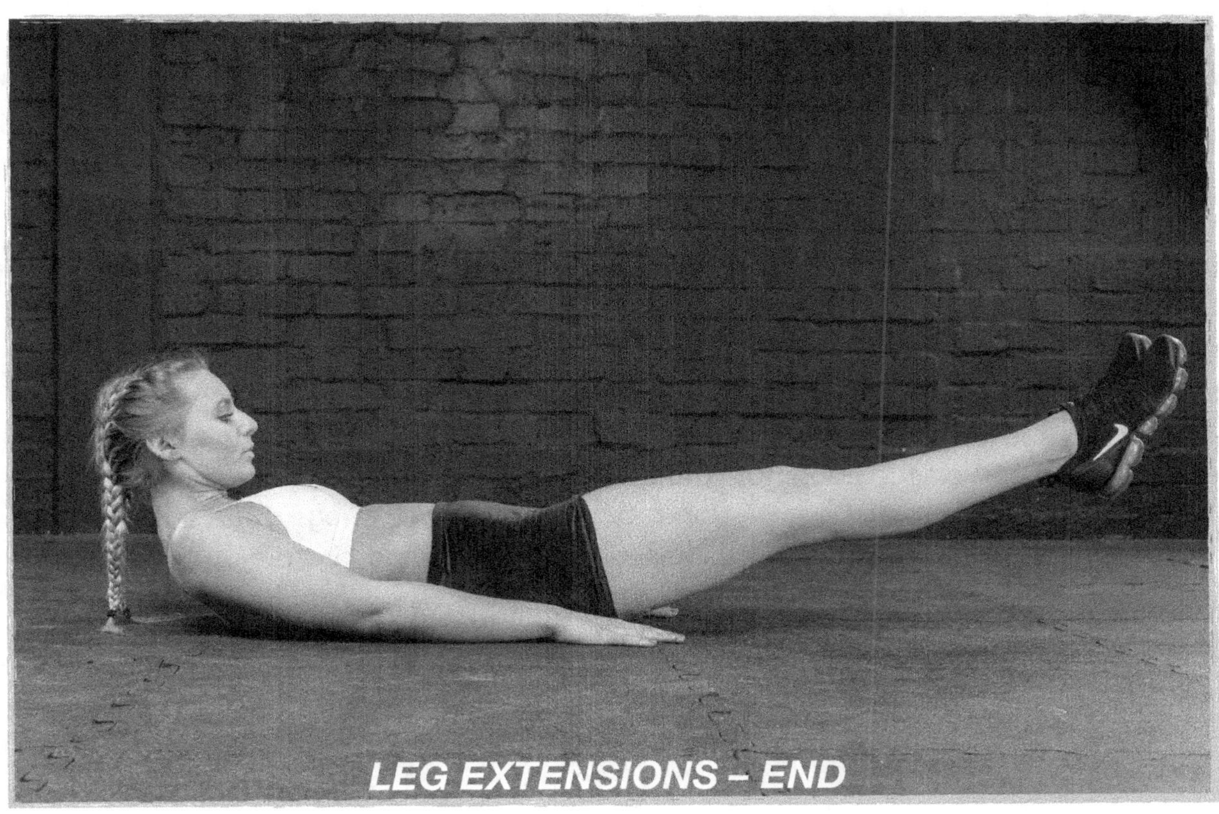

LEG EXTENSIONS – END

8.8 DISH

Everyone wants toned abs, and the dish is one way to get your core muscles in top shape. It's actually a very popular exercise in gymnastics, and we all know how toned gymnasts are! The full version is a little tough, but we show you how to make it easier, so don't worry!

HOW DO I SET THE EQUIPMENT UP?

For the dish you will need some floor space and a mat to cushion your back.

HOW DO I DO IT?

1. Lie on your back with your legs straight and your arms by your sides.

2. Lift your shoulders and upper back off the floor, and lift your hands off the ground.

3. Now lift your legs off the floor, ensuring that your lower back and middle back don't leave the ground. Think about pressing your spine down as hard as you can, or drawing your belly button towards the ground.

4. Now hold this position for as long as possible.

HOW MANY SETS AND REPS?

You should be looking to perform 3 to 5 sets of 20 to 30 second holds. This will no doubt be tough at first, so read on to see how to adjust the challenge!

HOW DO I ADJUST THE DIFFICULTY?

The dish is a tough exercise, no question about it. There are ways of making it easier, however. To make the dish easier simply draw your knees in to your chest, whilst keeping the upper body position the same. So, your shoulders and upper back should be lifted off the floor, but your knees will be drawn into your chest. This will be noticeably easier. As you get stronger, simply extend the legs out a little at a time, until they are fully stretched out as described in the method before.

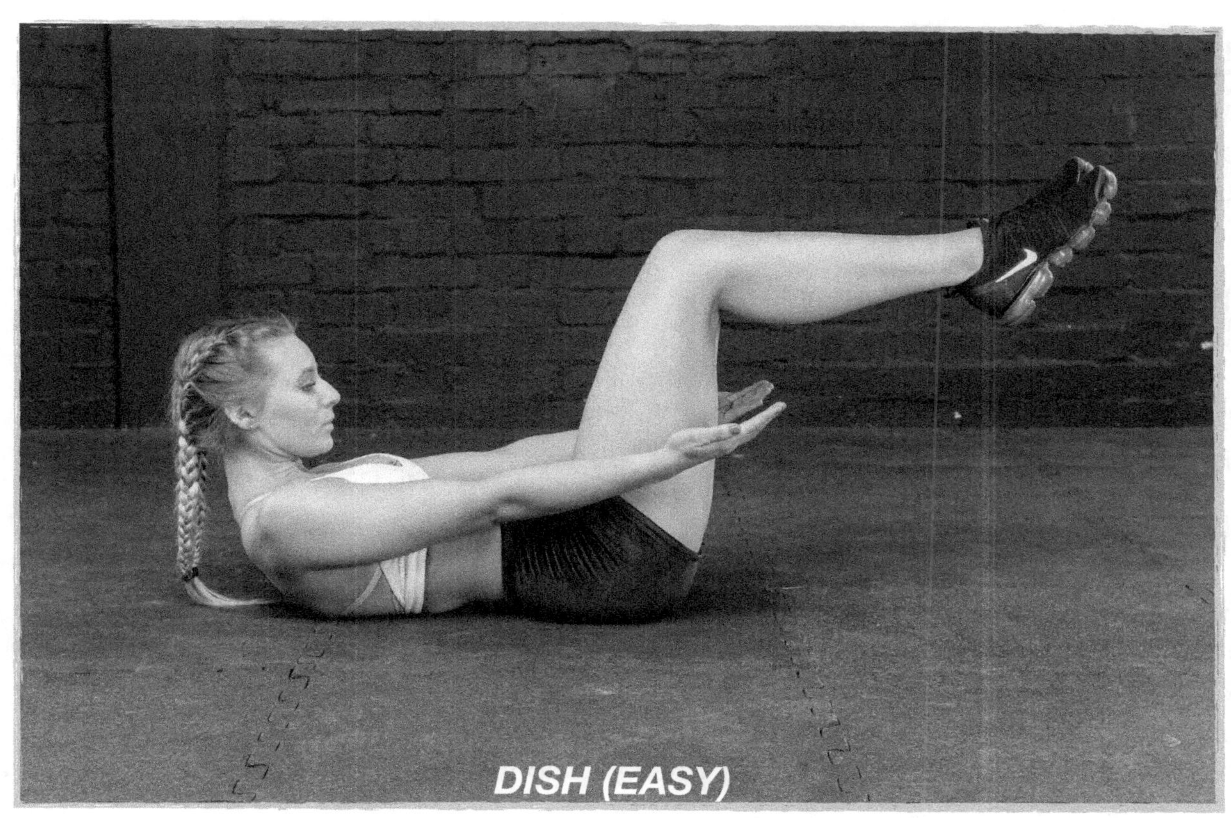

DISH (EASY)

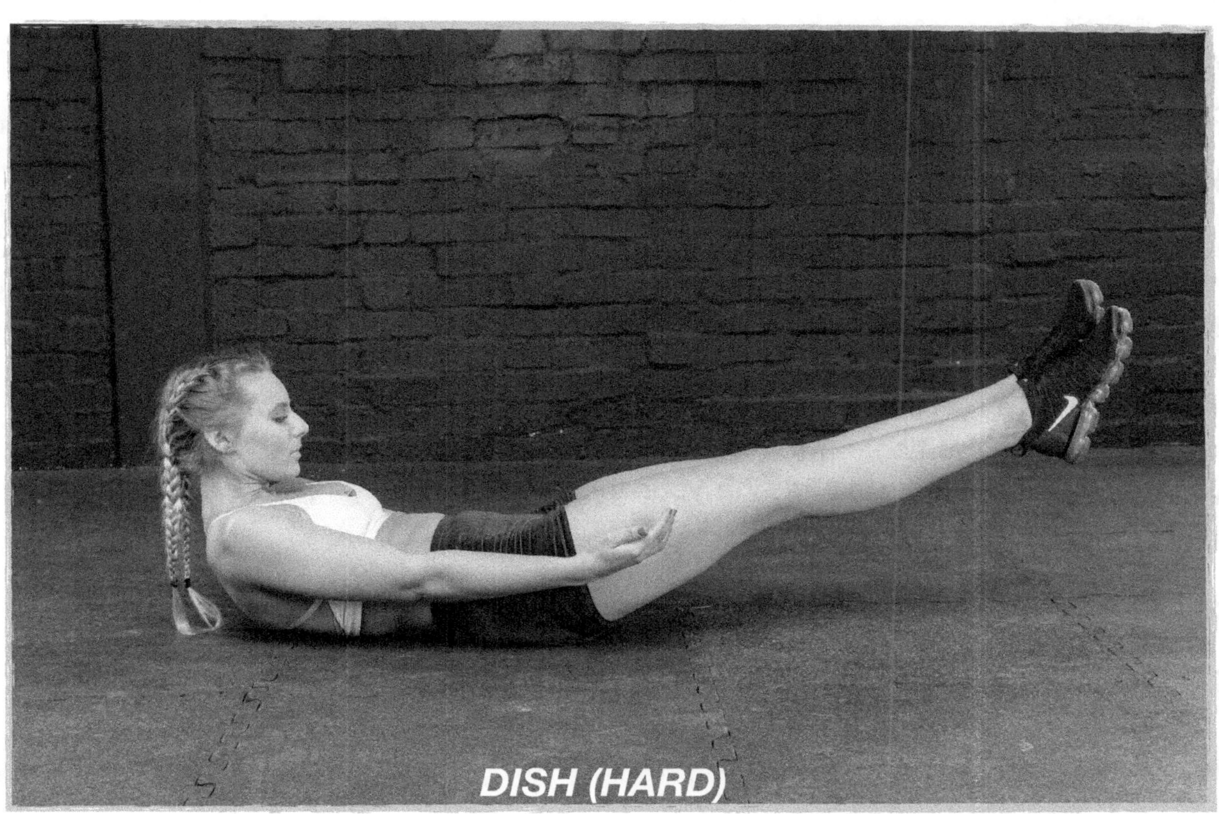

DISH (HARD)

8.9 *Hanging Knee Raise*

This exercise is great for those looking for a more whole-body core exercise, as it requires good strength from the upper body as well. It can also be adjusted to make the difficulty easier or harder, by either raising the knees or the legs.

HOW DO I SET THE EQUIPMENT UP?

For this exercise you will need access to a pull-up bar of some kind, either the one that is by itself, bolted to a wall, or one that is part of a larger machine (like the assisted pull-up and dip station).

HOW DO I DO IT?

1. Hang from the bar with an overhand grip (palms facing forwards), with your legs straight. Make sure that your entire body is straight.

2. Use your core muscles to draw up your thighs, bending your knees at the same time. Try and keep your elbows straight when you do this!

3. Keep raising your knees up until your thighs get as close as possible to your stomach. If you cannot do this, just make sure that your thighs are horizontal.

4. Pause for a second, and then return your legs to the starting position. This counts as one rep.

HOW MANY SETS AND REPS?

You should be looking to perform 3 to 5 sets of 8 to 12 reps.

HOW DO I ADJUST THE DIFFICULTY?

We're not going to lie; knee raises are tough! One way to make them easier is to swing a little, using momentum to help raise your knees. You can also work with a reduced range of motion, only raising your thighs so that they reach a horizontal position, before letting them down again.

Once knee raises become too easy, you can move onto hanging *leg* raises. These are exactly the same, except that you don't bend the knees, and raise the legs up when they're straight. The ultimate goal here is to raise the legs up high enough so that your toes touch the bar, but this is very tough, and may take you a little while to achieve.

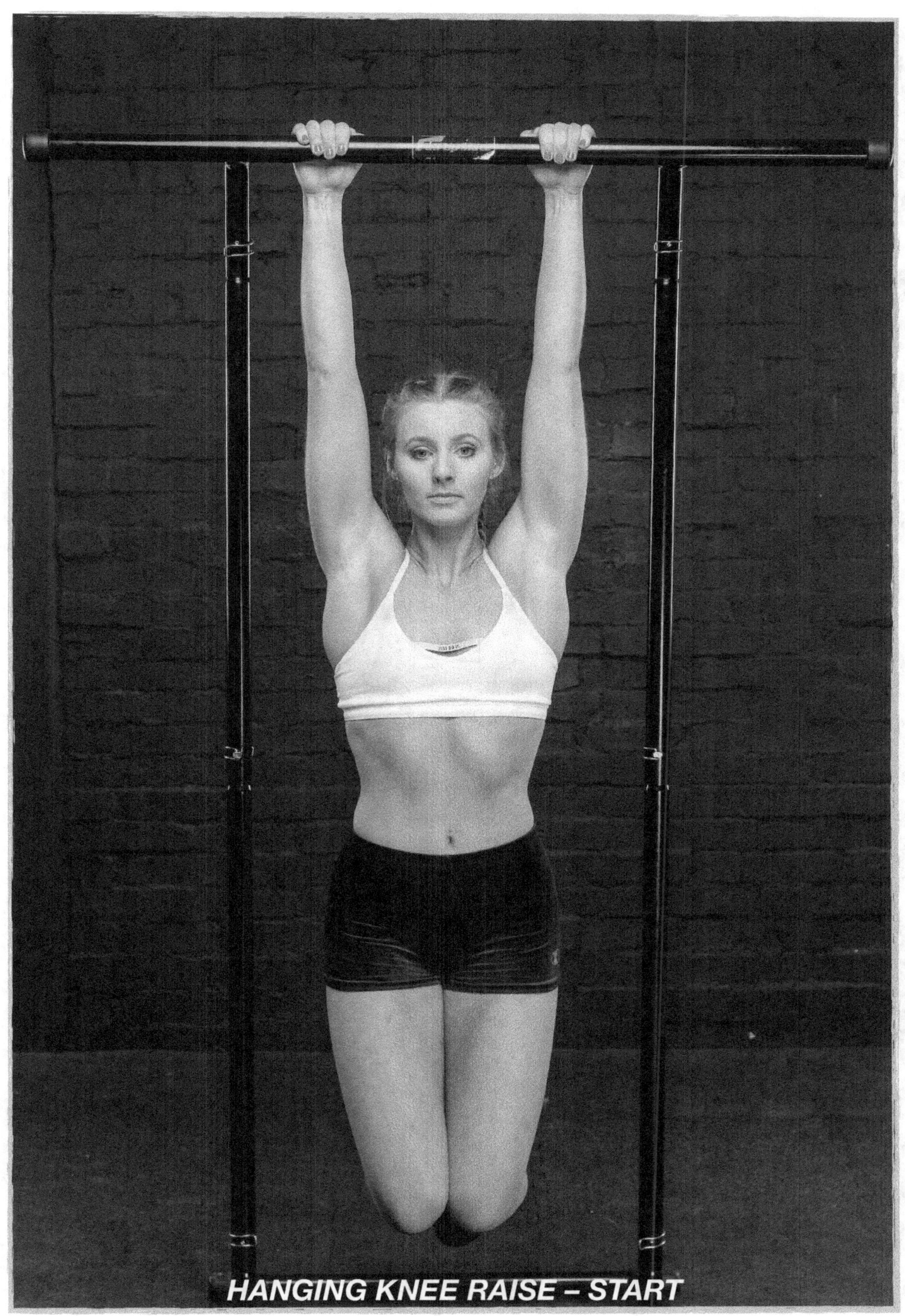

HANGING KNEE RAISE – START

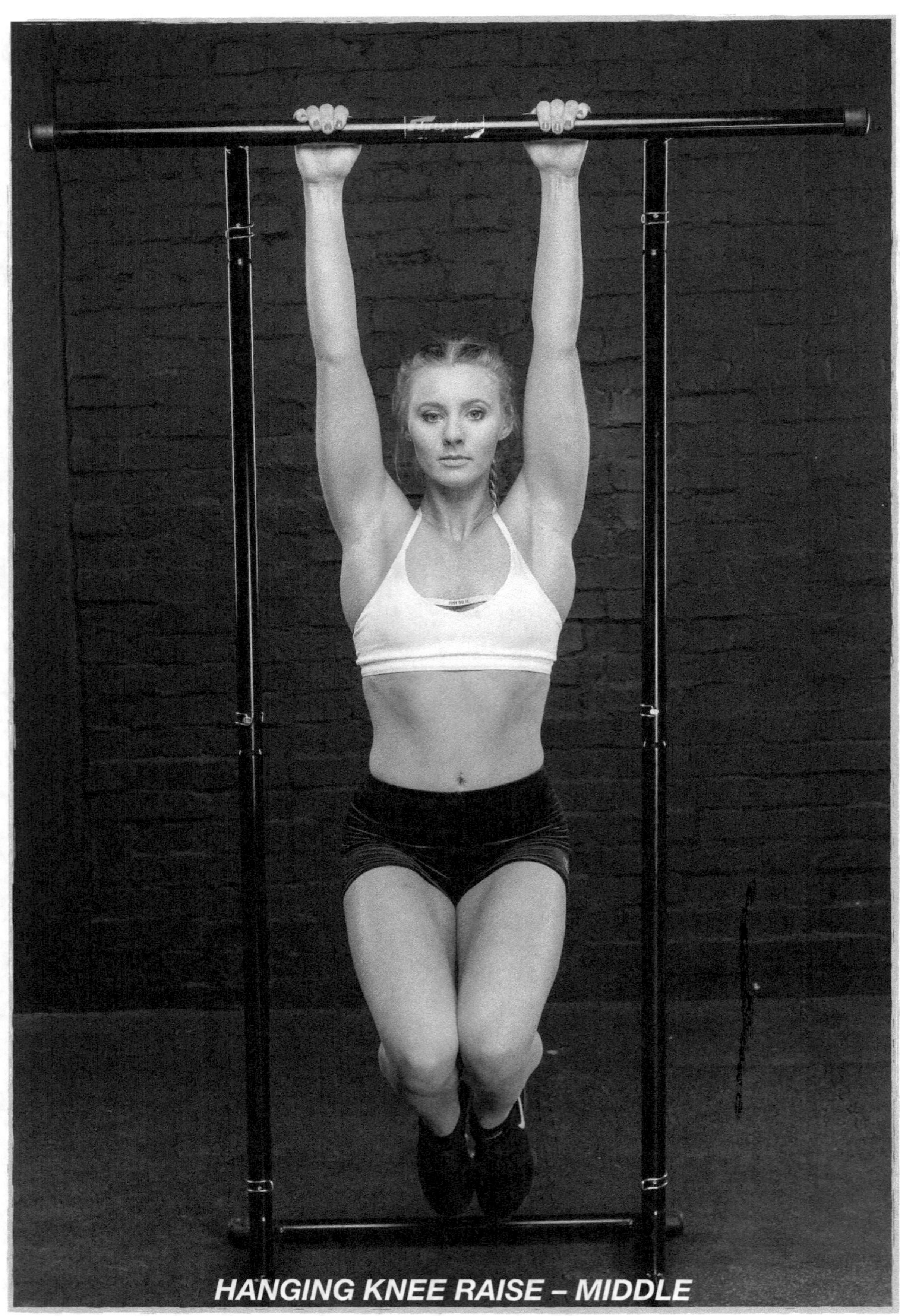

HANGING KNEE RAISE – MIDDLE

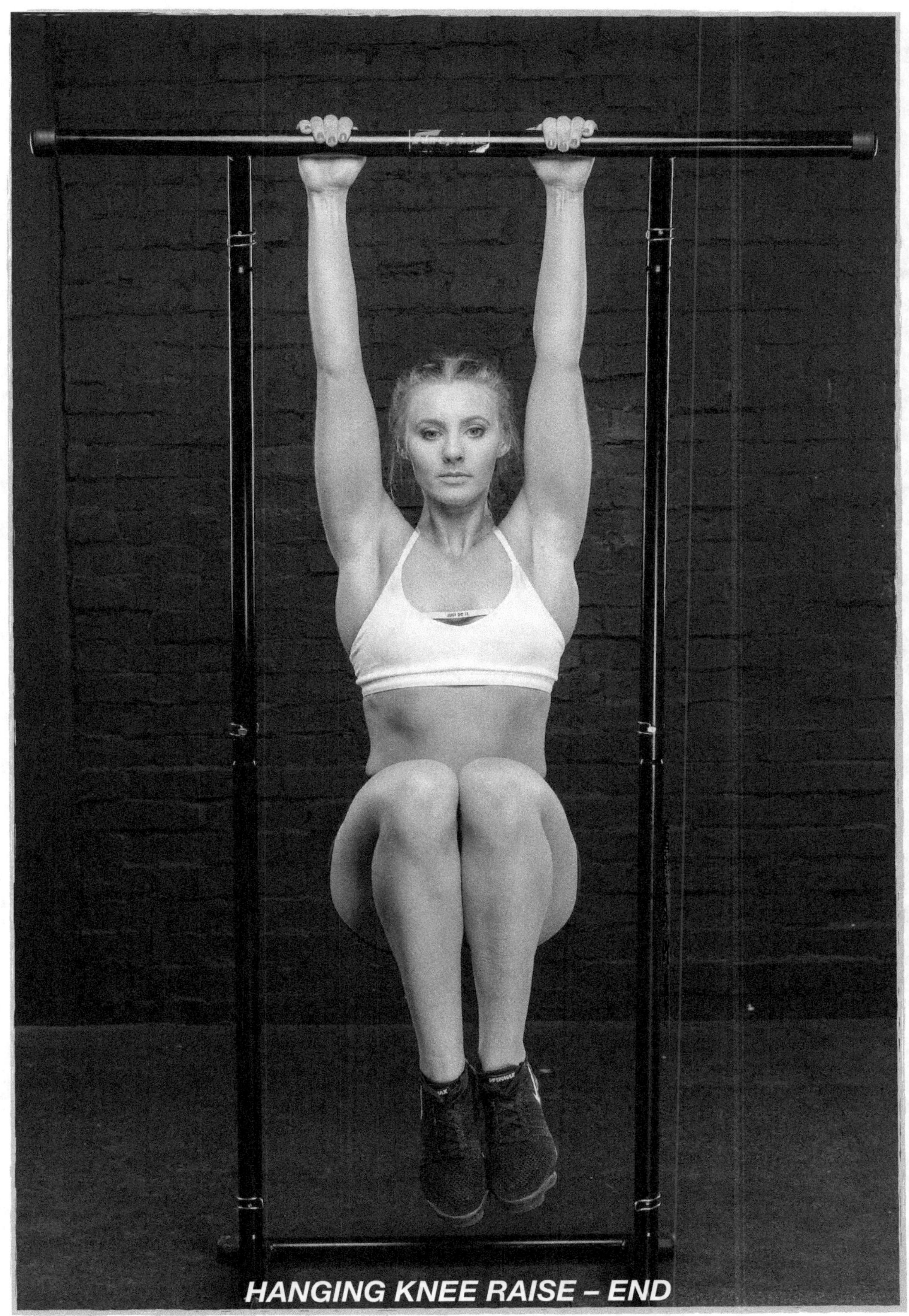

HANGING KNEE RAISE – END

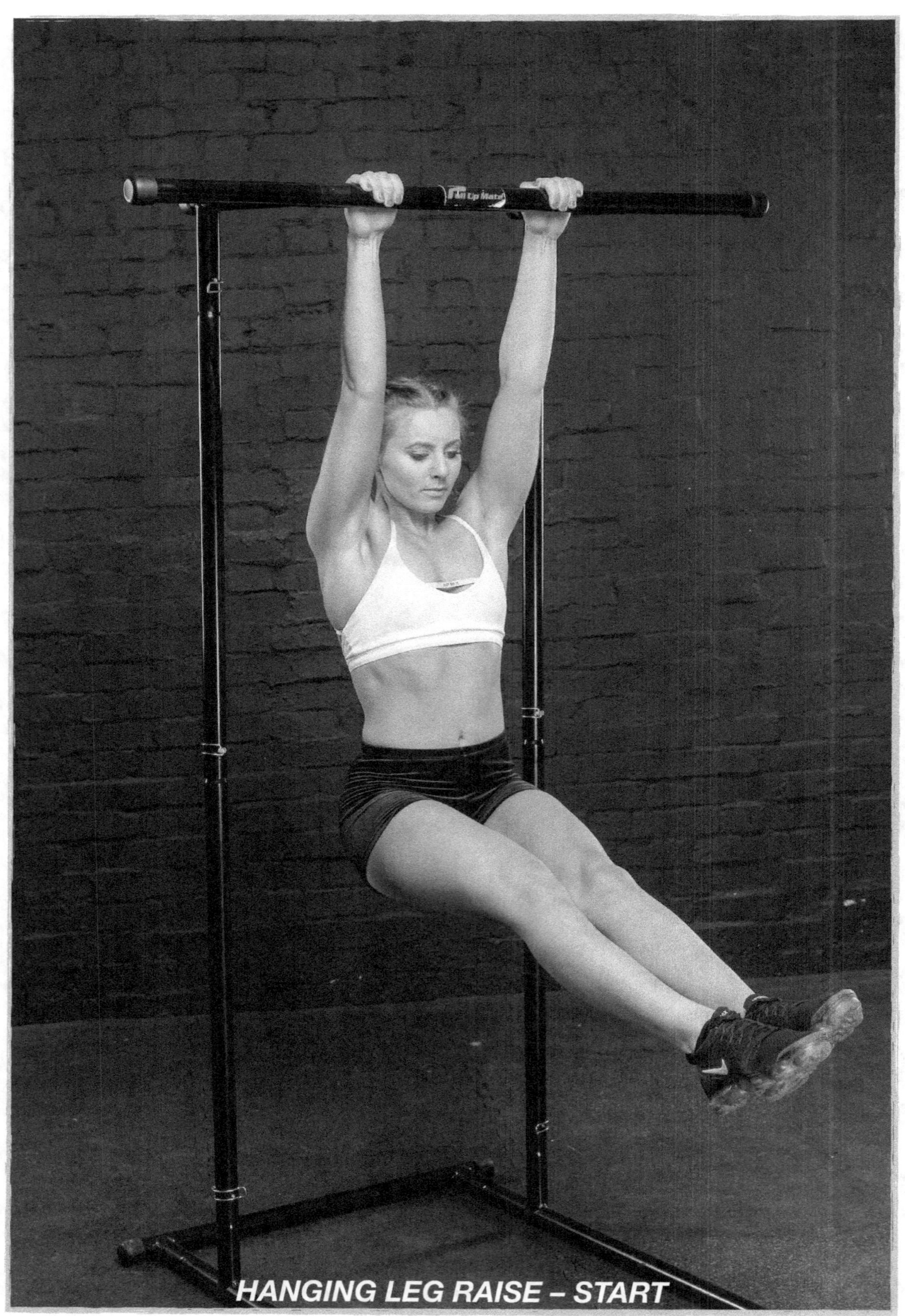

HANGING LEG RAISE – START

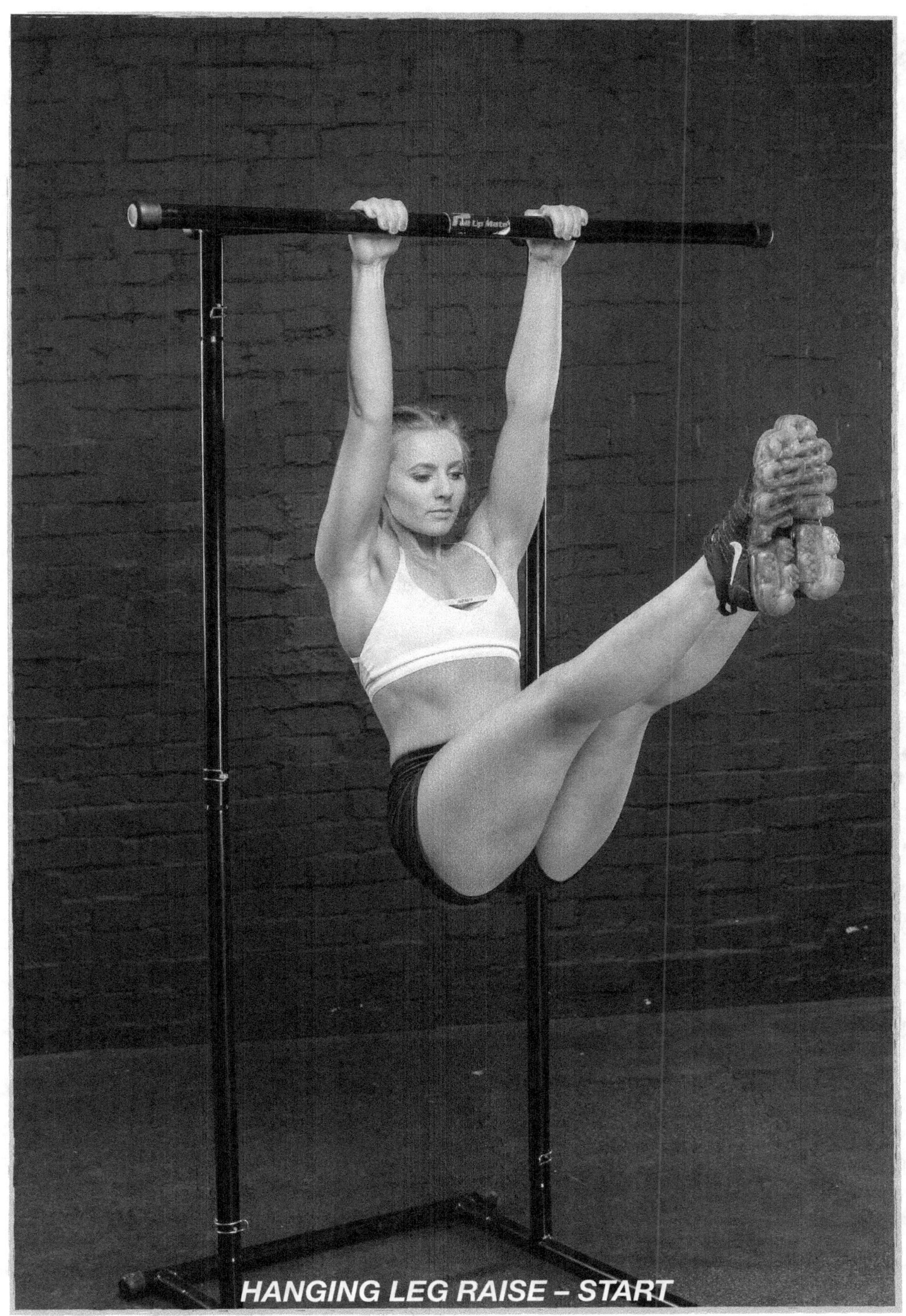

HANGING LEG RAISE – START

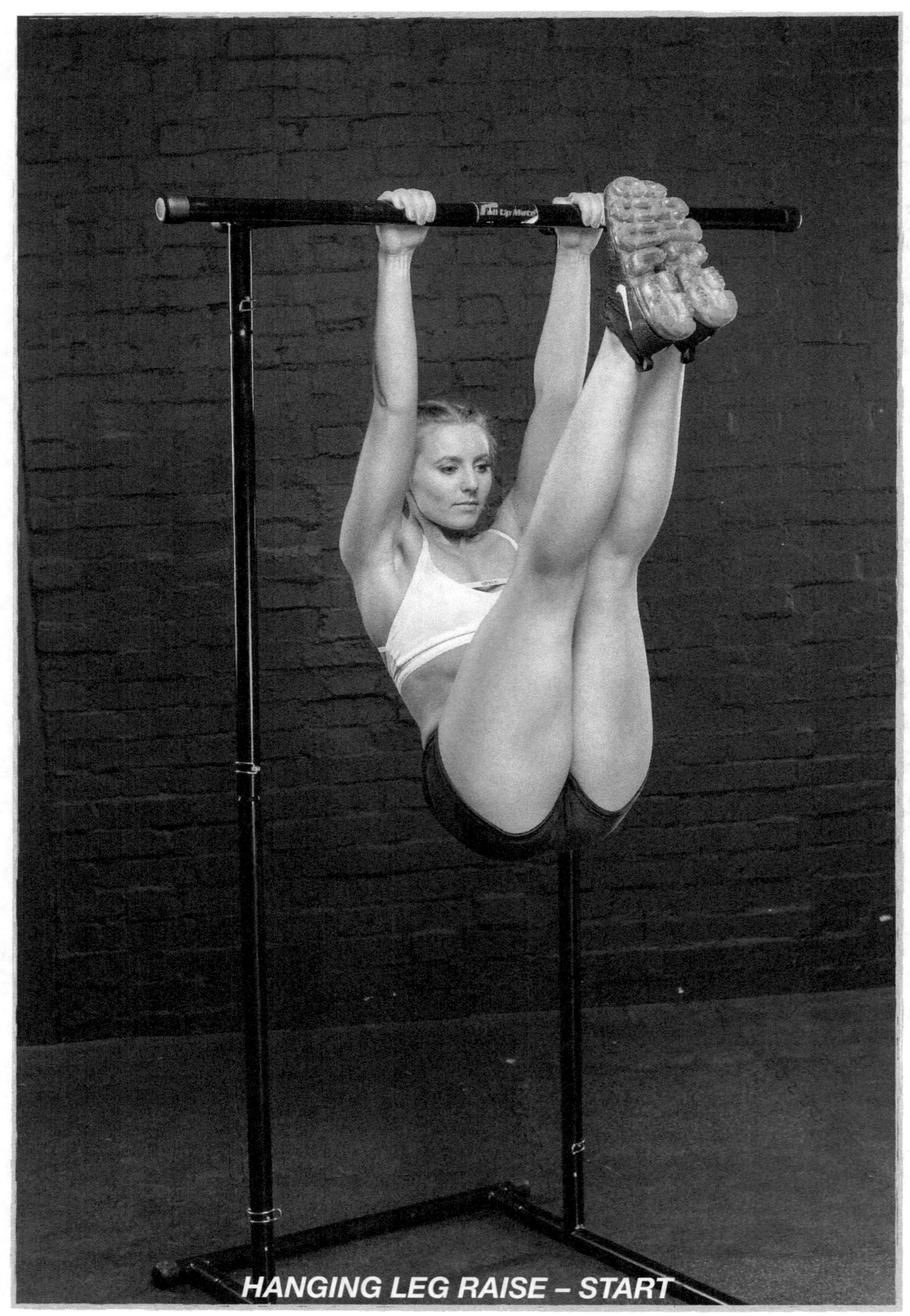

HANGING LEG RAISE – START

8.10 ROLLOUT

So, here we are! The rollout is by far the toughest core exercise in this book, but also the best in terms of the benefits that it brings. Like we said earlier, any exercise that stretches out the core is great for strengthening and improving muscle tone, and the rollout takes that approach and runs with it!

HOW DO I SET THE EQUIPMENT UP?

You will need an ab wheel for this exercise: one that is in good condition and rolls easily. Ideally it will have cushioned handles and a wide wheel that is stable and easy to use. You will also need some floor space, a mat to cushion your knees, and a weight or wall to roll the ab wheel into.

HOW DO I DO IT?

1. Kneel down with the ab wheel held with both hands. Place the weight about 2 feet away, or face a wall, again with the ab wheel 2 feet away from the base.

2. Keeping your arms straight start to roll the wheel forwards.

3. Keep rolling forward, aiming to keep your back horizontal at all times. Your arms and thighs will want to be the same angle as each other as you do the exercise.

4. Keep rolling forward until the ab wheel hits the weight or the wall.

5. Pause for a second, and then use your abs to pull the wheel away from the weight/wall and roll it back to the start position. This counts as one rep.

HOW MANY SETS AND REPS?

You should be looking to perform 3 to 5 sets of 8 to 12 reps.

HOW DO I ADJUST THE DIFFICULTY?

Making the rollout more or less difficult is straightforward. To make the exercise easier start closer to the weight/wall, and to make it more difficult start further away from the weight/wall.

The aim of the rollout is to be able to perform it without the weight/wall there, with the abs rolling the wheel away from you and back towards you. This is very tough, and may take you many weeks (or months!) to accomplish. Even though getting to this stage is desirable, don't worry if you don't! Even the easy versions of the rollout are beneficial, and will give your core a real workout!

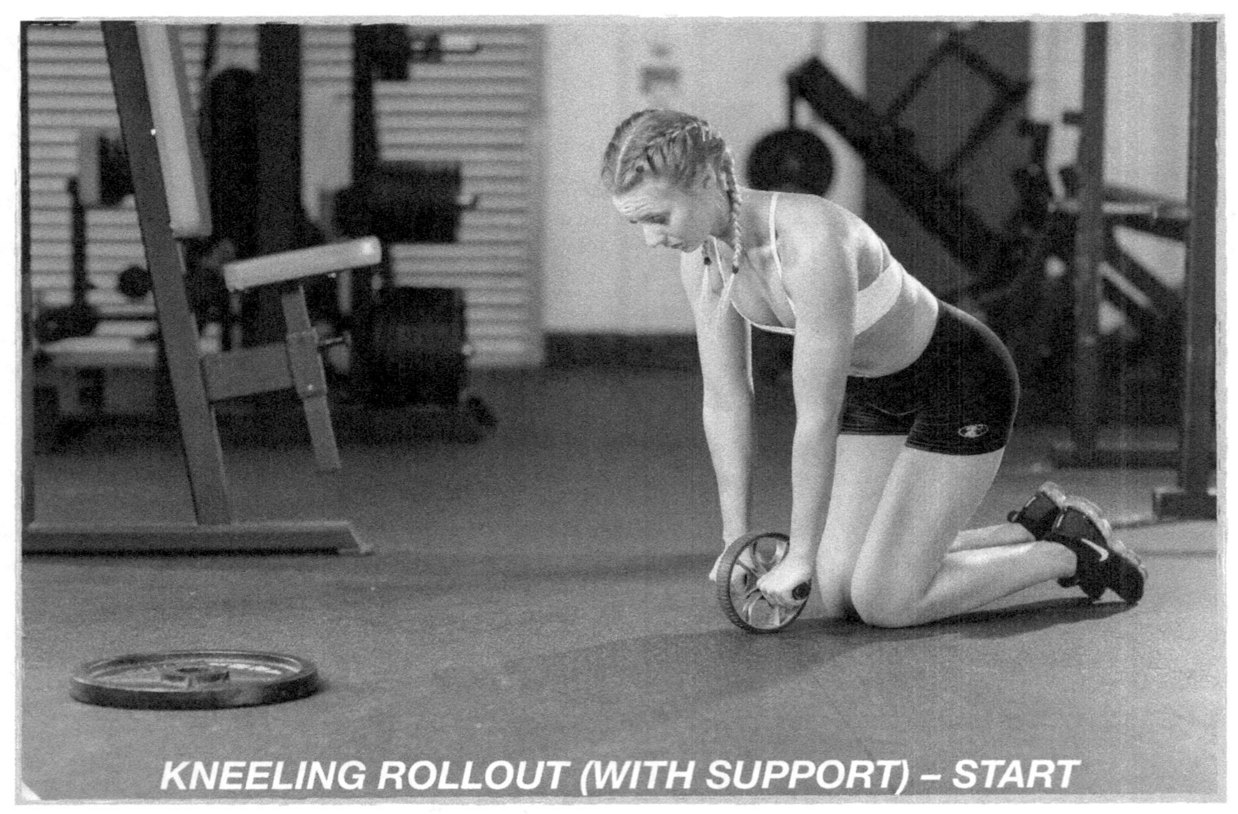

KNEELING ROLLOUT (WITH SUPPORT) – START

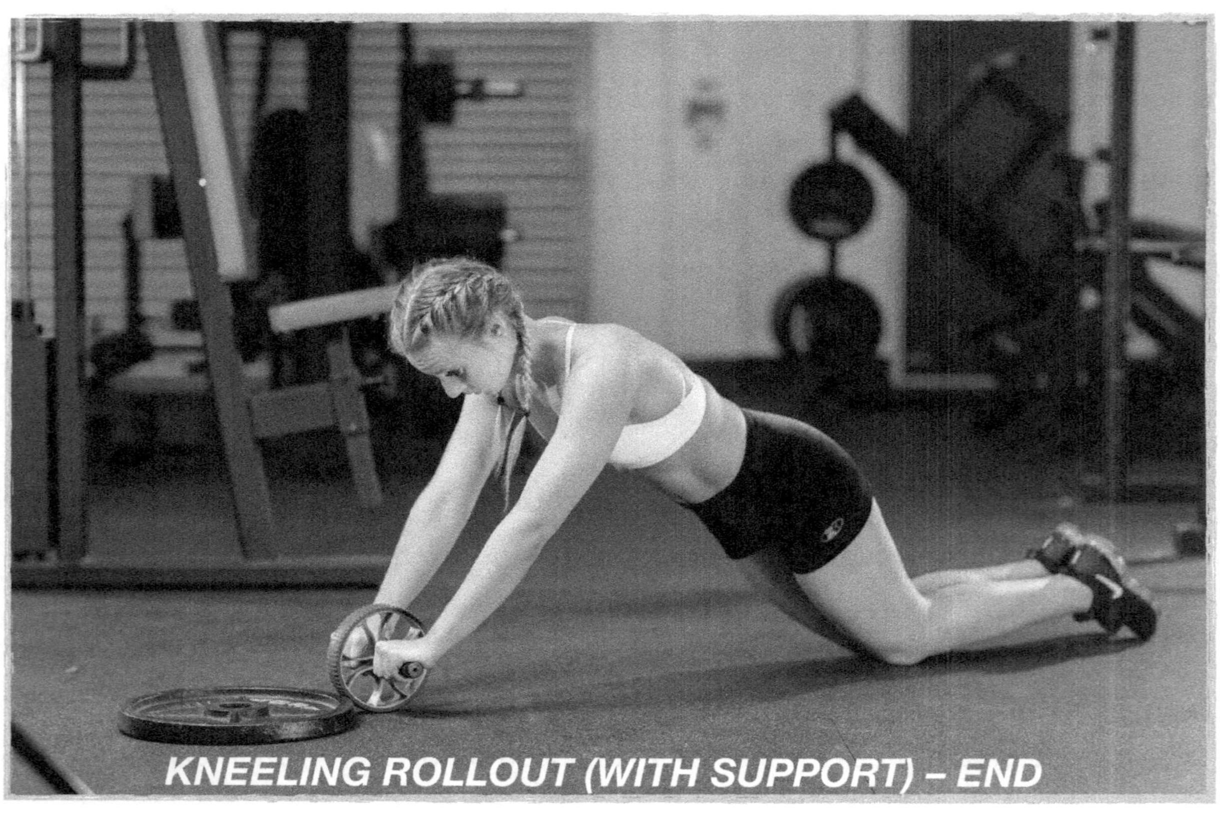

KNEELING ROLLOUT (WITH SUPPORT) – END

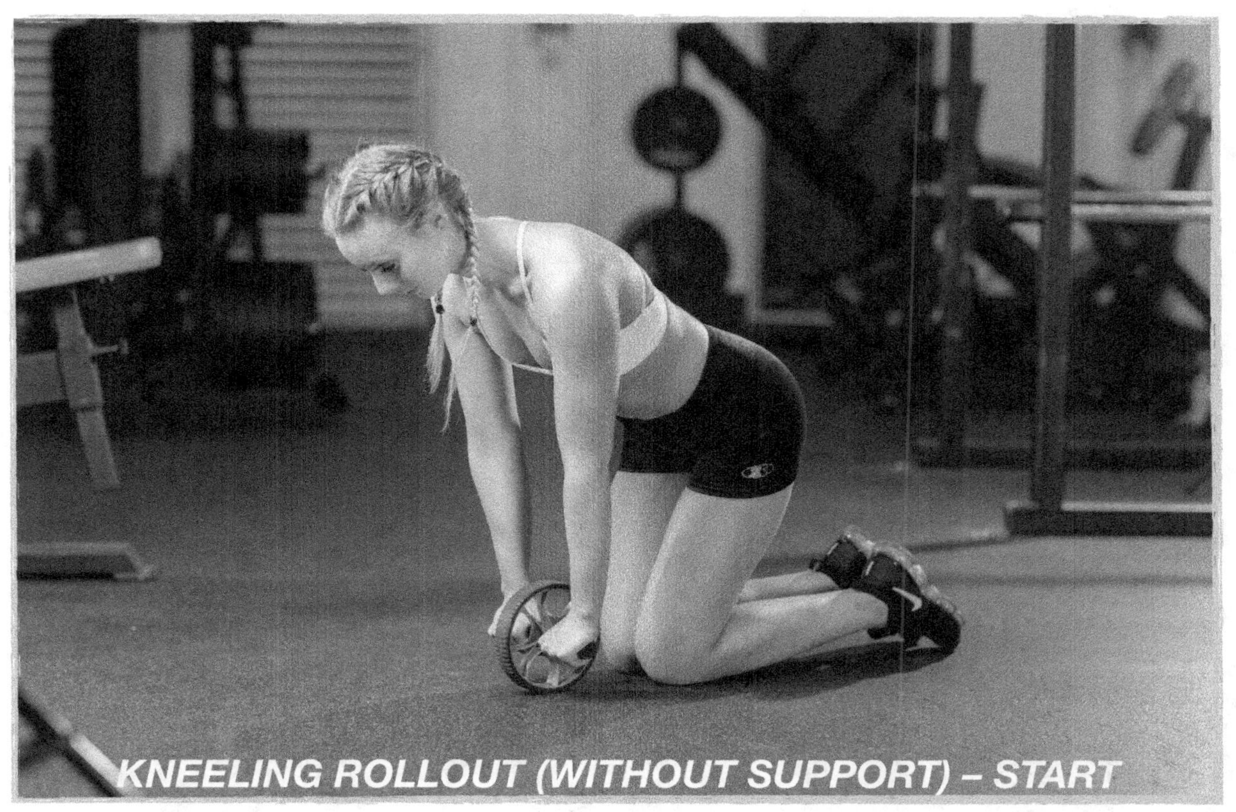

KNEELING ROLLOUT (WITHOUT SUPPORT) – START

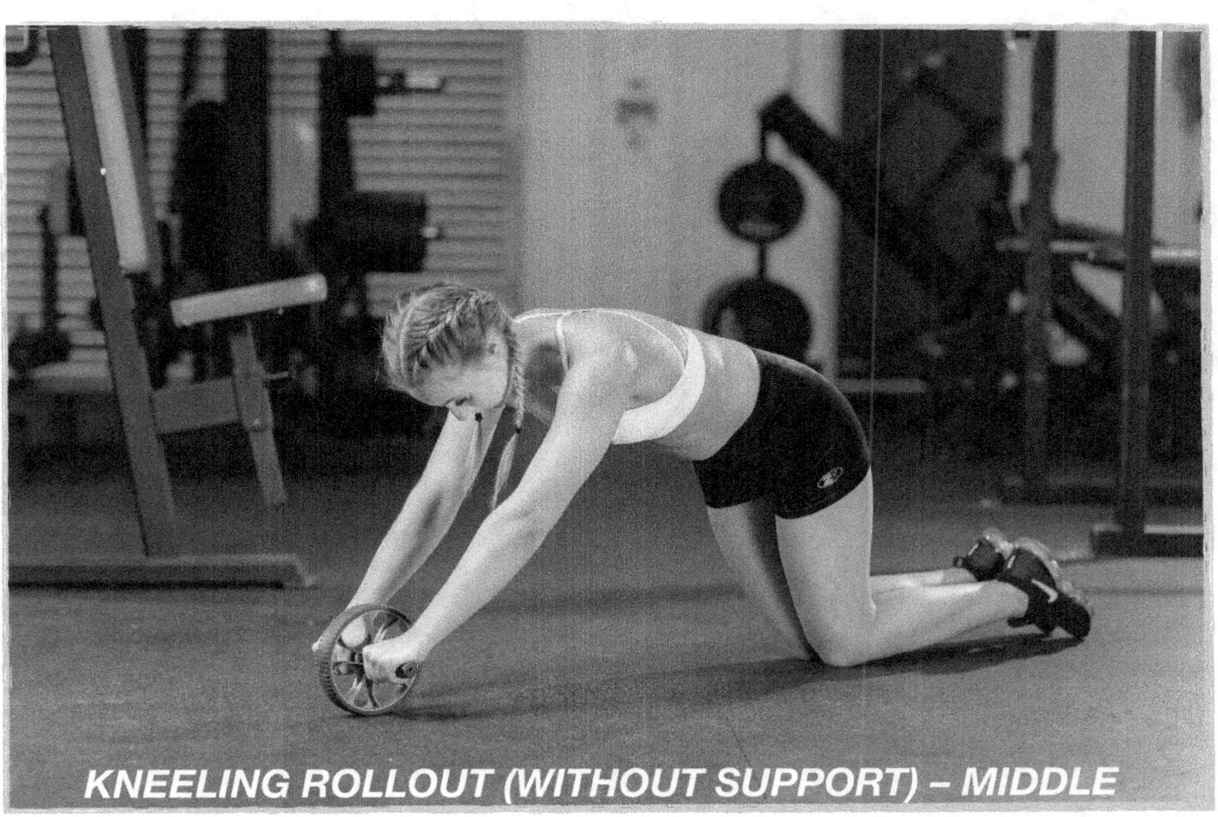

KNEELING ROLLOUT (WITHOUT SUPPORT) – MIDDLE

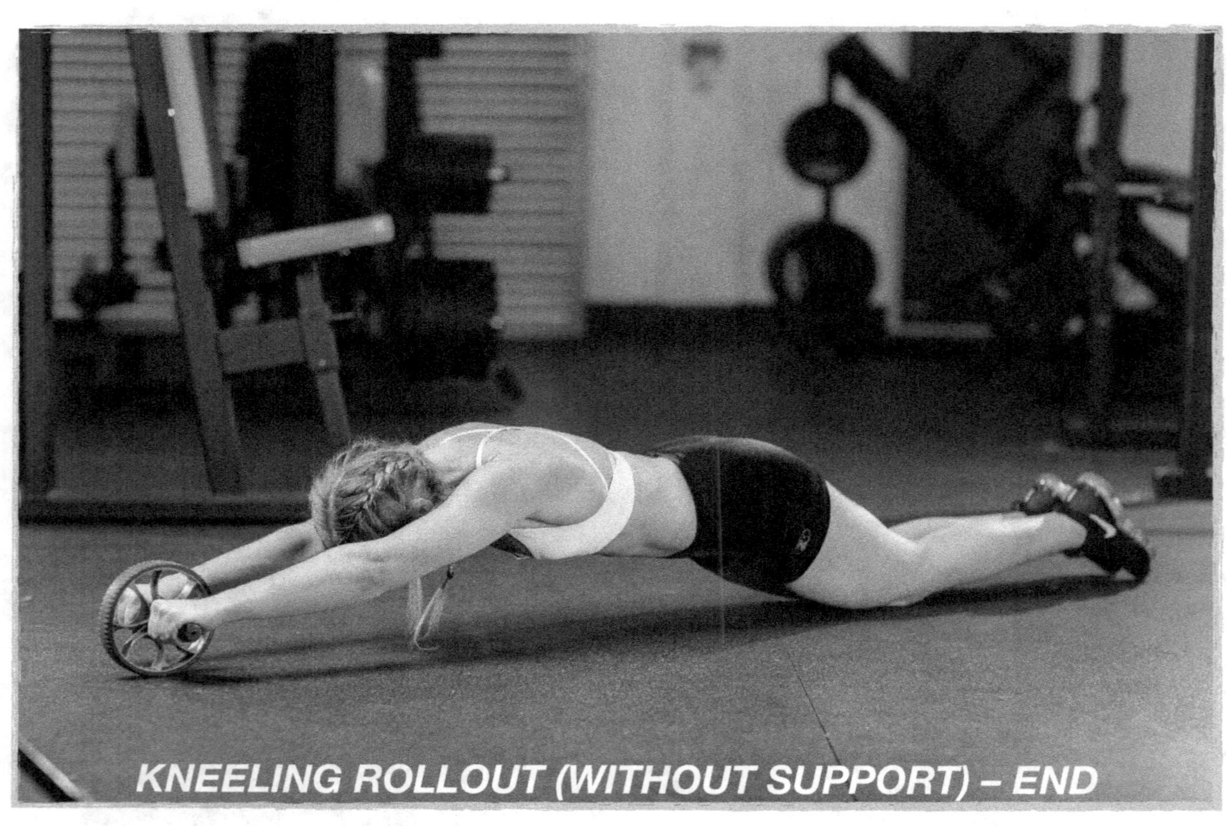

KNEELING ROLLOUT (WITHOUT SUPPORT) – END

SECTION THREE: LEGS AND BUM

The aesthetics of the legs and bum have come into vogue in the last few years, with some women even reverting to surgery to keep up with the fashion! We're here to tell you that you don't need to take drastic measures like surgery to get the legs and bum you want. Good, simple, resistance exercises will work wonders for your lower body, and combined with the abs and core training section, will give you any degree of hourglass shape that you want.

A word on leg and bum training; as the muscles are the largest in the human body, you are likely to feel very tired after a good workout. This is a good thing!

9.1 BODY WEIGHT SQUAT

If you want glutes, you have to squat, it's that simple! It won't have escaped your attention that having good glutes is in fashion, and has been for the past few years, especially with the rise of the Kardashians and their substantial behinds. But, whilst there are some that claim those glutes are fake, the squat will help you get the real deal. This version is the body weight squat, which is where we recommend everyone start regardless of your level of experience. Doing a proper squat with proper technique is not as easy or as straightforward as you might think, but follow our instructions and you should have no trouble perfecting them!

HOW DO I SET THE EQUIPMENT UP?

For the squat you will need some floor space.

HOW DO I DO IT?

1. Stand with your feet shoulder width apart, toes pointing out slightly, arms relaxed by your sides, head and neck in a neutral position.

2. Start to bend your knees, pushing your hips back and down at the same time.

3. Aim to keep your back straight, raising your arms into the air in front of you to aid balance if needed.

4. Keep bending your knees and pushing your hips back and down as you squat lower.

5. Descend until your thighs are at least horizontal, then pause for a second.

6. Push up and return to the standing position. This counts as one rep.

HOW MANY SETS AND REPS?

You should be looking to perform 3 to 5 sets of 8 to 12 reps.

HOW DO I ADJUST THE DIFFICULTY?

Some common problems with the squat are mainly to do with not being flexible enough to get into the bottom position, and this is the result of tight hips, knees, and ankles. The best way to practice this and get more flexible is to keep squatting, and perform the stretches that we outlined in the flexibility section.

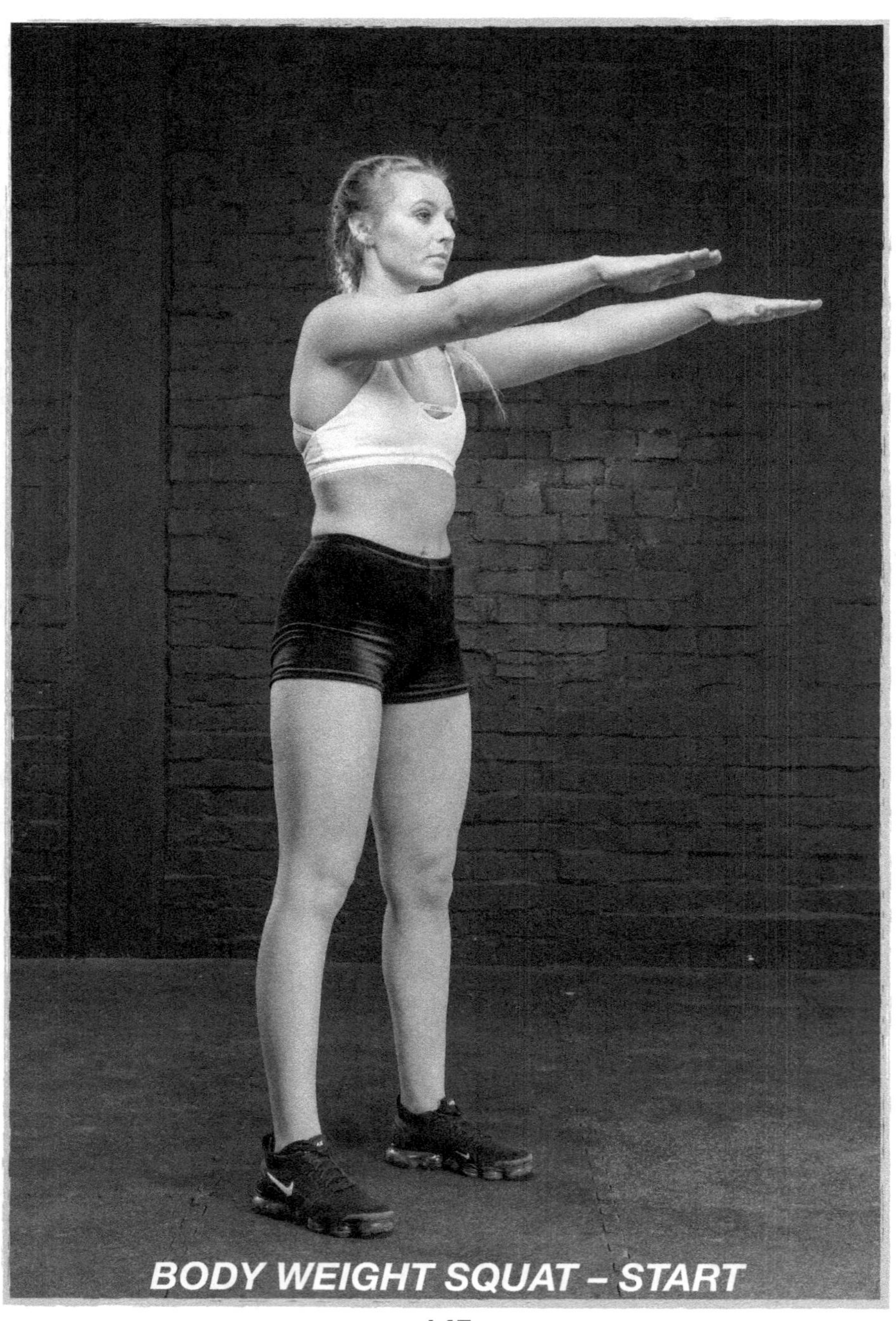

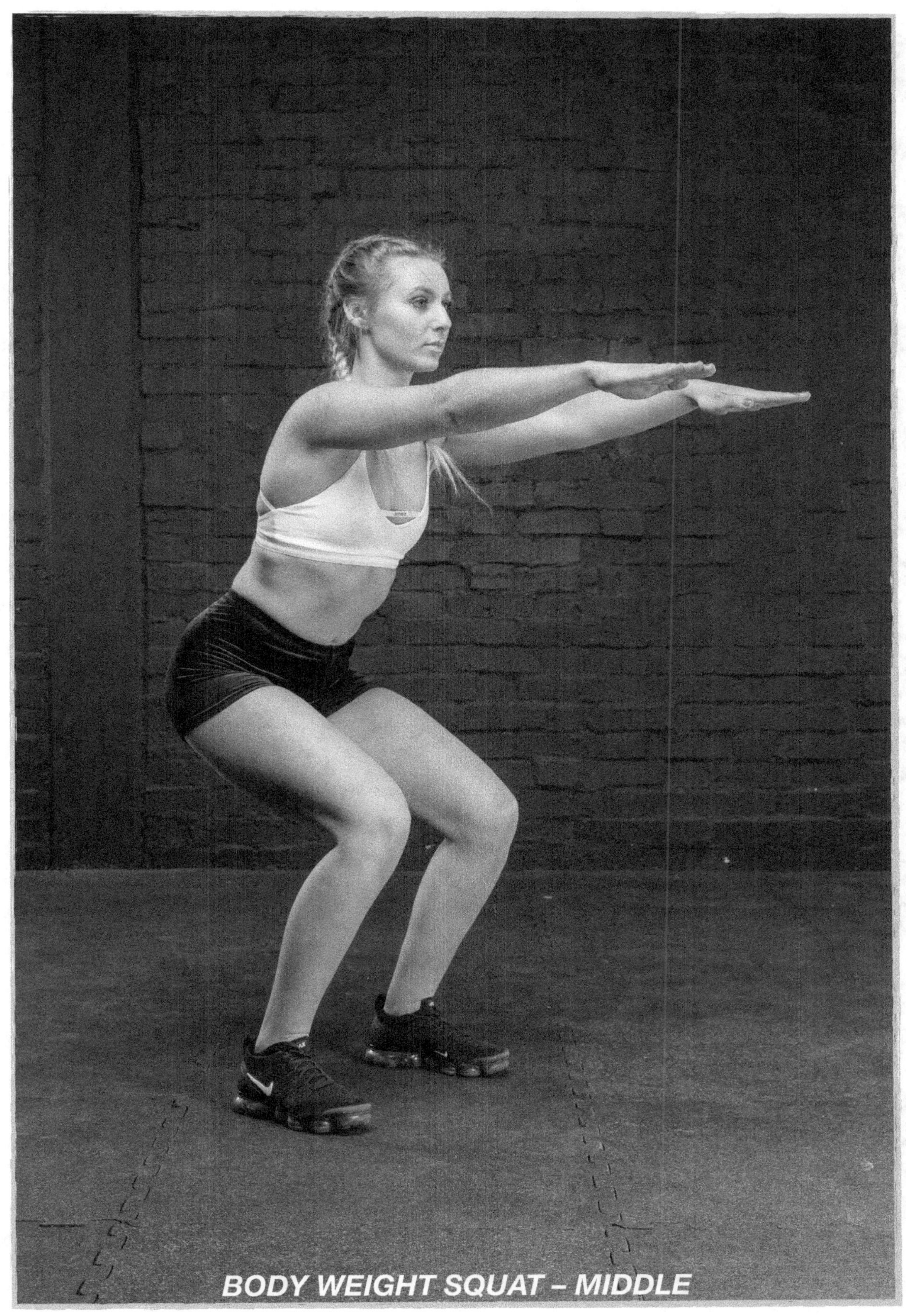

BODY WEIGHT SQUAT – MIDDLE

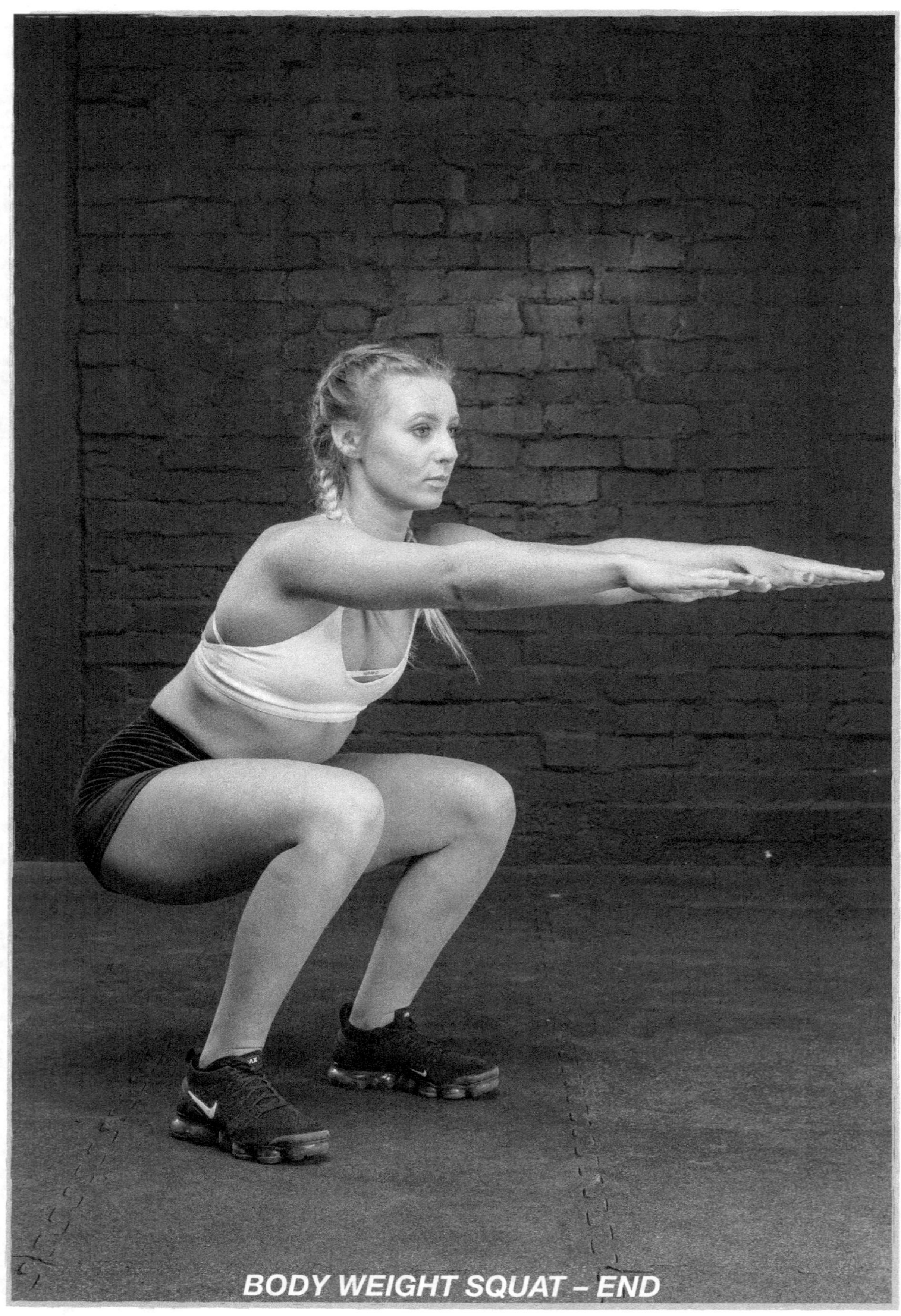

BODY WEIGHT SQUAT – END

9.2 LUNGE

Along with the squat, the lunge is one of the go to exercises to get your glutes fired up. They also work the hamstrings and quads as well, so as an all round lower body exercise they cannot be beaten.

HOW DO I SET THE EQUIPMENT UP?

For lunges you will need some floor space, with room in front of and behind you to step forwards and backwards.

HOW DO I DO IT?

1. Stand with your feet shoulder width apart, arms hanging loosely by your sides.

2. Take a large step forward with your right foot, bending your knee as your foot hits the ground.

3. Keep bending both knees at an equal rate so that you sink towards the floor.

4. Keep going until both knees are bent at ninety degrees, or your rear knee is almost touching the ground.

5. Pause for a second, and then get ready to push back up. There are two options here:
- Push off hard with the rear leg to step forward, OR
- Push off hard with the front leg to step backward

6. Once you return to the standing position this counts as one rep.

HOW MANY SETS AND REPS?

You should be looking to perform 3 to 5 sets of 8 to 12 reps.

HOW DO I ADJUST THE DIFFICULTY?

To adjust the difficulty of the lunge is easy. To make the lunge easier don't bend your knees as much, and to increase the difficulty bend your knees the full amount, or until your rear knee touches the ground.

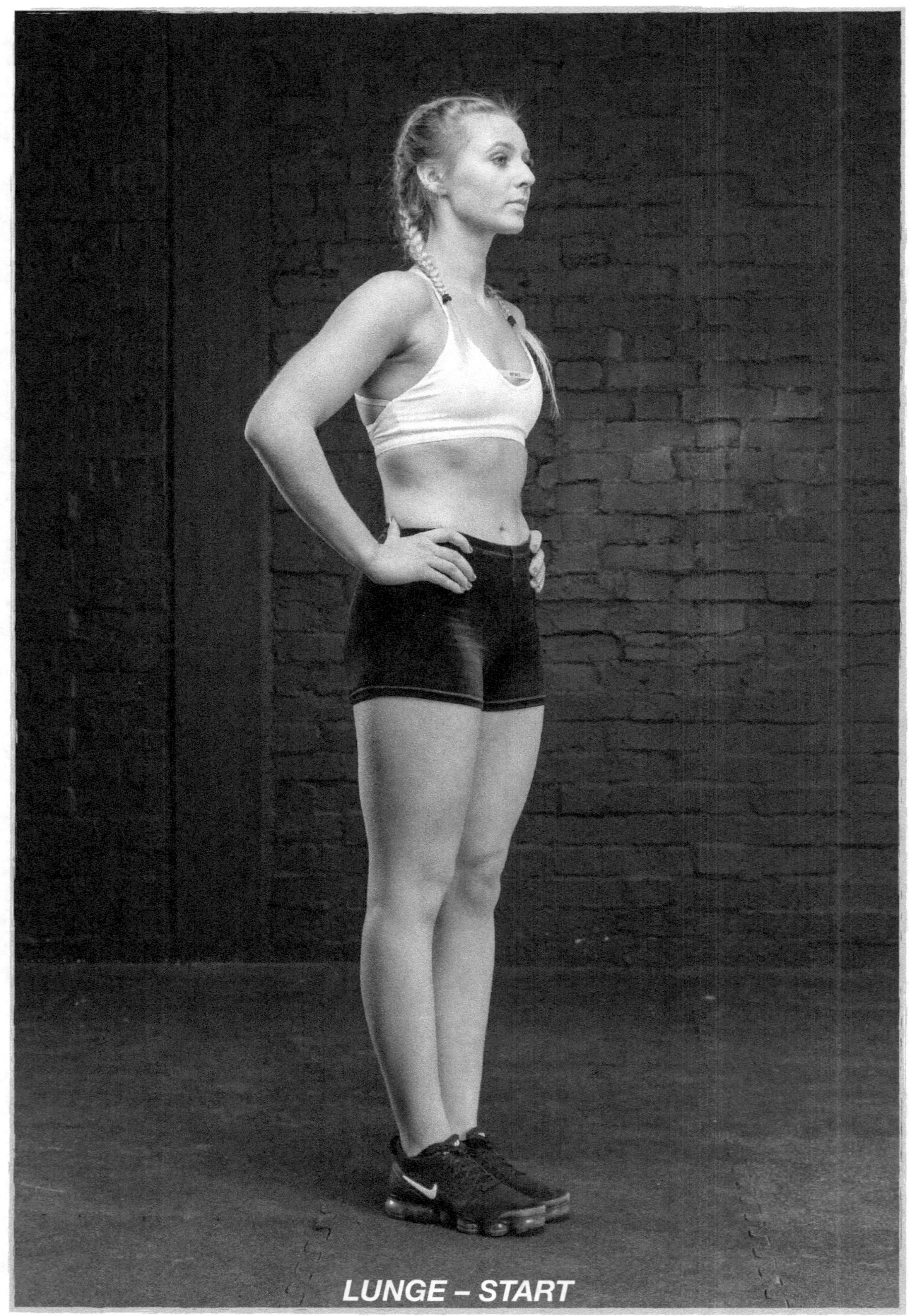

LUNGE – START

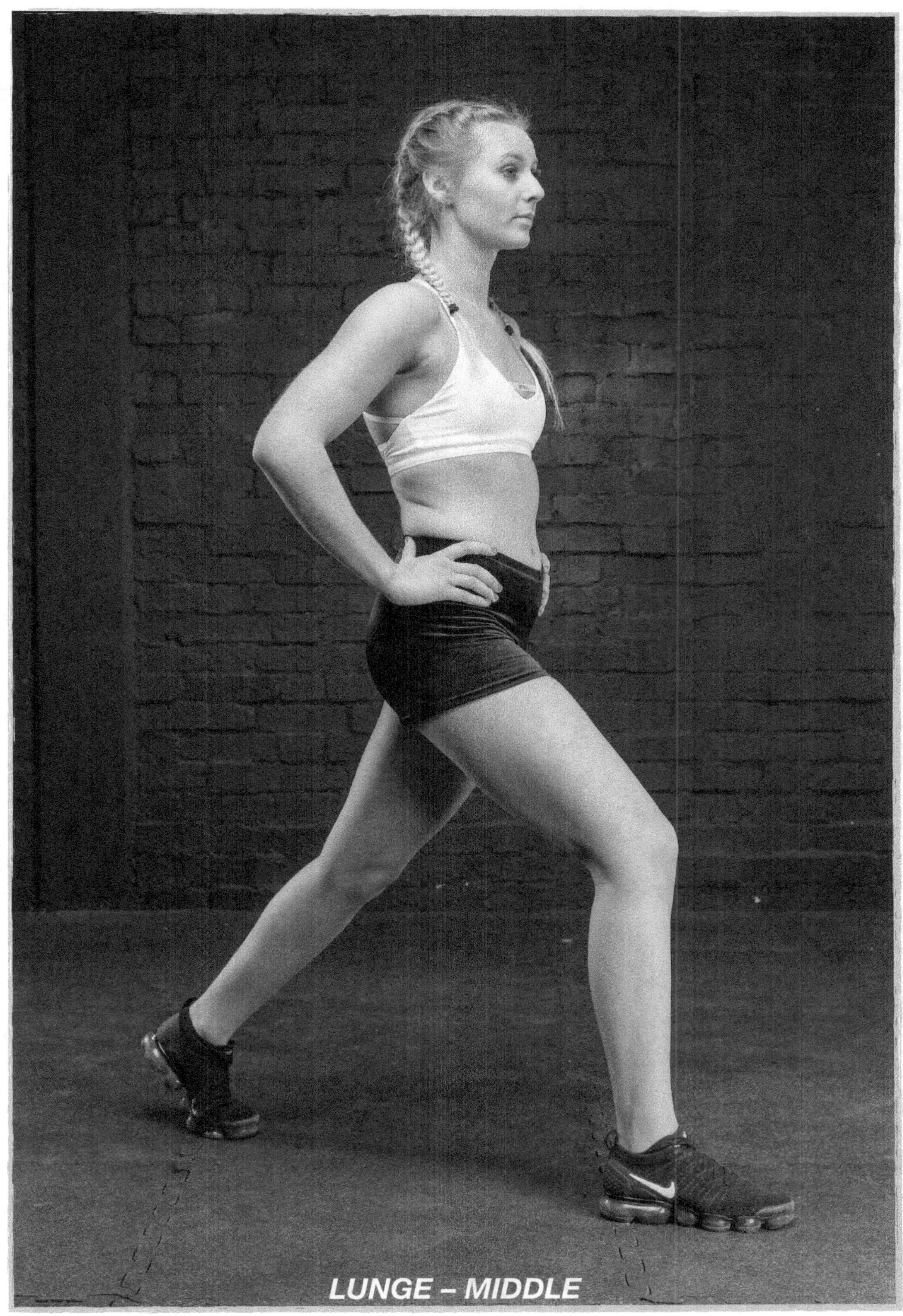

LUNGE – MIDDLE

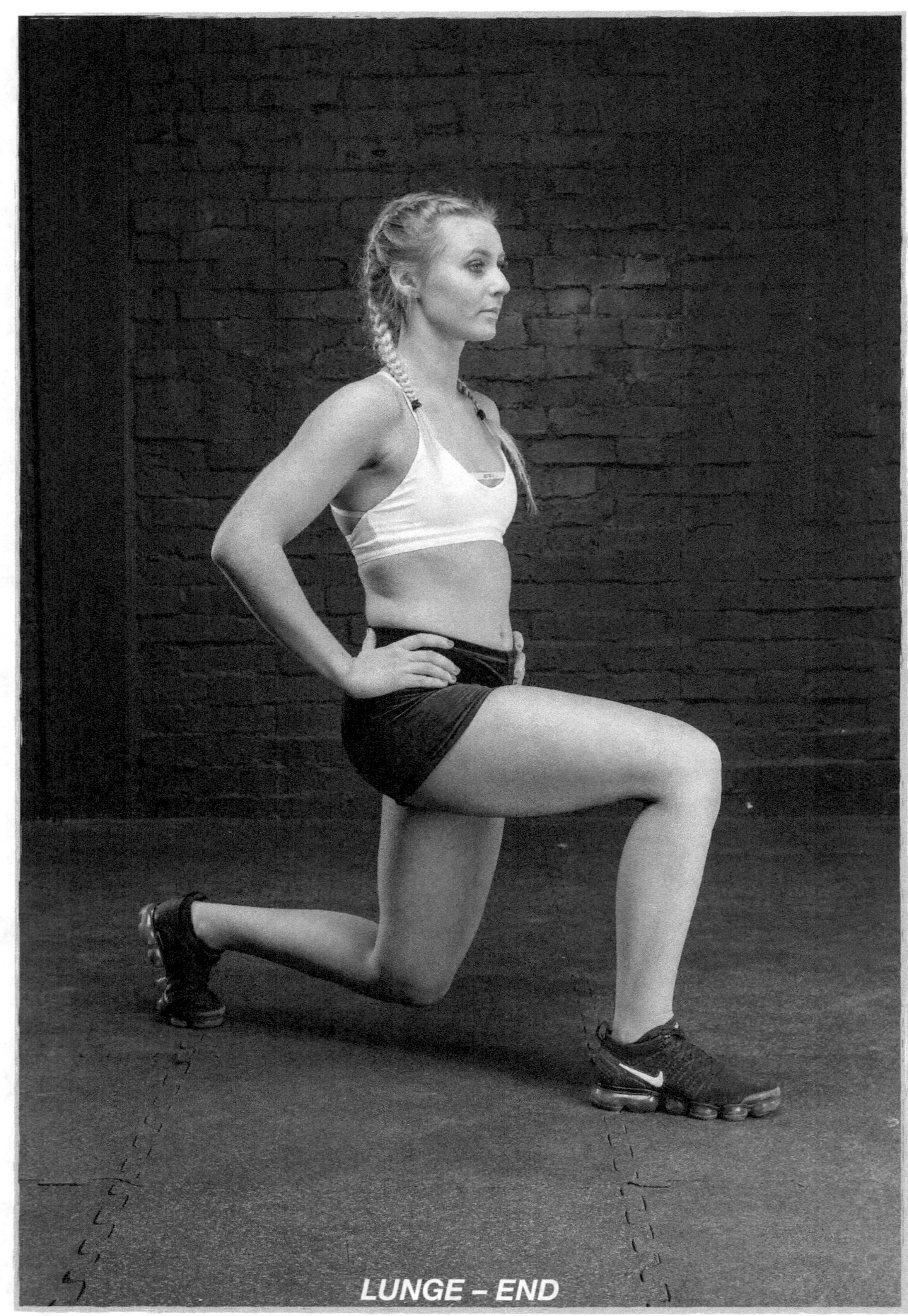

LUNGE – END

9.3 LATERAL LUNGE

Lateral lunges are a great alternative to the squat and normal lunge, and are a kind of hybrid of the two. As well being good for the thighs and glutes, they are also good for the adductors, which are the muscles on the insides of the thighs. If you want a good thigh gap, then these will help to tighten and shape those muscles effectively!

HOW DO I SET THE EQUIPMENT UP?

For the lateral lunge you will need some floor space, and room to move sideways. For the more advanced reader you may also need some form of weight, such as a dumbbell, kettlebell, or weight plate to hold, in order to make the exercise more difficult.

HOW DO I DO IT?

1. Stand with your feet together, toes pointing out slightly. You can raise your arms to help with balance.

2. Lift your right foot into the air, and move it 24 inches/2 feet to the right. As your foot hits the ground bend both knees and descend into a squat.

3. Your lower back should stay straight, head and eyes looking forward, and hips pushed down and back. Keep descending until your thighs are horizontal, or as low as your strength and flexibility allow.

4. Pause for a second, and then push back up. As you do so lift your left foot off the ground and move it to the right, so that you end up in the starting position again. This counts as one rep.

5. You can now either keep moving right, or step left with the left foot, and move back to your original starting location. Either method is fine, and will depend on how much room you have!

HOW MANY SETS AND REPS?

You should be looking to perform 3 to 5 sets of 8 to 12 reps.

HOW DO I ADJUST THE DIFFICULTY?

If you find the lateral lunge too difficult, then try reducing the range of motion so that you don't drop down as low for each rep. To make them more difficult, you can add a pause in the bottom position, or even hold a small weight in the hands as you do them.

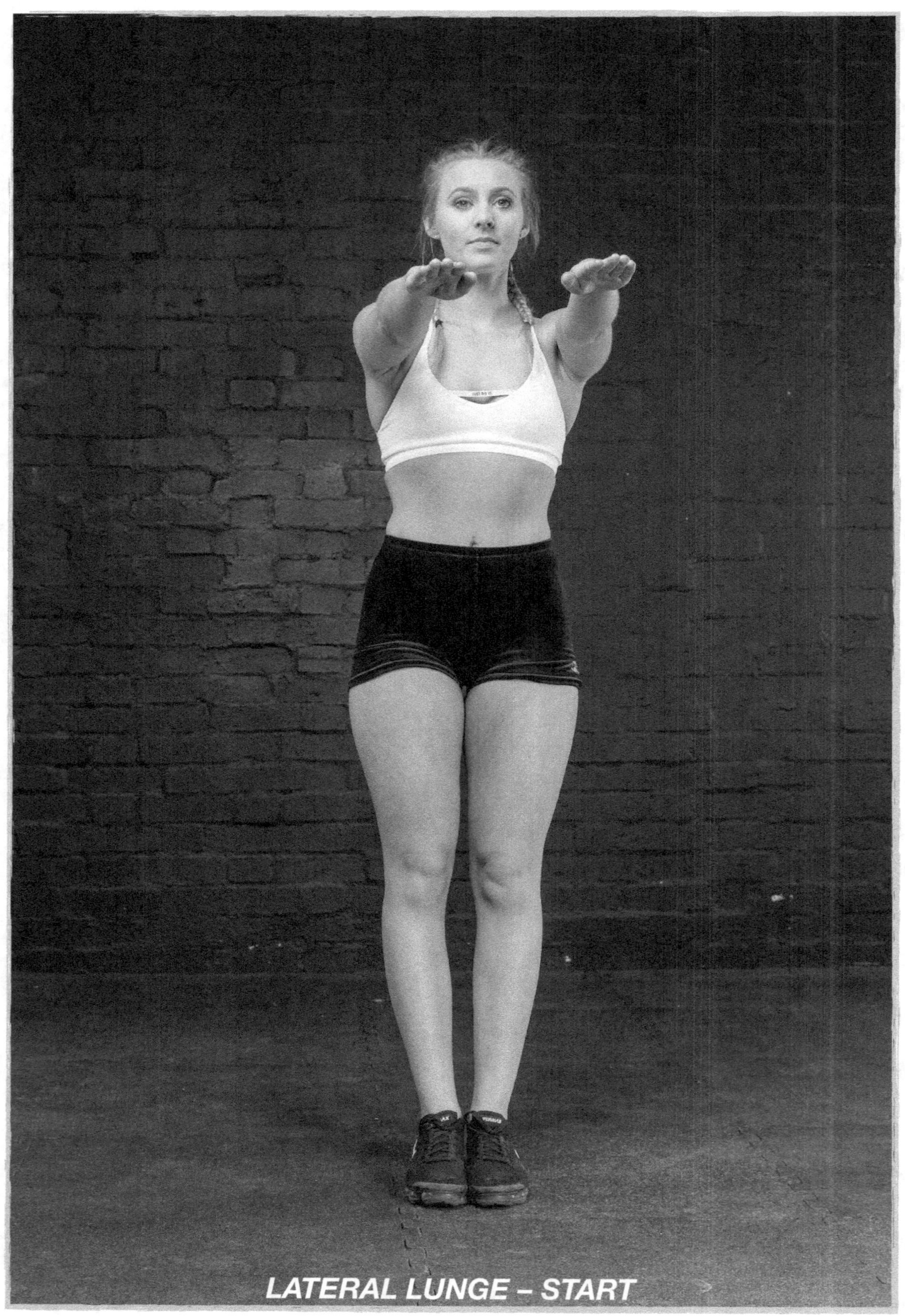

LATERAL LUNGE – START

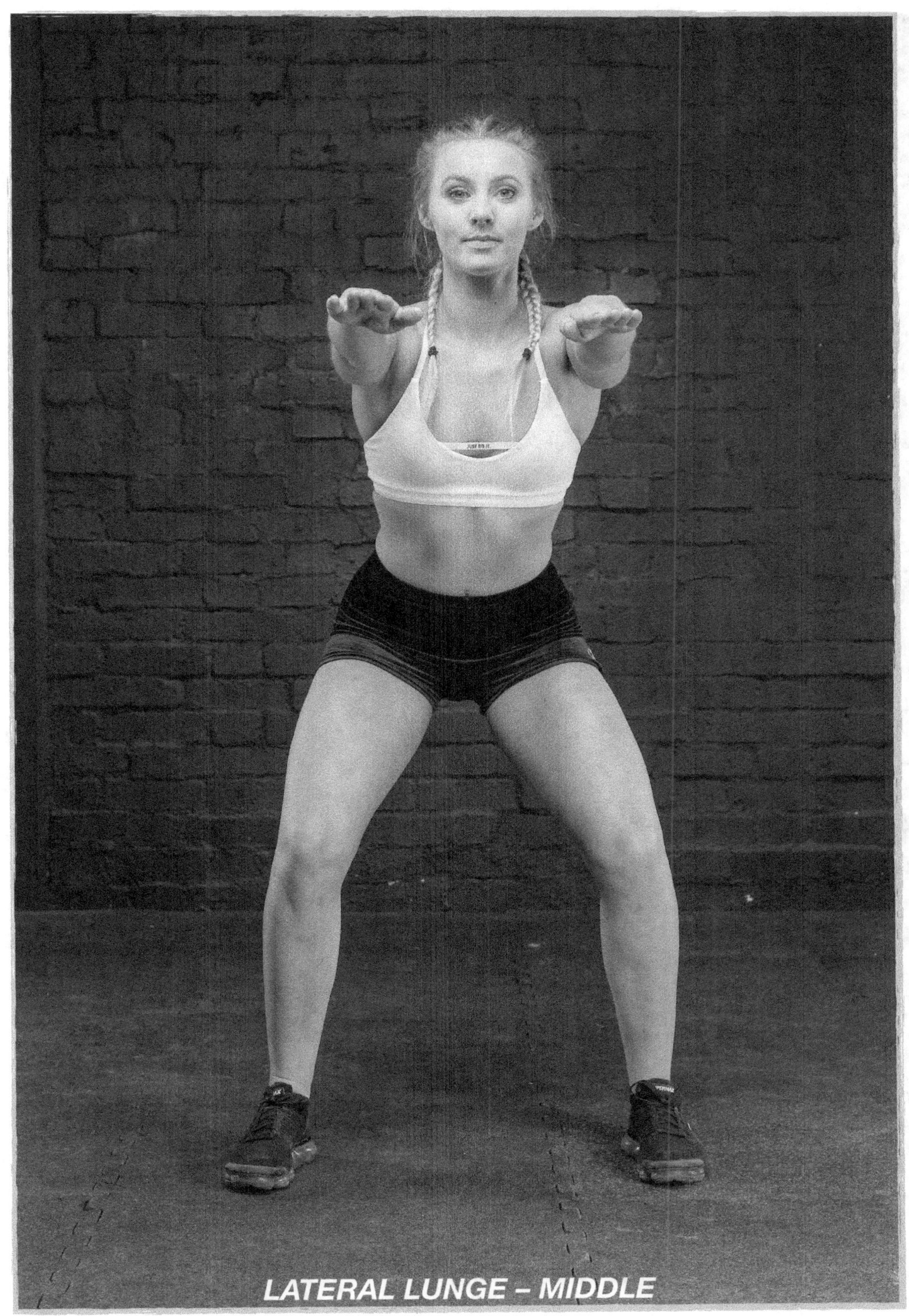

LATERAL LUNGE – MIDDLE

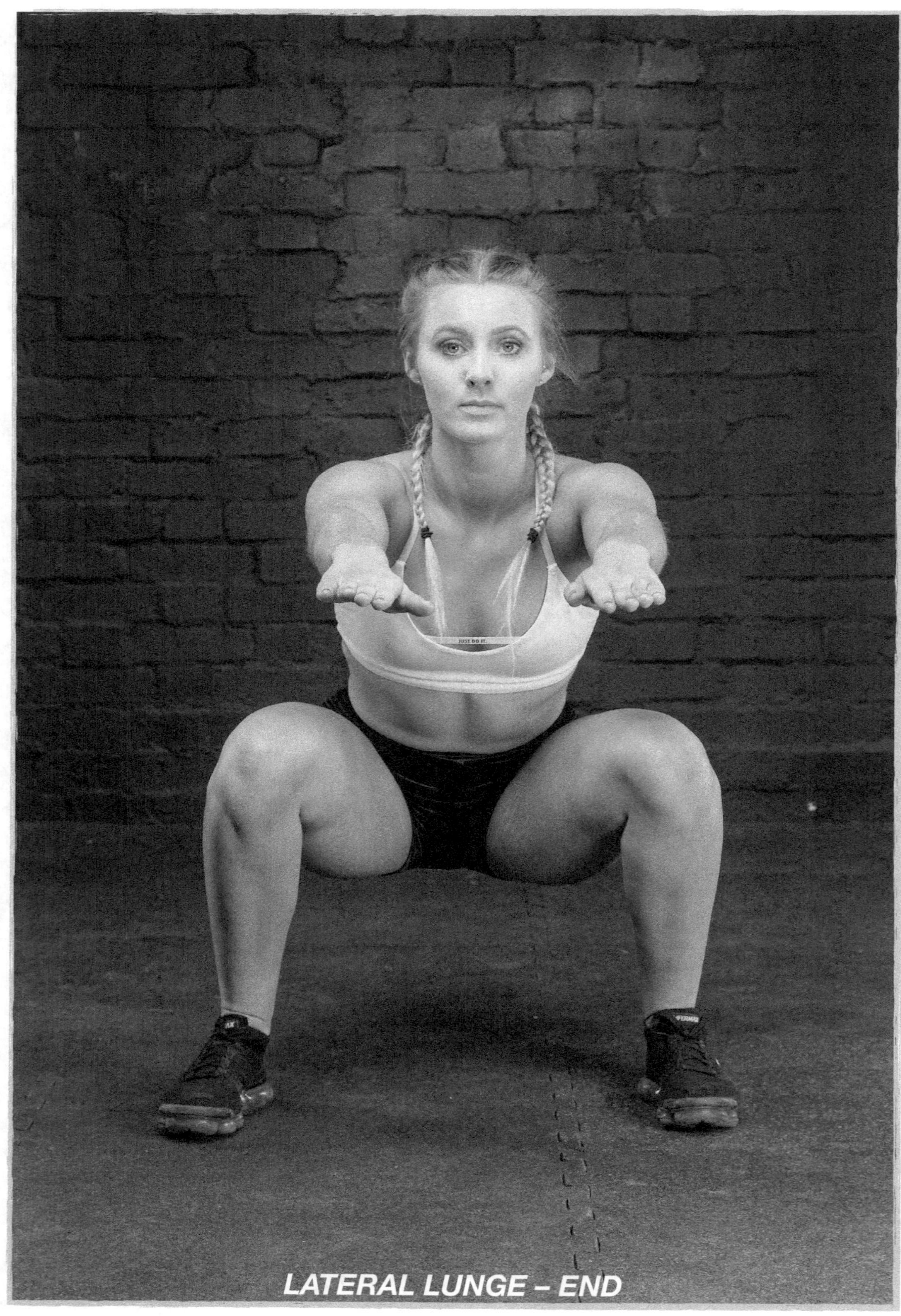

LATERAL LUNGE – END

9.4 BRIDGE

The bridge is similar to the hip thrust that appears later, but is performed with only your body weight, and is good for those who are new to leg and glute training. They can be performed either on the floor or with the aid of a bench, but we've shown the floor version here, as it is more accessible and doesn't require any equipment!

HOW DO I SET THE EQUIPMENT UP?

You will need some floor space and a possibly a mat to cushion your back and shoulders.

HOW DO I DO IT?

1. Lie down on your back with your arms by your sides and your knees bent at 90-degrees, feet flat on the floor.

2. Contract your glutes and hamstrings and raise your hips up into the air. Keep your shoulders and upper back in contact with the ground.

3. Keep raising your hips up until your shoulders, hips, and knees form a straight line.

4. Hold this position for a second, and then return to the start position. This counts as one rep.

HOW MANY SETS AND REPS?

You should be looking to perform 3 to 5 sets of 8 to 12 reps.

HOW DO I ADJUST THE DIFFICULTY?

To make the bridge easier you can reduce the range of motion, or move your feet closer to your bum.

To increase the difficulty of the bridge you can hold the raised position for longer, move your feet further away from your bum, and even extend one leg out to introduce a balance element to the exercise. If you do this make sure to do reps with each leg raised as to work both sides equally.

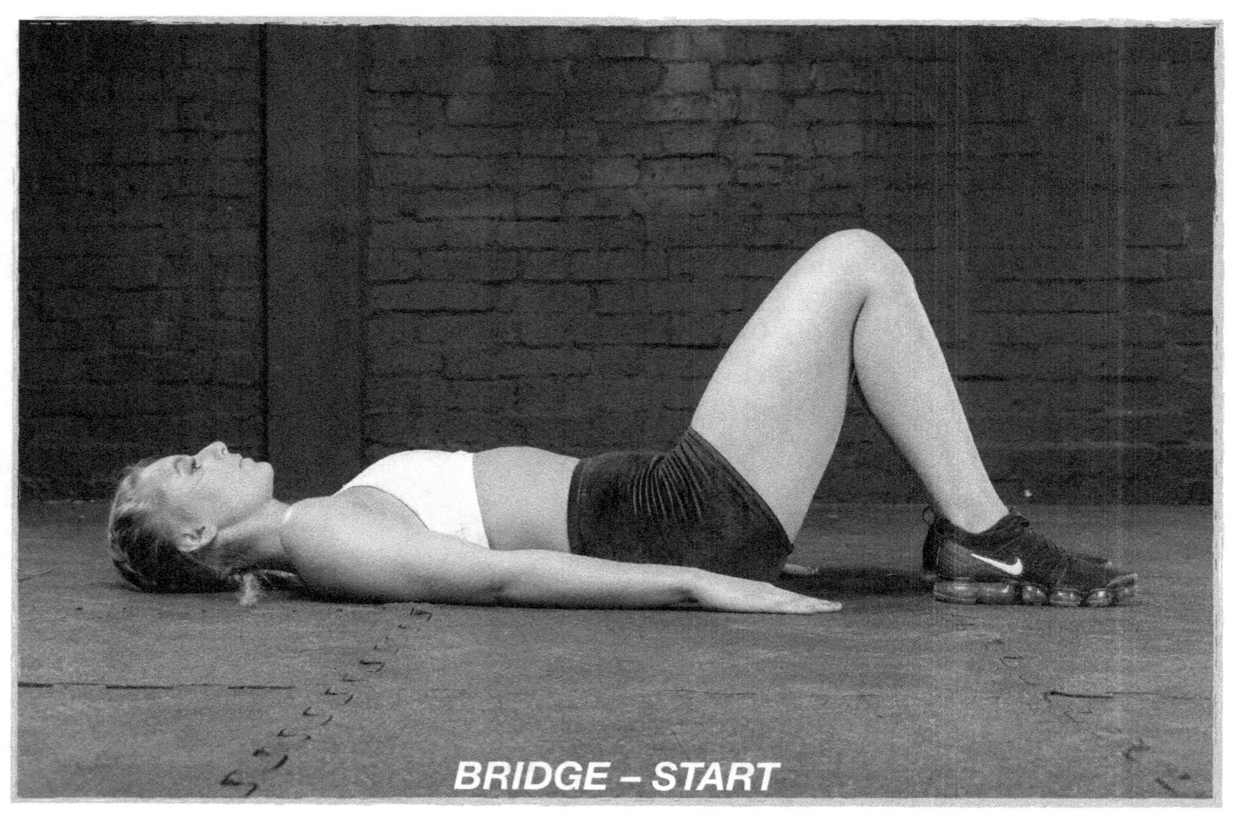

BRIDGE – START

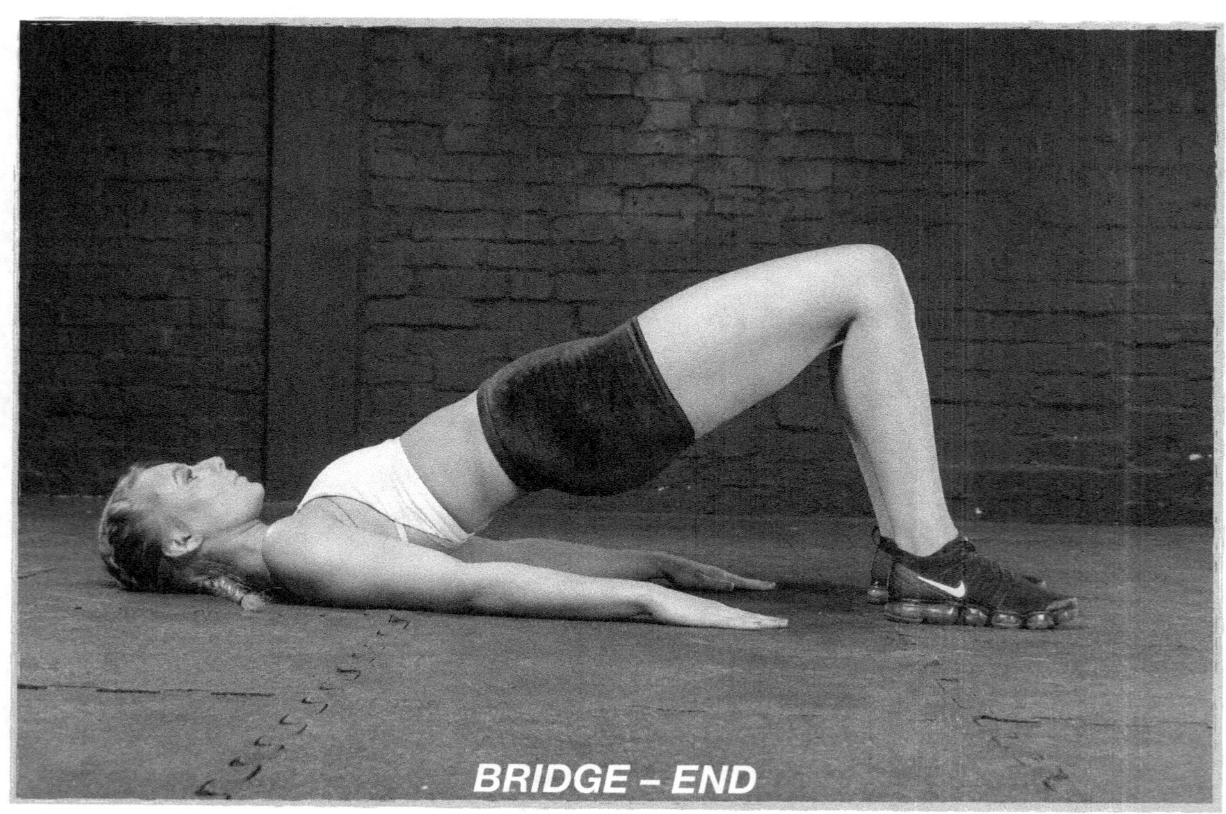

BRIDGE – END

9.5 SINGLE LEG SQUAT

We know what your thinking; normal squats are tough enough, so why on earth would you do single leg squats?! Well, they're not as difficult to perform as you might think, especially with certain methods of assistance, and they're great for developing strength and shape throughout all of the lower body.

HOW DO I SET THE EQUIPMENT UP?

To do the single leg squat you'll need some floor space, and something to secure an exercise band or suspension trainer to. A doorframe, a squat rack (which we have used), or anything else that will allow you to pull against it will do the trick.

HOW DO I DO IT?

1. Stand on one leg, with the other lifted so that your foot is just above the ground.

2. Hold onto the band or suspension trainer and start to bend your knee, squatting down slowly.

3. As you descend lift your free leg so that it doesn't touch the ground.

4. Keep squatting down as low as possible, or until your knee is bent over 90 degrees.

5. Pause for a second, and then push back up to the start position. Use your arms to help you pull back up. This counts as one rep.

HOW MANY SETS AND REPS?

You should be looking to perform 3 to 5 sets of 3 to 5 reps.

HOW DO I ADJUST THE DIFFICULTY?

No doubt you will find the exercise as described above difficult, but don't worry! There are easy ways to make single leg squats accessible. The first method is to only bend your knee a small amount, so that you can still stand back up again. The second method is to use your arms a lot to pull with. As you get stronger you can use your arms less and less, until you are doing most of the work with your legs.

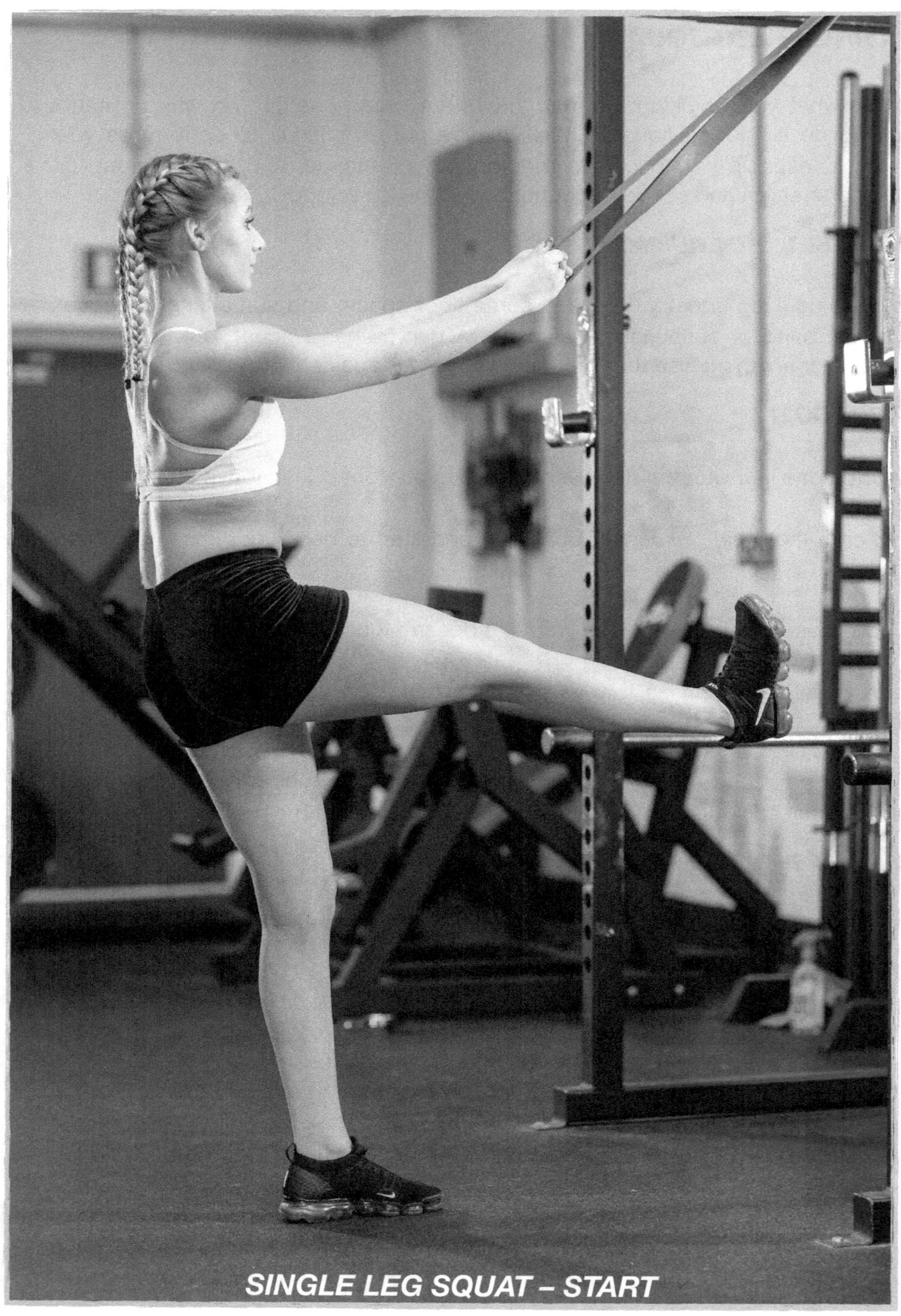

SINGLE LEG SQUAT – START

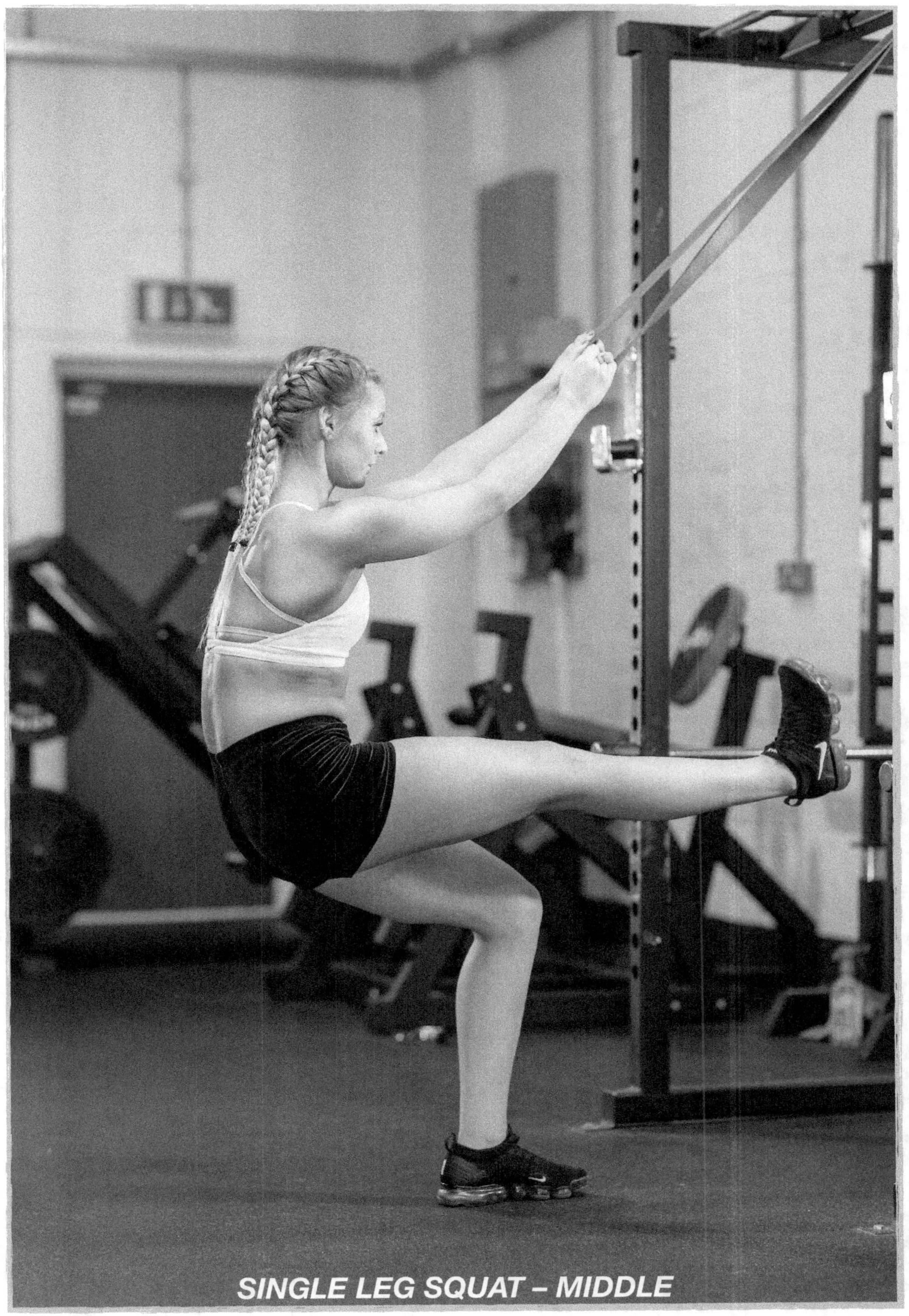

SINGLE LEG SQUAT – MIDDLE

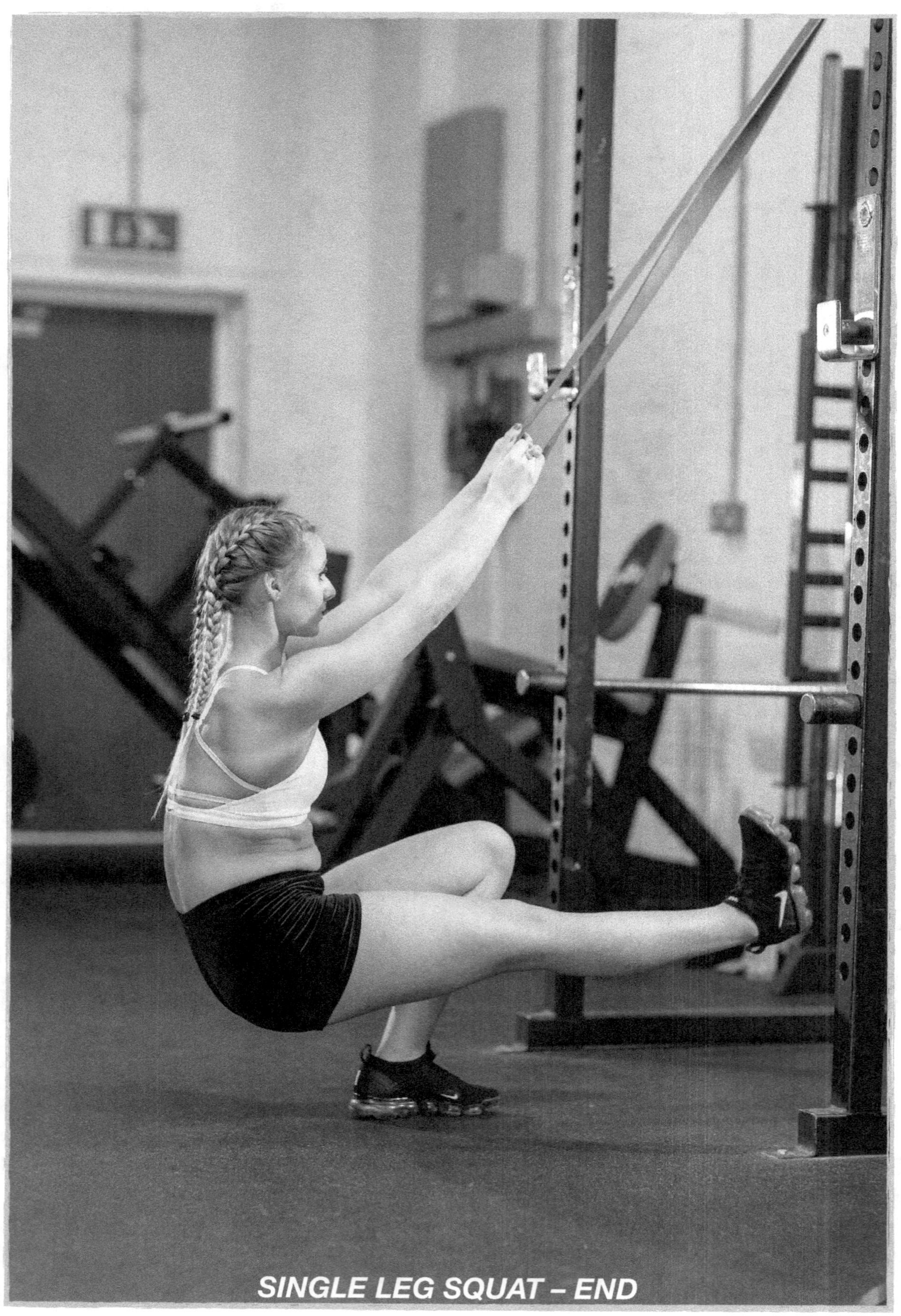

SINGLE LEG SQUAT – END

9.6 BARBELL SQUAT

The squat is one of the best bum and leg building exercises that there is! If you want glutes, then you need to squat, it's that simple. Normal body weight squats are great to get your technique dialled in, but soon you'll want to start adding some weight, and the best way to do that is to use a barbell and a squat rack.

Most gyms will have a squat rack or two, and some will also have a Smith machine or other piece of equipment that will allow you to squat with weight. Personally we do not recommend the Smith machine version. It is easier to do, but will not teach you to squat properly, and that is the main aim here. The Smith machine is also very two dimensional, as the bar is guided up and down on tracks. This recruits less muscle and places less demand on the body as a result, diminishing your gains. We're all about the gainz!

This demonstration section is a little more involved than other exercises (like the body weight ones), but this is because safety is a priority here.

HOW DO I SET THE EQUIPMENT UP?

The squat rack should be set up so that the supports (that the bar is placed on) are a few inches lower than your shoulder height. This is so that you can lift the bar off the rack safely, and are not forced to tiptoe out of the rack. How the hooks are moved will differ depending on what squat rack your gym has. If you are unsure, then ask a Personal Trainer or someone that works in the gym.

For the barbell you will need one that is long enough to sit on the hooks on the squat rack. This is likely to be an Olympic style barbell. As said before, these come in two basic weights: 15 kg (30 lbs) and 20 kg (45 lbs). They should be long enough so that the smaller diameter part of the bar sits comfortably on the supports.

HOW DO I DO IT?

1. Make sure the squat rack is set up properly and the barbell is secure on the supports.

2. Load the bar with the correct amount of weight. If you are just starting then use the bar with no added weight! 15 kg (30 lbs) or 20 kg (45 lbs) will be plenty to start with.

3. Grab the bar with both hands in an overhand grip (palms facing the floor) with your hands slightly wider than shoulder width apart. Step forward under the bar.

4. Place the bar on the top of you back, tensing your upper back muscles to create a strong platform for the bar to rest on. Raising your elbows up and back can help to do this.

5. Making sure that your feet are directly under the bar, stand up so that the bar lifts off the supports.

6. Pause a second to make sure that bar is centred and secure and then take a step back with one foot. Take another step back with the other foot, and pause.

7. Use this opportunity to make sure that you are comfortable, the bar is centred and secure, and that you are ready to start squatting.

8. Now bend your knees and push your hips back at the same time, keeping your eyes looking forward and your head and neck in a neutral position.

9. Keep descending, under control, until your thighs reach a horizontal position, or your hips are lower than you knees.

10. Ensure that your knees push outwards and open up, and that your back stays as straight as possible. Keep your core tight.

11. Pause for a second, and then push back up to the start position. This counts as one rep.

12. Once you have completed your set, take two steps forward until the barbell comes into contact with the vertical face of the squat rack supports. Then lower the bar until you feel it come into contact with the supports. You can then let go of the bar and step out from the squat rack.

HOW MANY SETS AND REPS?

You should be looking to perform 3 to 5 sets of 8 to 12 reps.

HOW DO I ADJUST THE DIFFICULTY?

Adjusting the difficulty of the squat is easy, but even if you're experienced with exercise, always start with just the bar. This goes for warming up as well. ALWAYS do a good number of reps with just the bar to warm up properly.

Obviously, lowering the weight will make the squat easier, and adding more weight will make the exercise more difficult. We don't recommend using a smaller range of motion to make them easier; the goal is to squat to a proper depth, as this will protect the knees much more than if you only do a limited range of motion.

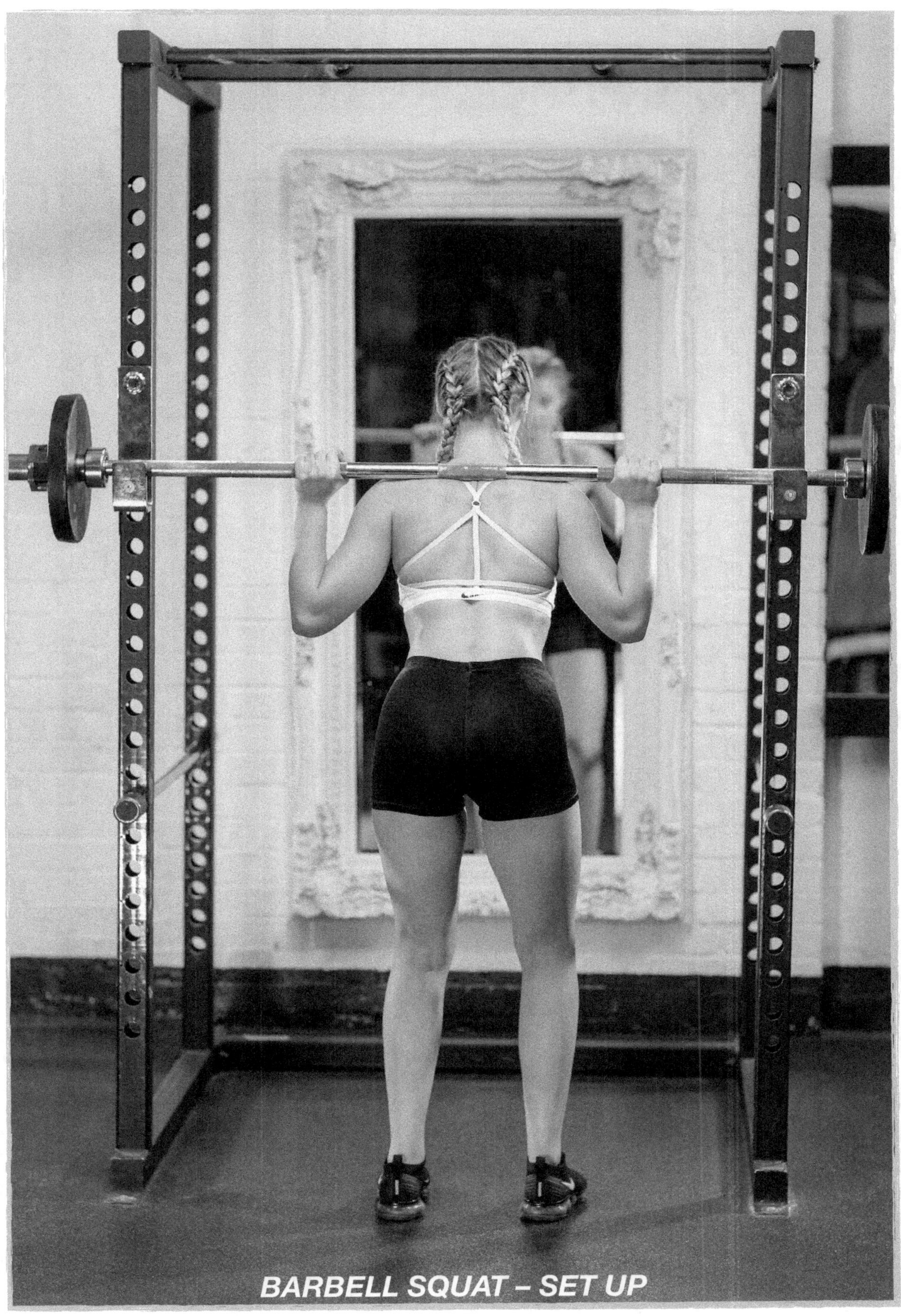

BARBELL SQUAT – SET UP

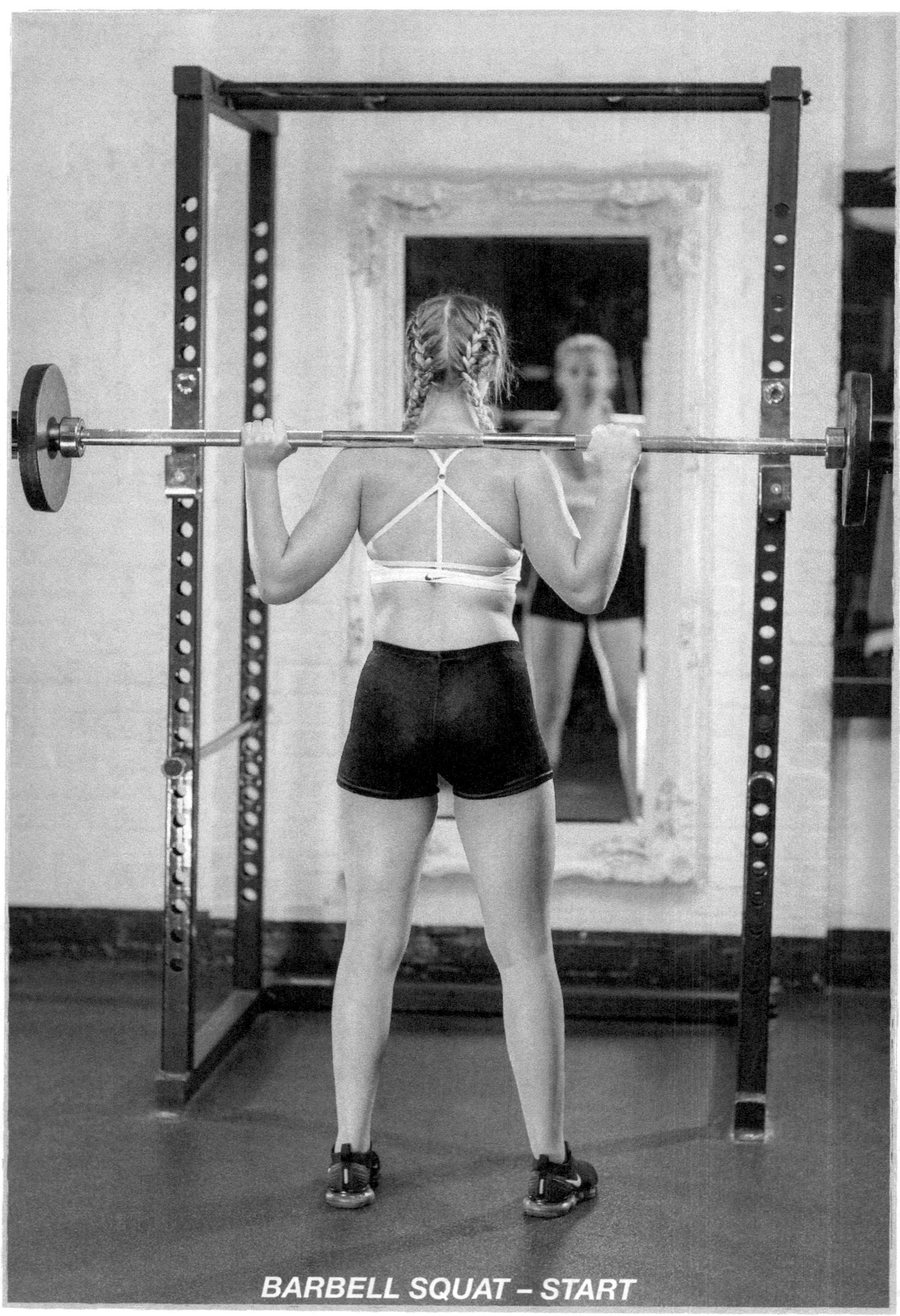

BARBELL SQUAT – START

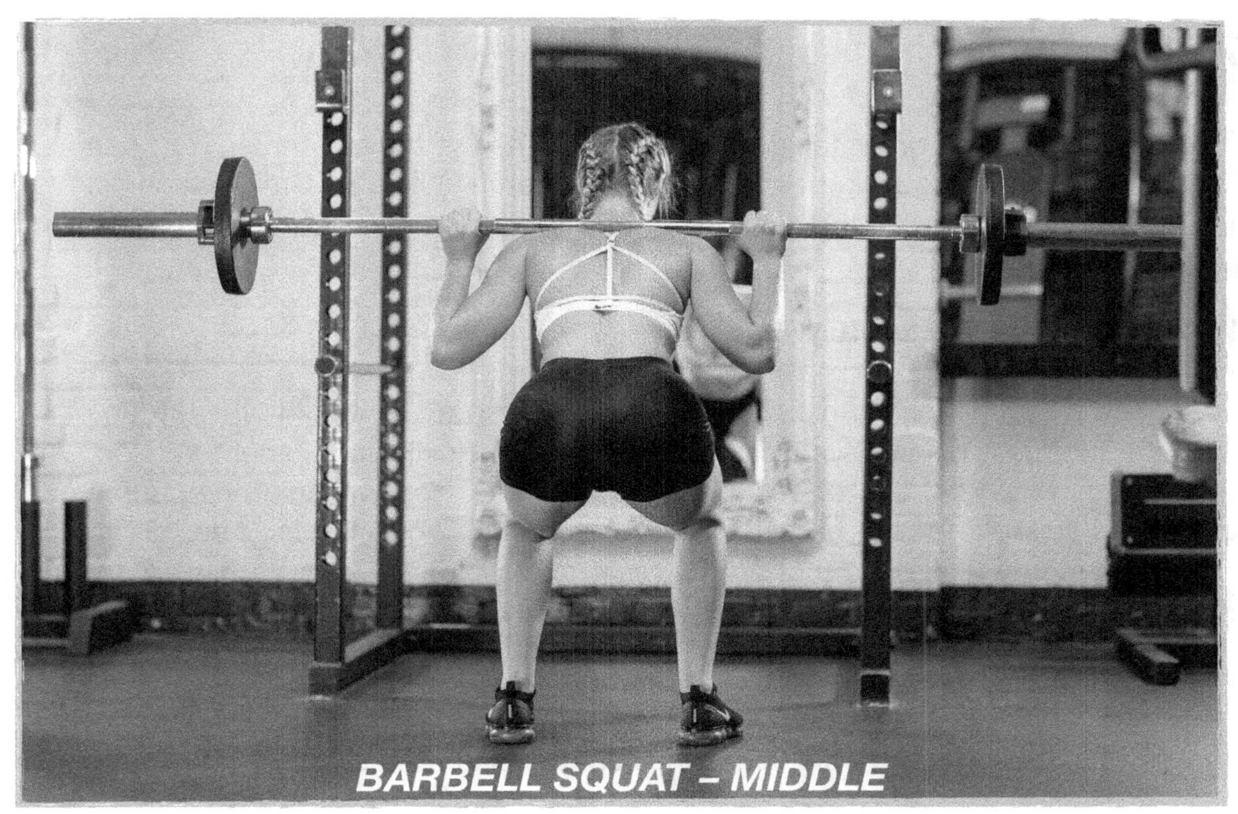

BARBELL SQUAT – MIDDLE

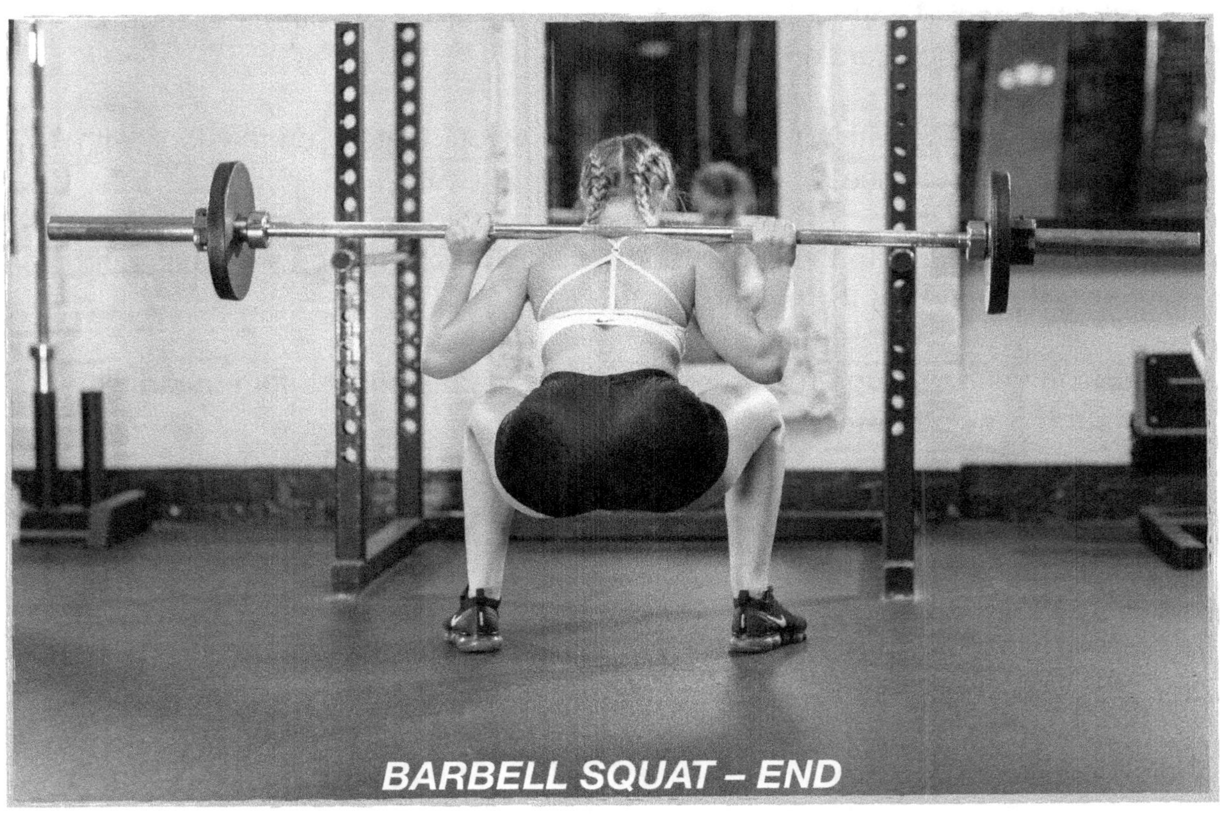

BARBELL SQUAT – END

9.7 HIP THRUST

Another exercise that is great for developing the glutes is the hip thrust. You can perform this free standing on a bench (which is preferable) or on a Smith machine. Combined with exercises like the squat and deadlift, this will give your lower body a real workout!

HOW DO I SET THE EQUIPMENT UP?

You will need a barbell for the hip thrust, either one with a set weight (like the one used in the pictures) or an Olympic style one. As said in the equipment section, these come in 15 kg (30 lbs) or 20 kg (45 lbs) variants. You will also need some weight plates suitable for the barbell that you are using. You will also need a flat bench that is sturdy. The ones that are found in gym weights areas are perfect for this.

HOW DO I DO IT?

1. Set-up the barbell with the weight, making sure the plates are secured in place.

2. Place the barbell in front of the bench, so that they are parallel to each other.

3. Slide under the barbell so that it comes to rest in the crook of your hips, and rest your upper back and shoulders on the bench.

4. Secure the bar in place with your hands, and place your feet flat on the floor, with a 90 degree bend in your knees.

5. Now drive your hips up into the air, supporting your upper body on the bench and keeping your feet planted on the ground.

6. Keep pushing your hips up until your knees, hips, and shoulders form a straight line and your torso is horizontal.

7. Pause for a second, and then lower your hips down to the floor. This counts as one rep.

HOW MANY SETS AND REPS?

You should be looking to perform 3 to 5 sets of 8 to 12 reps.

HOW DO I ADJUST THE DIFFICULTY?

If you struggle with the hip thrust then simply use less weight, or the bar by itself. If you really struggle then it can be performed just with body weight, similar to the bridge, but with a greater range of motion.

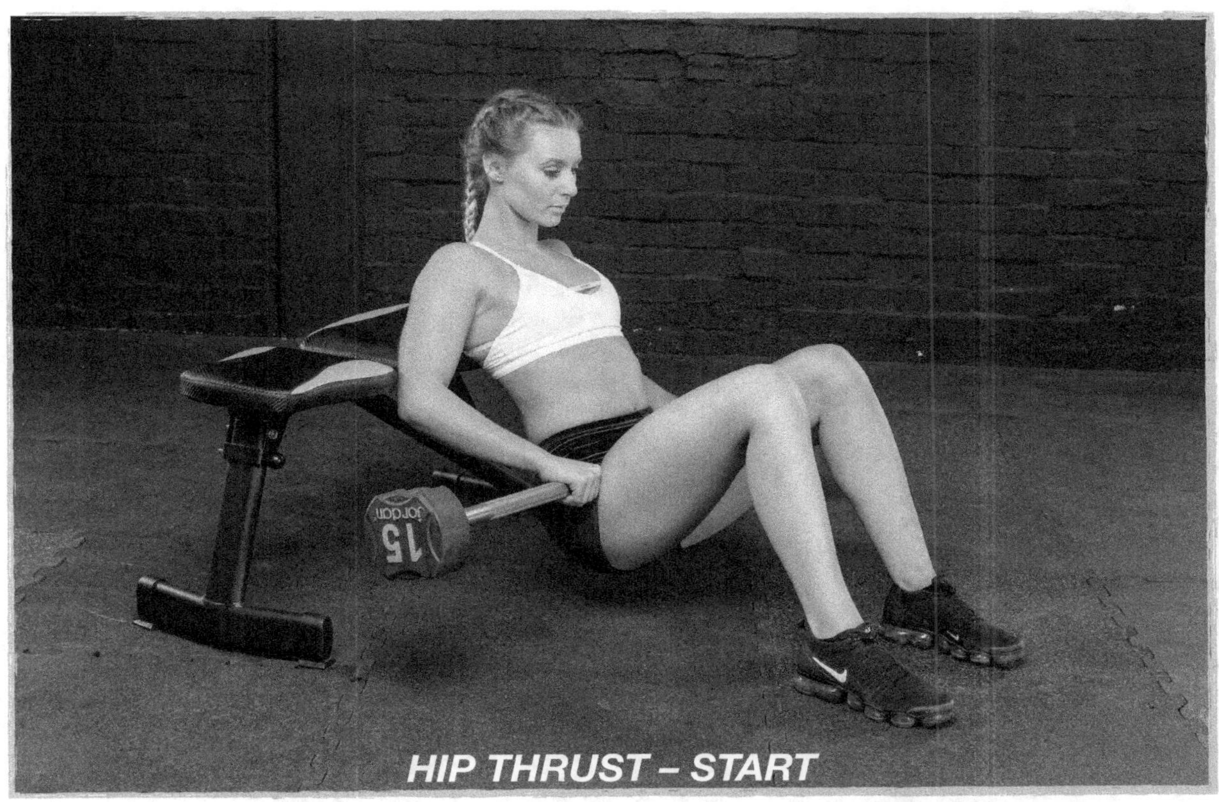

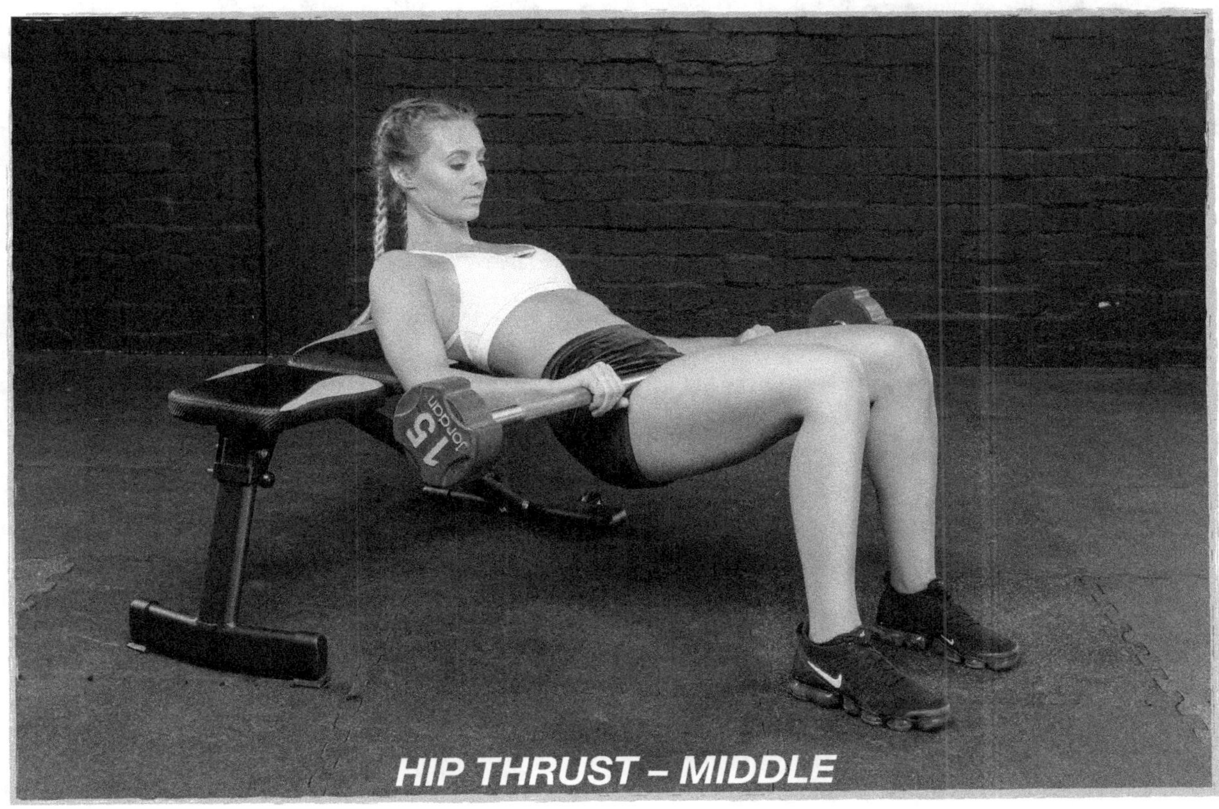

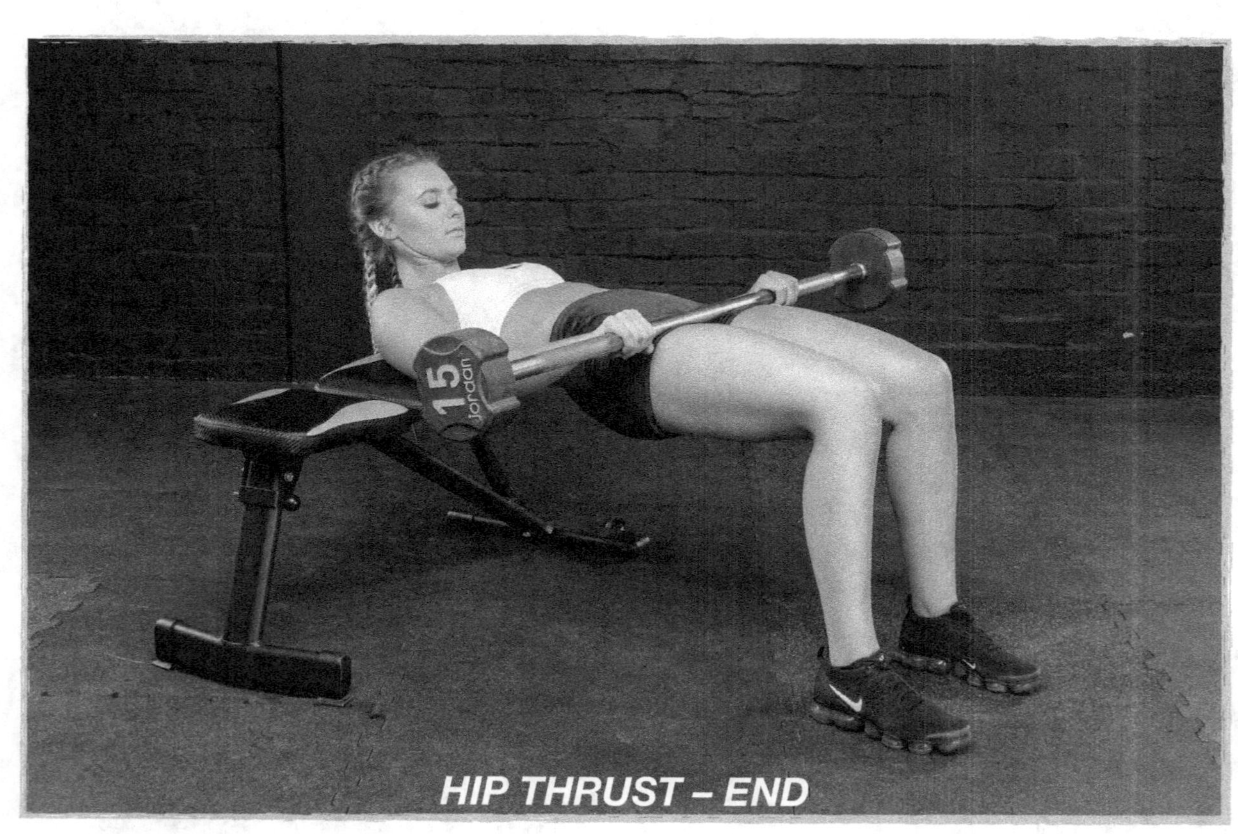

HIP THRUST – END

9.8 STEP-UPS

If there is one exercise that will get the legs burning more than anything else it is step-ups! These are hugely adjustable, and can be used as a strength exercise on their own, or even as part of a larger circuit. They are designed to be done with weights, normally dumbbells or kettlebells, but can also be performed with just your own body weight.

HOW DO I SET THE EQUIPMENT UP?

You will need a step or platform of some kind, preferably one that is solid and sturdy, with little chance of moving. A flat bench is suitable, and so are exercise steps used in exercise classes. When using weights try and use dumbbells or kettlebells, as these can be easily dropped onto the floor if you get into trouble.

HOW DO I DO IT?

1. Stand in front of the step, with your feet about 12 inches (one foot) away from the edge. Hold a dumbbell or kettlebell in each hand, arms hanging loosely by your sides.

2. Take a large step up onto the box, making sure your foot is planted firmly. Pause for a second to make sure you are balanced, and then push off hard with the foot that is still on the ground.

3. Use the foot that is on the box to push and pull your body forwards, bringing your other foot up onto the box.

4. Once both feet are on the box stand up fully, keeping your eyes looking forward and your head and neck in a neutral position.

5. Now step back carefully with the foot that stepped onto the box first, then follow with your other foot, until you arrive in the starting position. This counts as one rep.

HOW MANY SETS AND REPS?

You should be looking to perform 3 to 5 sets of 8 to 12 reps.

HOW DO I ADJUST THE DIFFICULTY?

It goes without saying that step-ups are tough, but their difficulty can be changed quite easily. To make them less challenging use a lower step, decrease the speed of your steps, use less weight, or no weight at all if you find them really tough. To make them harder use a higher step, use more weight, or increase the speed of your steps.

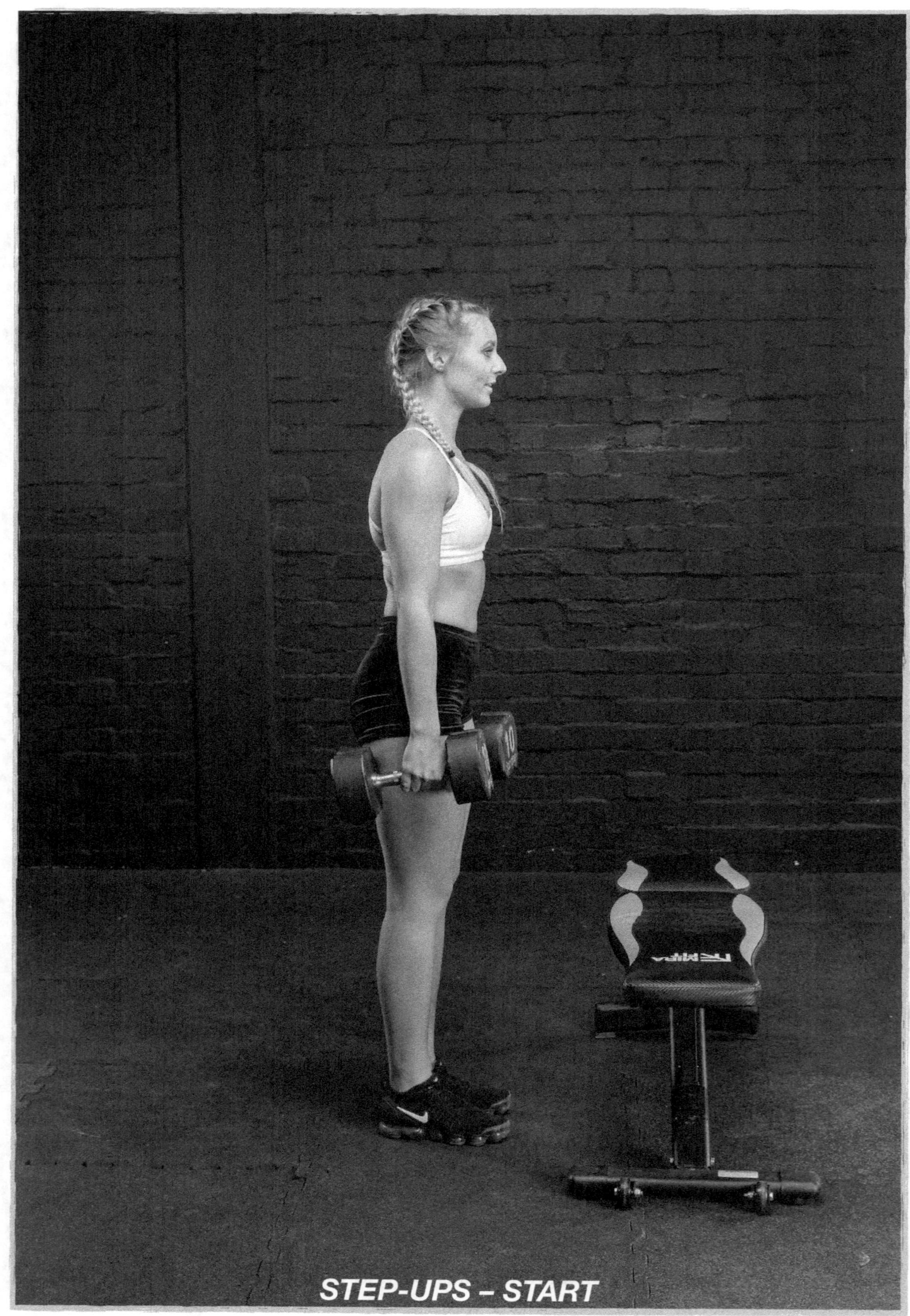

STEP-UPS – START

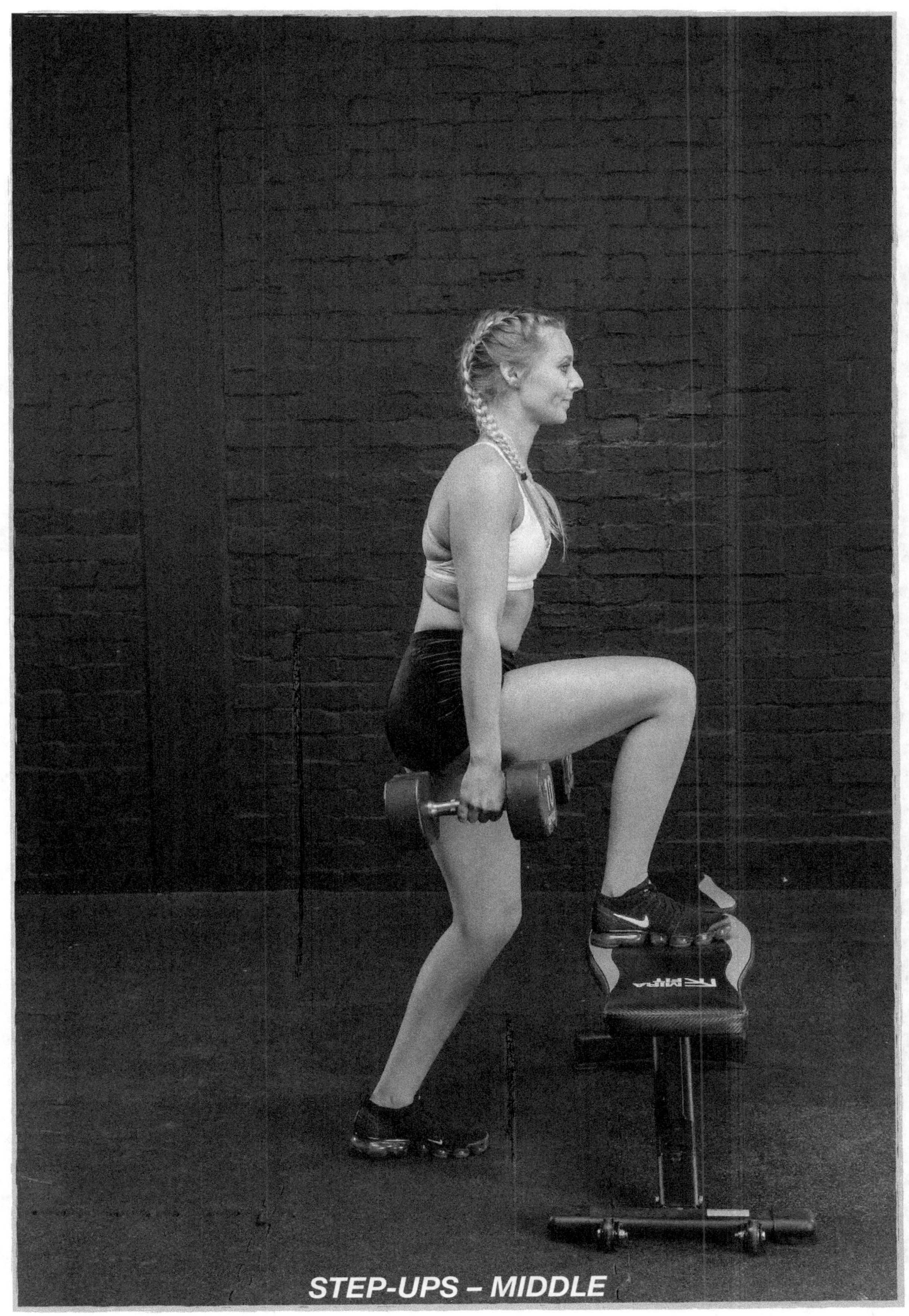

STEP-UPS – MIDDLE

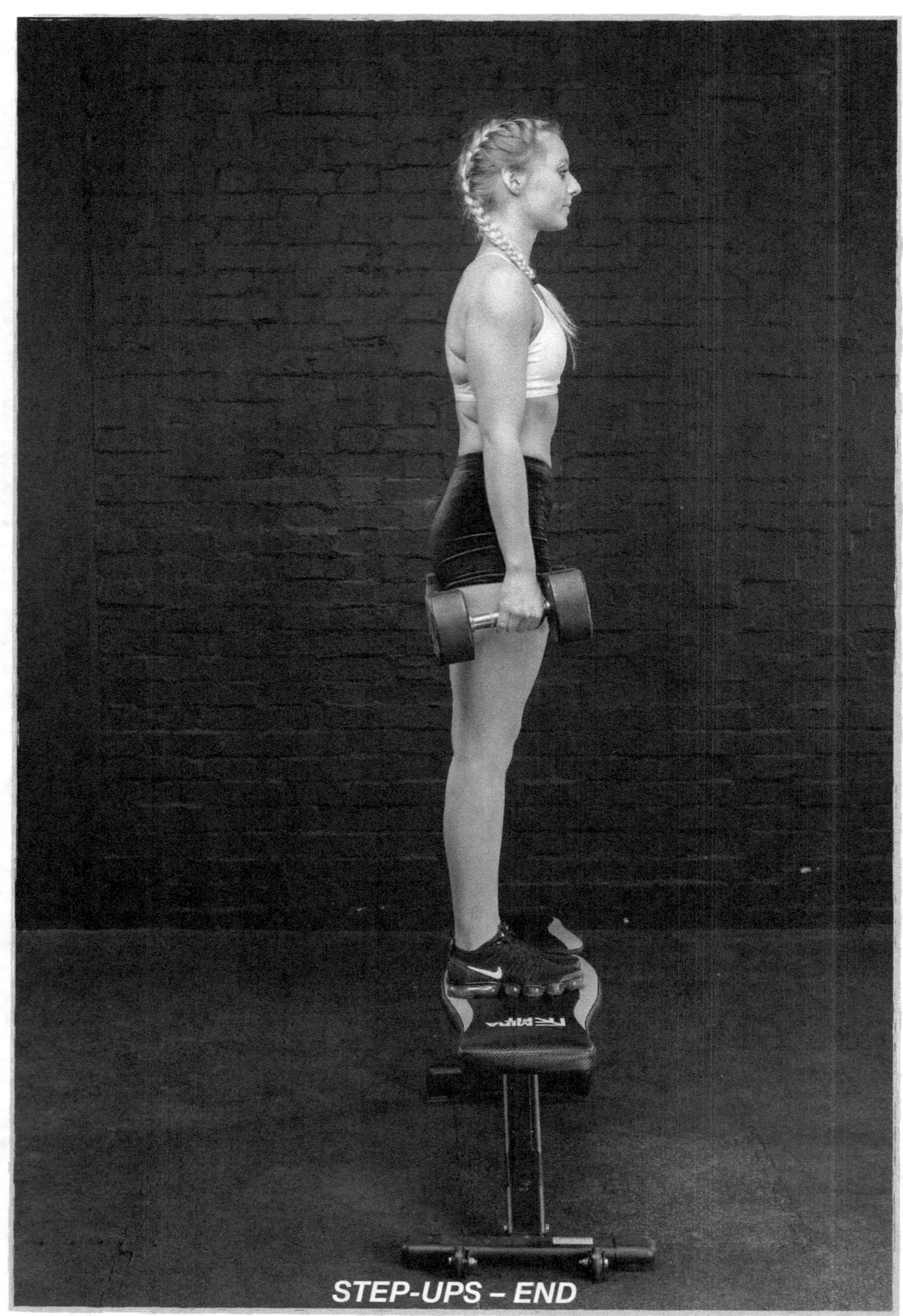

STEP-UPS – END

9.9 CALF RAISE

Everyone wants good calves; they make your legs look better in shoes, and make everyday activities like walking, running, and climbing stairs much easier. Calf raises are the exercise that you do if you want good calves. They can be done unweighted, using just your own body weight, but the calves are strong muscles, and so doing them weighted is much better, and even beginners will be able to perform them this way.

HOW DO I SET THE EQUIPMENT UP?

For calf raises you will need a small step or ledge of some kind. It only needs to be high enough to allow your heels to drop, so you use a single exercise class step if needed, or even a weight plate (as is shown in the pictures).

For the weight we recommend using a dumbbell in each hand, as these can easily be picked up and dropped when needed.

HOW DO I DO IT?

1. Set up your step so that it is secure and cannot move at all.

2. Grab the dumbbells in both hands, arms hanging loosely by your sides, and get onto the step with your toes on the edge.

3. Allow your heels to drop down lower than the step, so you feel a stretch in your calves.

4. Pause, and then push up, aiming to get your heels to rise as much as possible.

5. Hold this for a second, before letting your heels drop down below the level of the step. This counts as one rep.

HOW MANY SETS AND REPS?

You should be looking to perform 3 to 5 sets of 8 to 12 reps.

HOW DO I ADJUST THE DIFFICULTY?

As said before, calf raises are fairly straightforward, but you may need to adjust the difficulty. If you find the weighted version too tough, then simply drop the dumbbells and use just your body weight. If you want to make them harder then use more weight, or perform them with only one foot on the step. Obviously if you do this then make sure to work both legs equally.

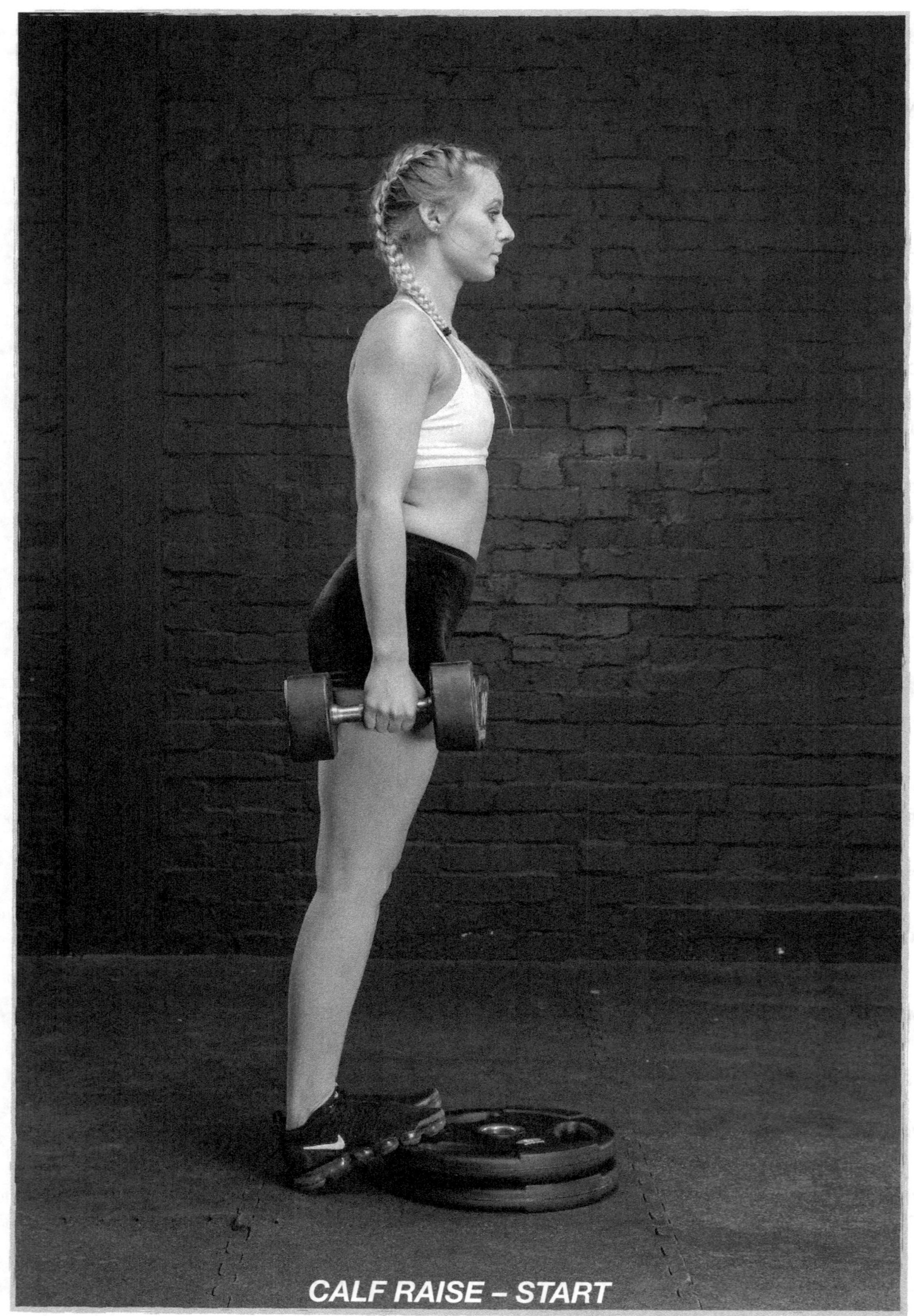

CALF RAISE – START

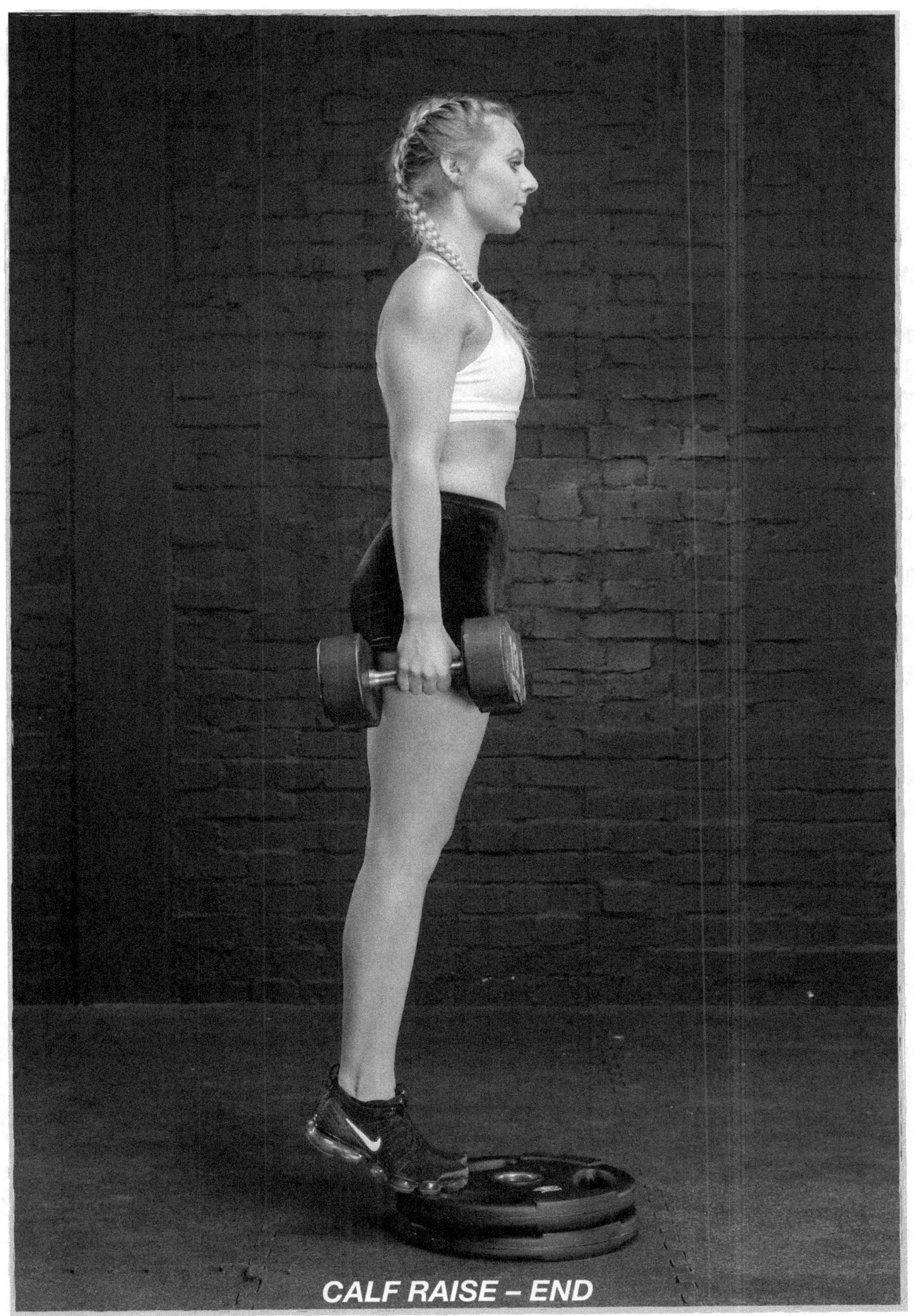

CALF RAISE – END

9.10 DEADLIFT

The deadlift is a great exercise, and will target pretty much every muscle group in your body. It will work your back, bum, legs, core, and entire upper body, and when done for a good number of reps, will also act as a good cardio workout. Also, you'll get a huge calorie burn both during and after your workout, which makes it the perfect exercise to do if you are looking to lose weight!

HOW DO I SET THE EQUIPMENT UP?

To do the deadlift you will need a barbell, preferably an Olympic style barbell that weighs either 15 kg (30 lbs) or 20 kg (45 lbs). You will also need various weight plates from light to heavy, and also collars or clips to secure the weights on the bar. You will also need some floor space, and room to manoeuvre around the barbell.

If you are only strong enough to lift the bar (or have never deadlifted before), it is a good idea to place the ends of the barbell on two exercise steps, or the supports found on the squat rack. Alternatively you can use an exercise class barbell, and the weights that go with it.

HOW DO I DO IT?

1. Set-up your barbell with a suitable amount of weight. If you are using the bar without any weight, place the bar on a support to get it at the right height.

2. Walk up to the bar, place your feet under the bar, so that the bar nearly touches your shins. Your feet should be shoulder width apart, and toes pointing out slightly.

3. Squat down with a straight back, and grab the bar with both hands. Your hands should be shoulder width apart, and in an overhand grip (palms facing backwards).

4. Now get into the start position. Your knees should be bent, back straight but at an angle, arms straight, and head and neck in a neutral position.

5. From here apply tension to the bar so that it lifts very slightly. Not off the floor, but just so there is tension there. This is very important for a safe lift!

6. Now pull with your upper body, push down hard with your legs, and try and move your hips forward. The bar should start to rise off the ground.

7. Keep lifting the bar by pushing down against the floor with your legs, pulling up with your arms, and pushing forward with your hips. Allow the head to rise naturally and keep your arms straight.

8. Keep going until you are standing up straight and your hips are pushed into the bar. Pause for a second, and then return the bar to the floor, using the same technique as used to lift the bar. This counts as one rep.

HOW MANY SETS AND REPS?

You should be looking to perform 3 to 5 sets of 8 to 12 reps.

HOW DO I ADJUST THE DIFFICULTY?

You can adjust the difficulty of the deadlift in a few ways. To make the lift easier you can reduce the amount of weight that you use, reduce the range of motion (by starting with the bar resting on a platform that is higher than the floor), and by reducing the number of reps and sets that you do.

To make the movement harder, you can add more weight, increase the range of motion (by standing on a low exercise step and placing the bar on the floor), and by increasing the number of reps and sets that you do.

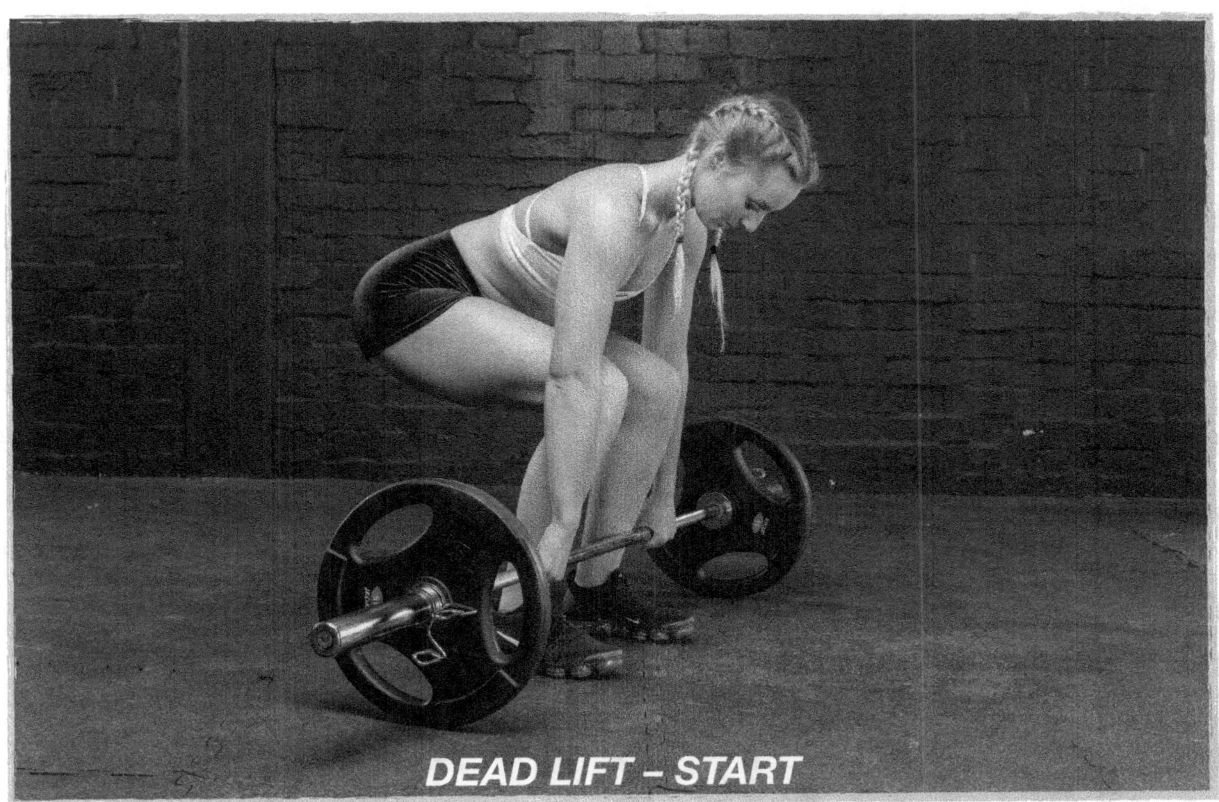

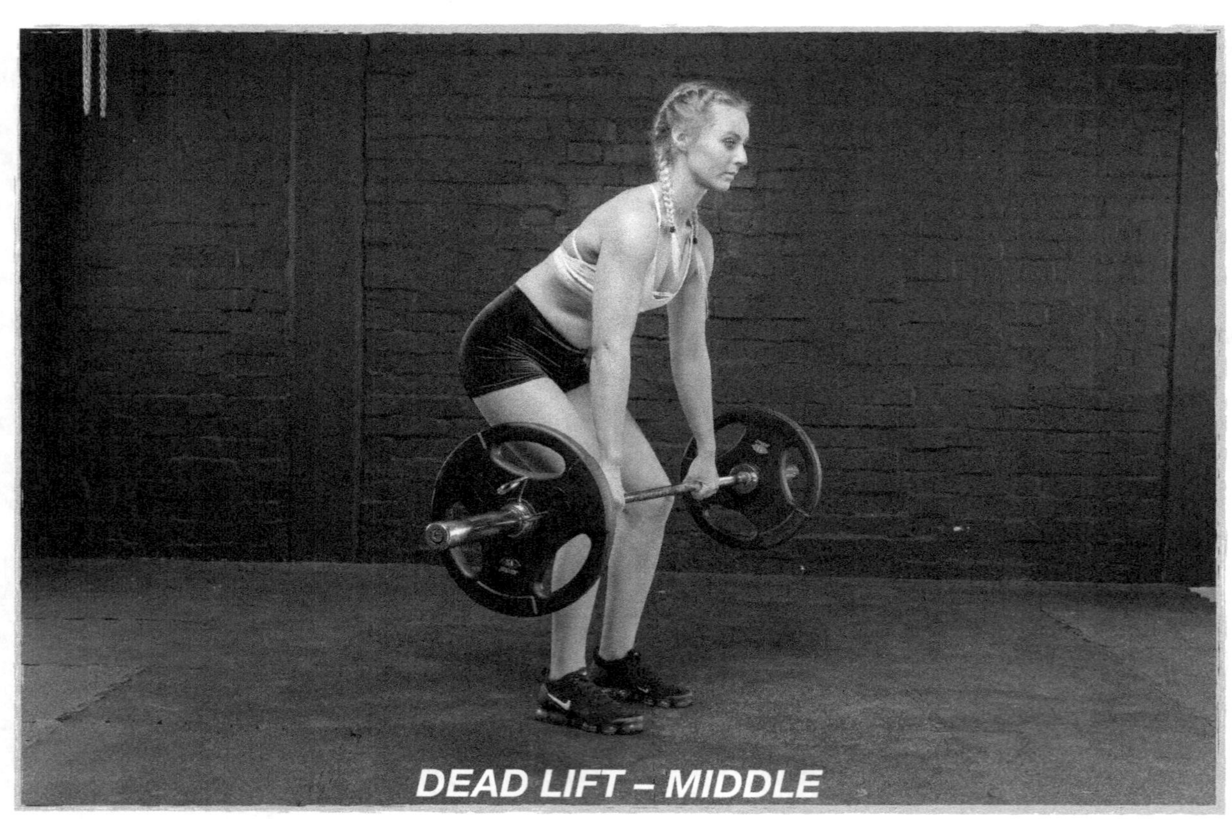

DEAD LIFT – MIDDLE

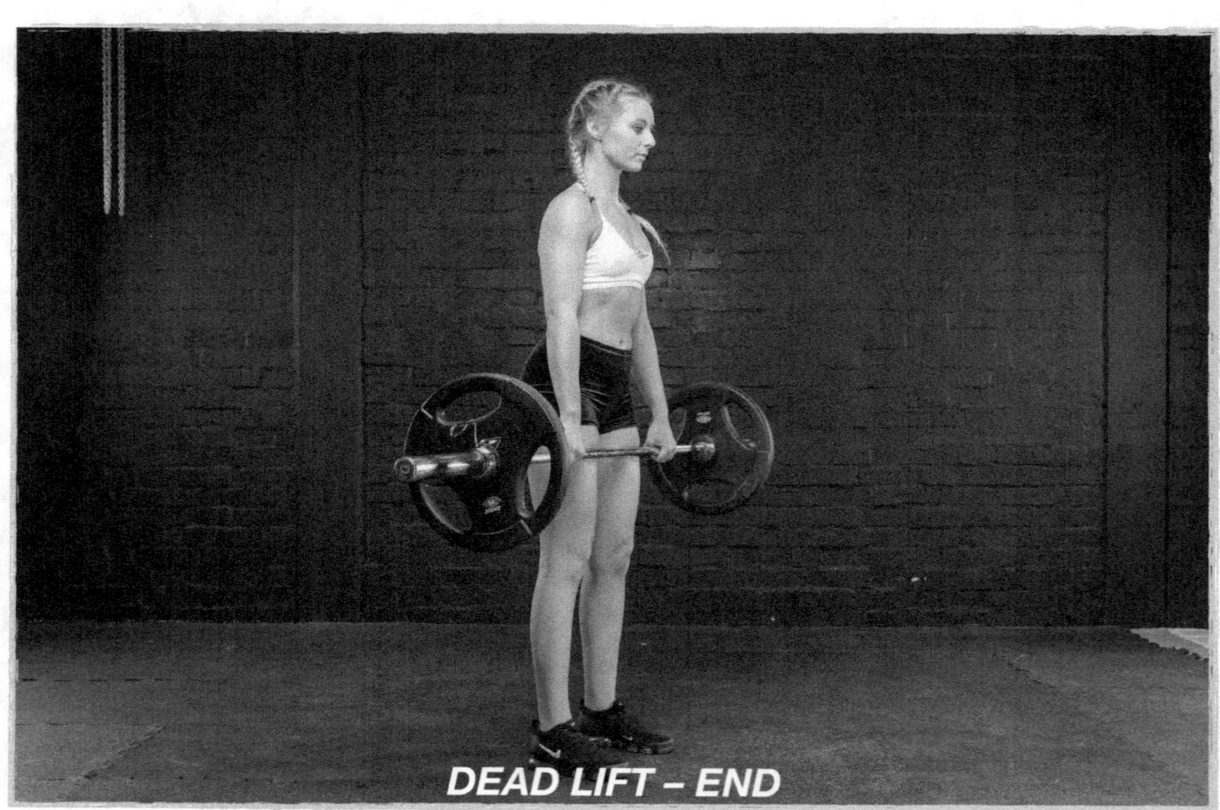

DEAD LIFT – END

SECTION FOUR: HIGH INTENSITY CARDIO

You'll love the exercises in this section... NOT!

High intensity cardio is pretty straightforward; you do exercises that use many muscles groups, for a short period of time, at super high intensity. We know that high intensity workouts are very tough, but because of this the benefits are awesome. In effect, these are the "cardio" workouts in this book, but they are miles away from the cardio that you might be familiar with, or the cardio that you see being performed at the gym.

10.1 STAR JUMP

The star jump is perhaps the simplest and easiest cardio exercise we've got here, but it's still good for getting the heart rate up and the calories burned. You may have seen them called jumping jacks, but it doesn't matter; the key is that they are a good cardio exercise that can be performed with very little space and require no equipment.

HOW DO I SET THE EQUIPMENT UP?

For star jumps you will need some floor space.

HOW DO I DO IT?

1. Stand with your feet together and your arms by your sides.

2. Jump up into the air, and move your feet and arms out the side as you do so.

3. Keep moving the feet and arms until you land on the ground again, by which point your feet will be widely spaced apart and your arms will be raised over your head.

4. From this position, jump again and bring your feet back to the centre and your arms back down towards your sides. This counts as one rep.

HOW MANY SETS AND REPS?

Like with other fat burning exercises there are a couple of ways of doing them. You can do them for sets of reps, or for specific time periods. Try 5 sets of 20 star jumps, or 5 sets of 30 seconds.

HOW DO I ADJUST THE DIFFICULTY?

To make star jumps more difficult you can jump higher into the air when moving the legs and arms in and out. To make them easier simply reduce the height of the jump.

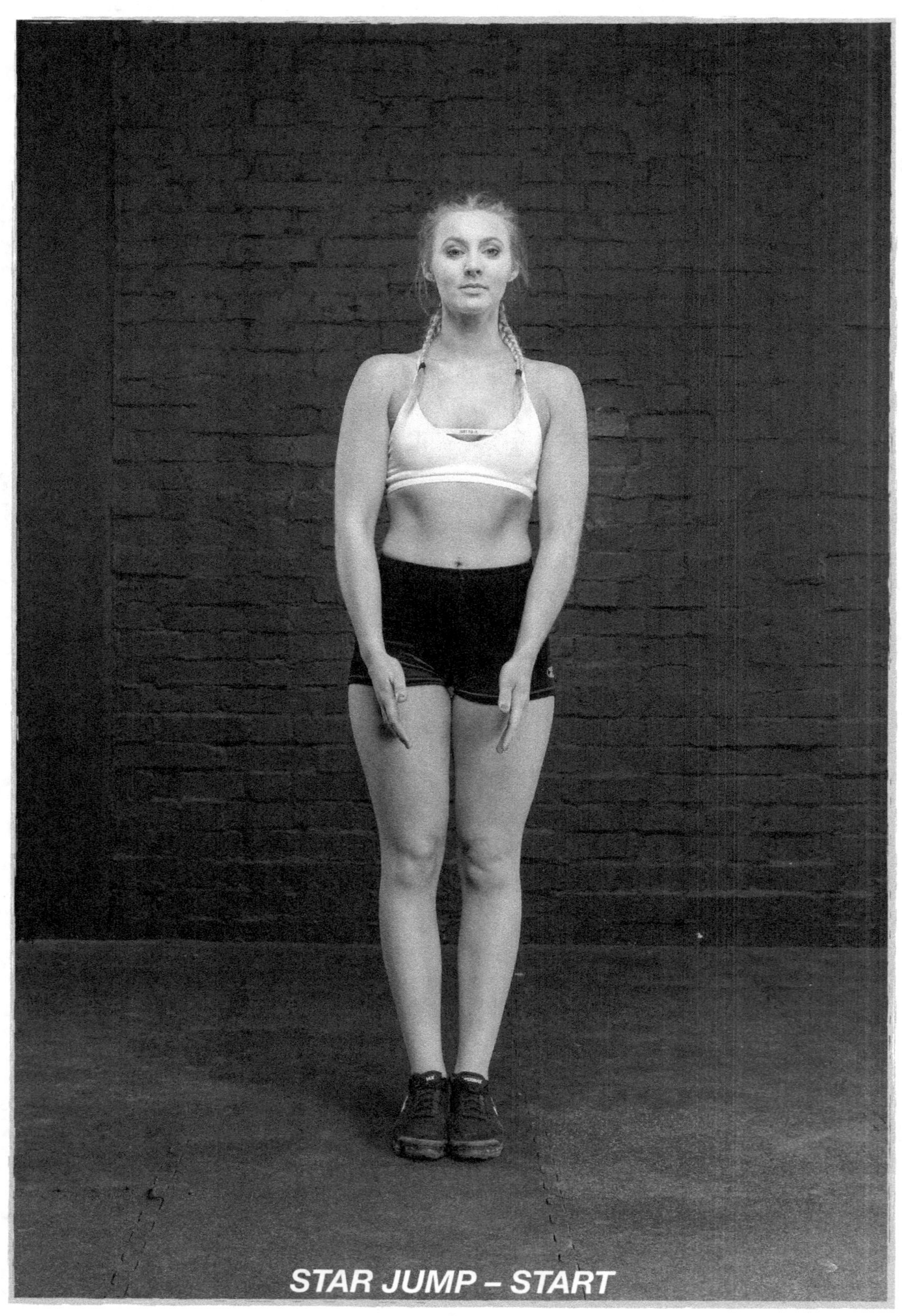

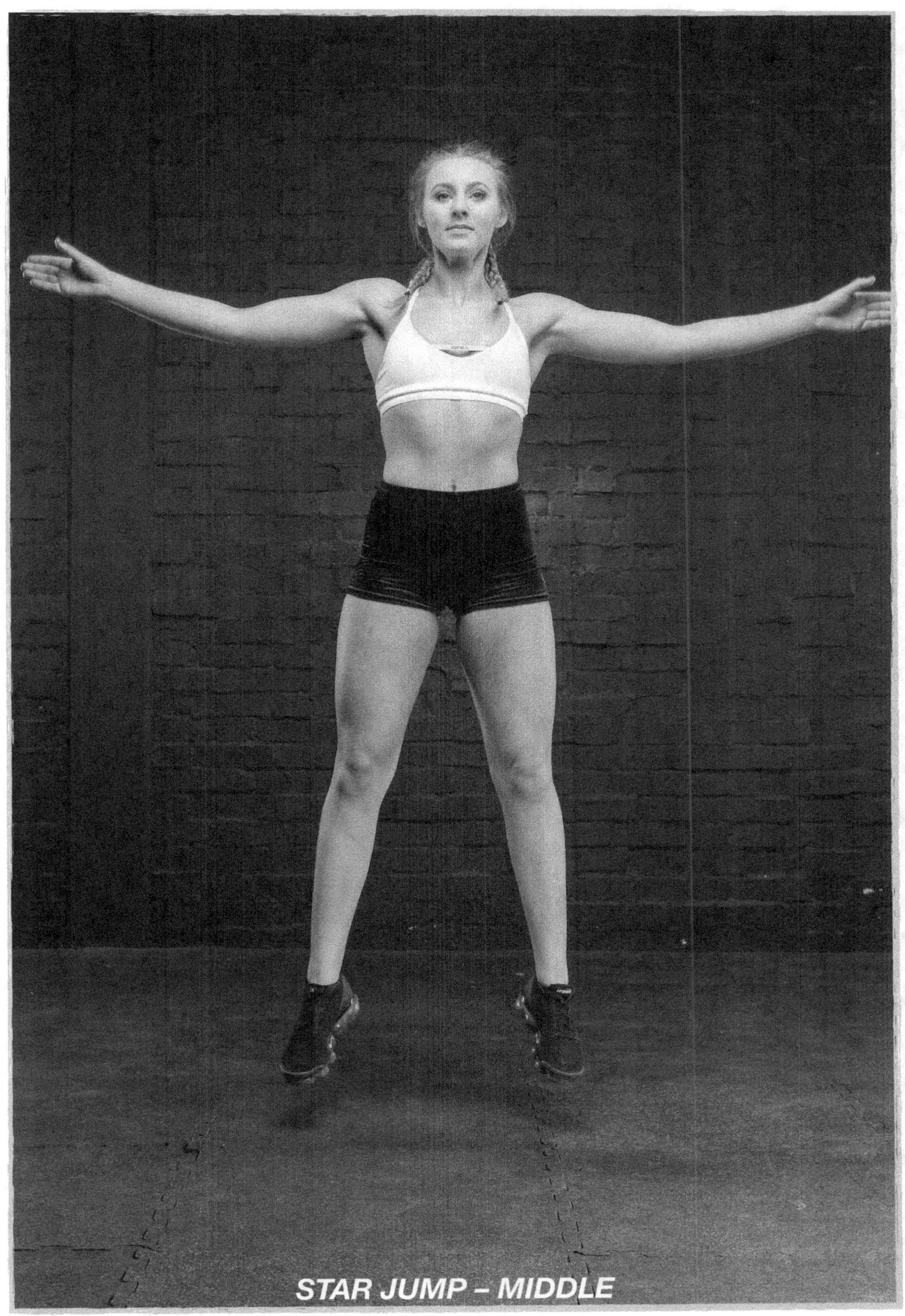
STAR JUMP – MIDDLE

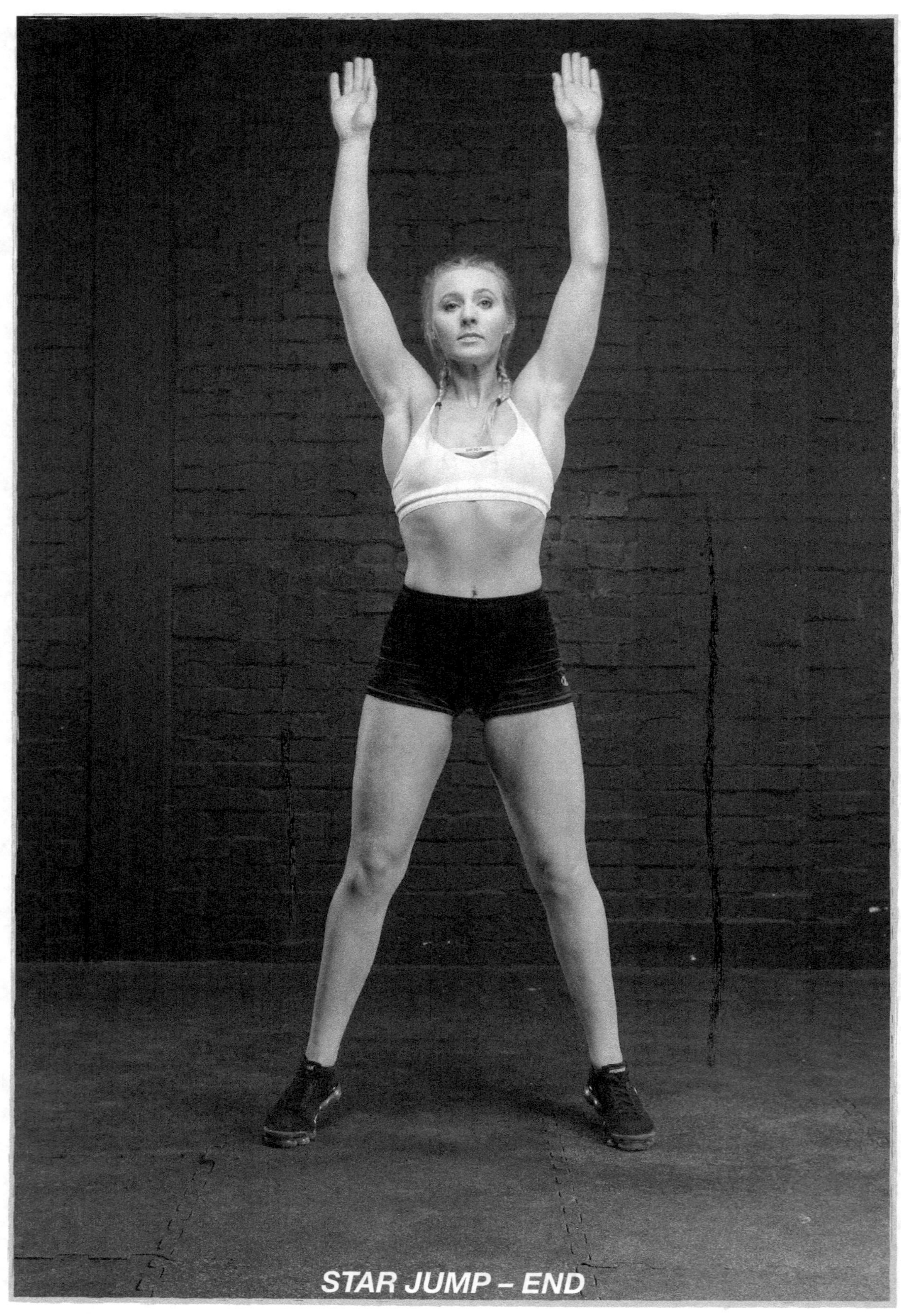
STAR JUMP – END

10.2 SKIPPING

Although skipping is something you see a lot of in the playground, it has been used by trainers and boxers for a long time, and for good reason! It's adjustable, can be made very challenging, and is suitable for inserting into circuits or acting as an exercise in its own right.

HOW DO I SET THE EQUIPMENT UP?

For skipping you'll obviously need a skipping rope, preferably one that allows you to adjust the length of the rope. Make sure that it's not too long or too short, as you don't want the rope fouling excessively on the ground, or for it to hit your feet when it passes beneath you. You'll also need some floor space and plenty of room both in front and behind you.

HOW DO I DO IT?

1. Stand with your feet shoulder width apart, and the skipping rope held firmly in both hands. The rope should be on the floor, behind you.

2. Swing the rope around until it gets near to your feet and then jump into the air.

3. Timing it right will allow the rope to clear the bottom of your feet.

4. Keep swinging the rope and continue skipping.

HOW MANY SETS AND REPS?

Skipping is best done for time, as counting reps will either be impossible or drive you mad! Try doing 5 sets of 60 seconds, or once you get good, 1 set for as long as you can without the rope hitting your feet.

HOW DO I ADJUST THE DIFFICULTY?

To make skipping easier you can jump less high, or slow down the speed at which you're skipping. To increase the difficulty you can jump higher or increase the speed you're skipping.

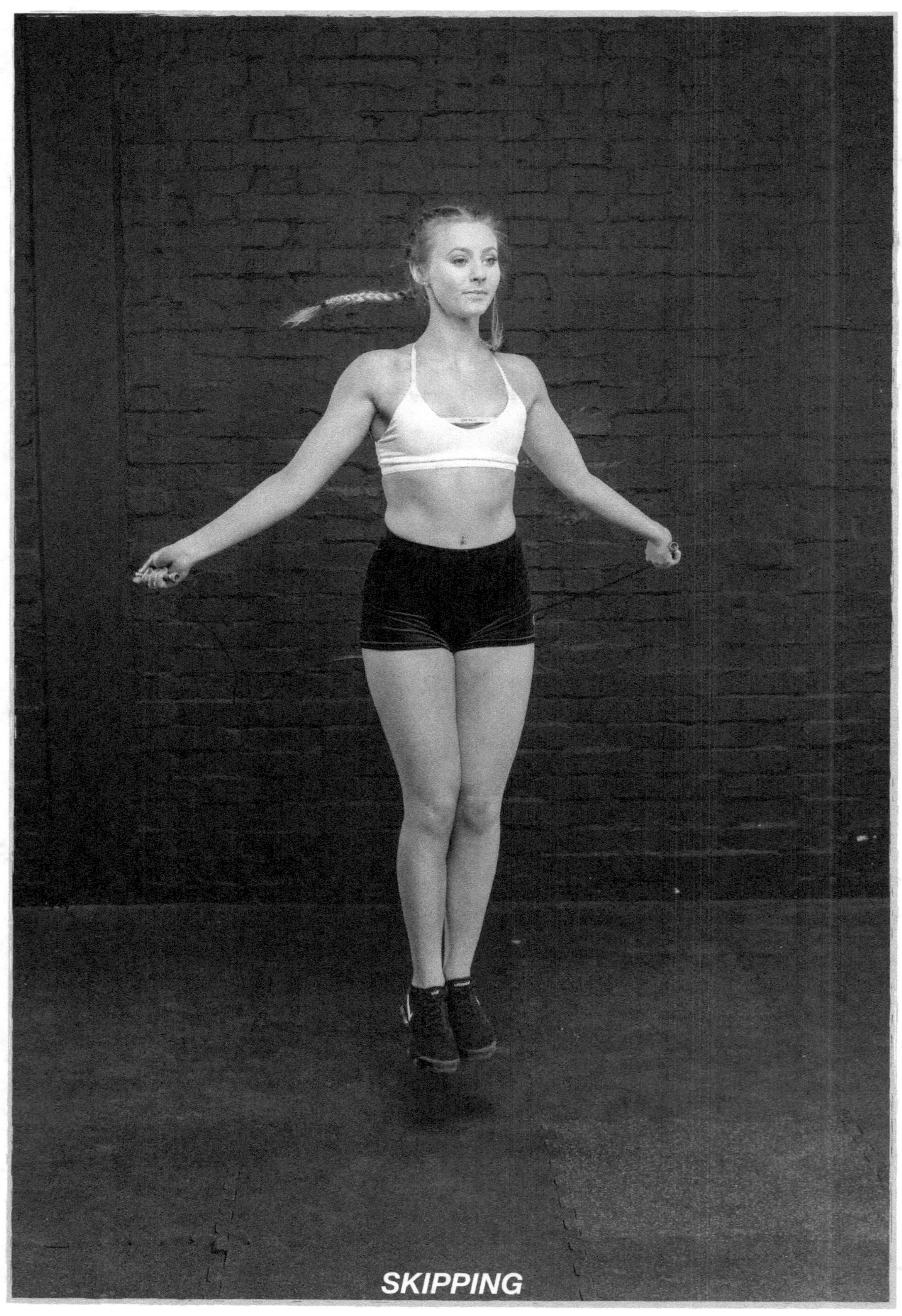

SKIPPING

10.3 MOUNTAIN CLIMBER

The mountain climber is another great movement, that's simpler and easier than the burpee. It still burns loads of calories and uses most muscles in the body, but is more suitable for an end of workout blast, or as a pulse raiser as part of a circuit.

HOW DO I SET THE EQUIPMENT UP?

For mountain climbers you will need some floor space, and an exercise step or platform if you need to raise the hands.

HOW DO I DO THEM?

1. To perform the mountain climber, start in a push-up position, but with one foot stretched out behind you and the other near your hands. Keep your arms as straight as you can.

2. From here, jump into the air and switch legs, so that the front leg goes to the back and the back leg goes to the front.

3. From here, jump up and repeat the action so your legs end up in the start position. This counts as one rep.

HOW MANY SETS AND REPS?

For doing sets and reps try 5 sets of 10 reps. For sets and time do 5 sets of 20 seconds.

HOW DO I ADJUST THE DIFFICULTY?

To make mountain climbers easier you can move your feet backwards and forwards by stepping them and not jumping. You can also raise your hands by placing them on a platform. This will reduce the amount of weight felt by the upper body.

To make them harder you can try and move your feet as wide apart as possible, getting the front foot right next to your hands, and you rear leg as far back as possible. You can also jump a little higher, and try supporting your body weight on your hands for a little longer.

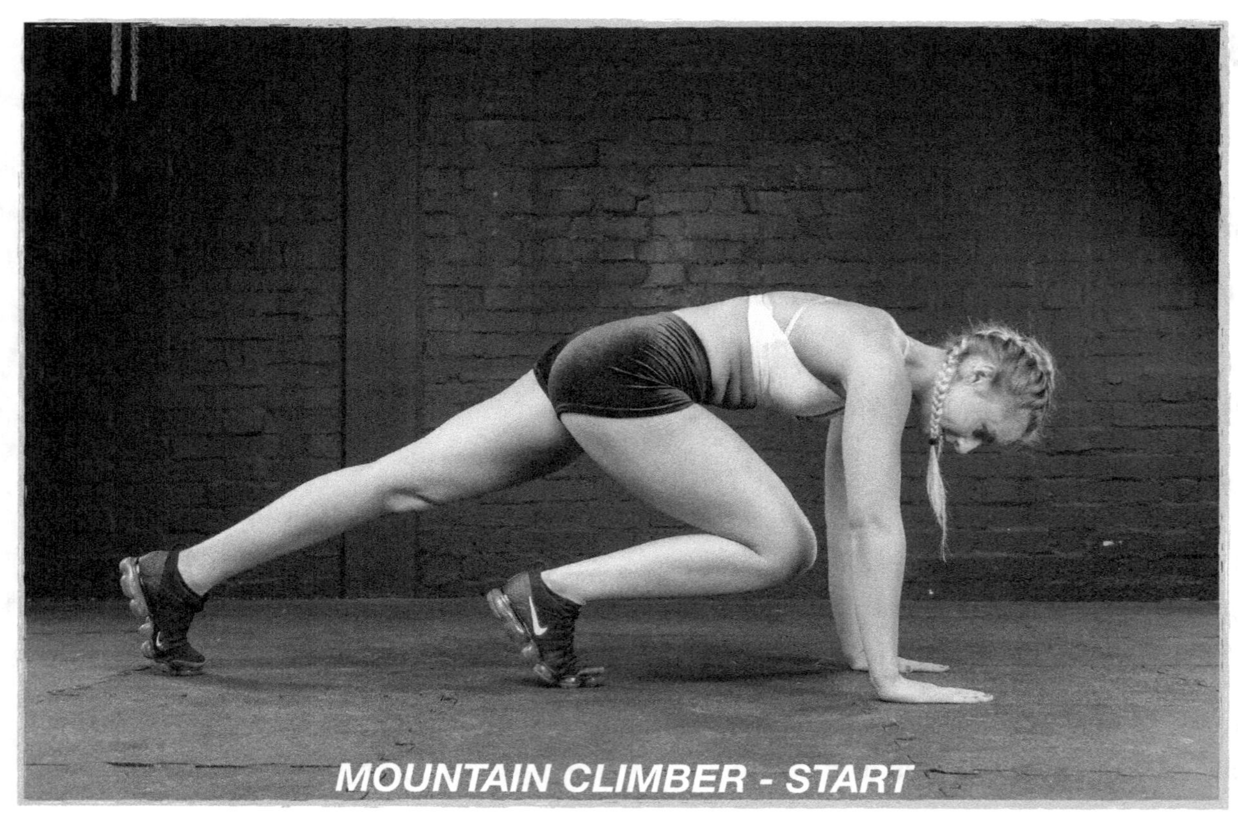

MOUNTAIN CLIMBER - START

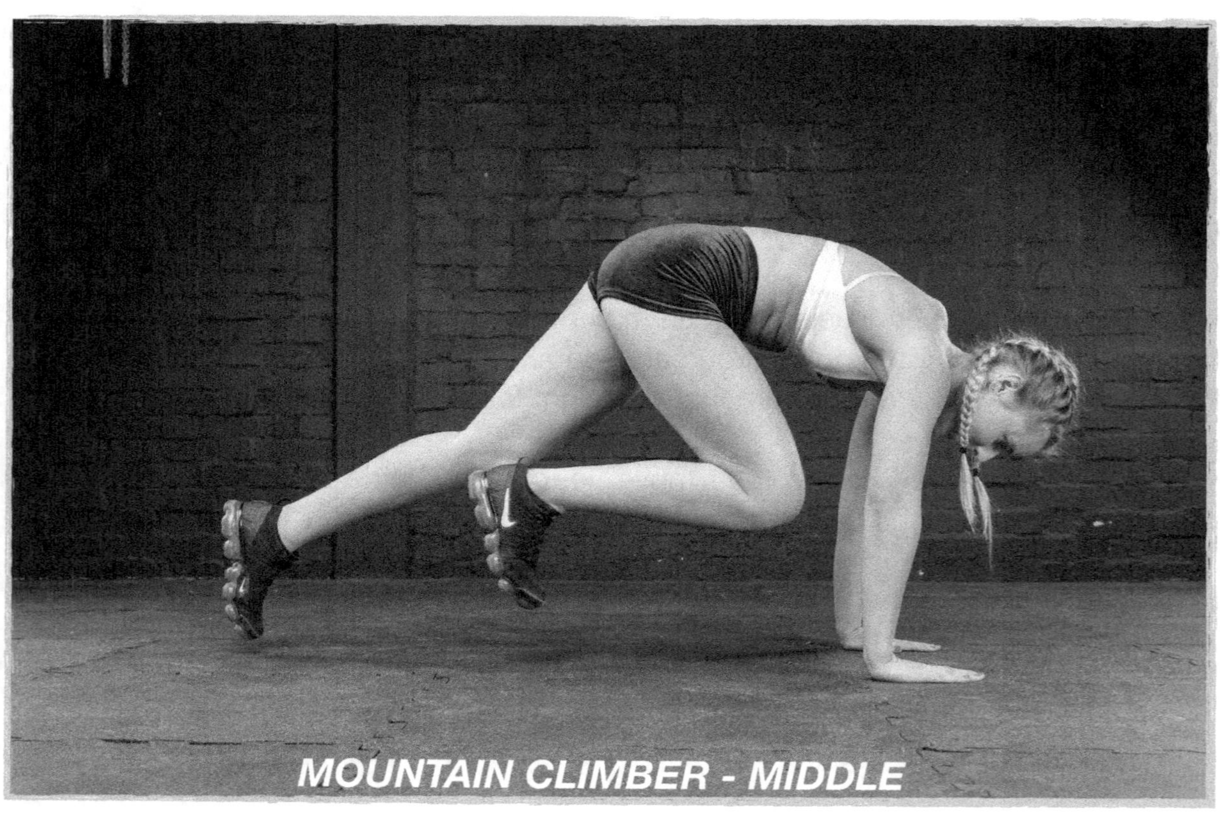

MOUNTAIN CLIMBER - MIDDLE

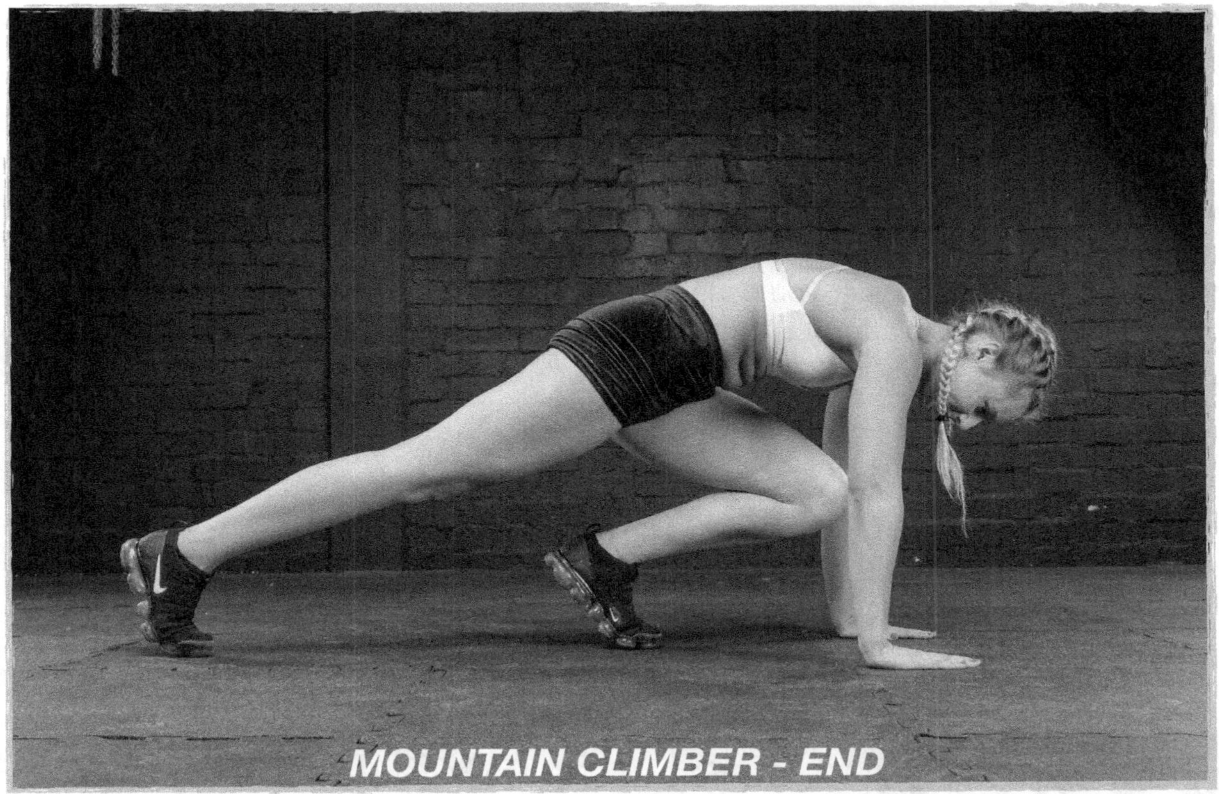

10.4 SQUAT THRUST

The squat thrust is basically a simpler version of the burpee, without the standing up part or the jump at the top.

HOW DO I SET THE EQUIPMENT UP?

For the squat thrust you will need some floor space, and if needed, an exercise step or platform to raise the hands.

HOW DO I DO THEM?

1. To perform the squat thrust, crouch down and place your hands flat on the floor. This is the start and finish position.

2. From here, jump your feet into the air and extend your legs out backwards until you land in the top of a push-up position.

3. From here, jump your feet into the air and return them to the crouched position that we started with. This counts as one rep.

HOW MANY SETS AND REPS?

Like the other exercises in this section, you can do them for sets of reps, and for sets of time. Try 5 sets of 15 reps or 5 sets of 25 seconds.

HOW DO I ADJUST THE DIFFICULTY?

To make the squat thrust easier you can reduce the distance that you jump, or place your hands on a raised platform. To make them harder increase the distance that you jump.

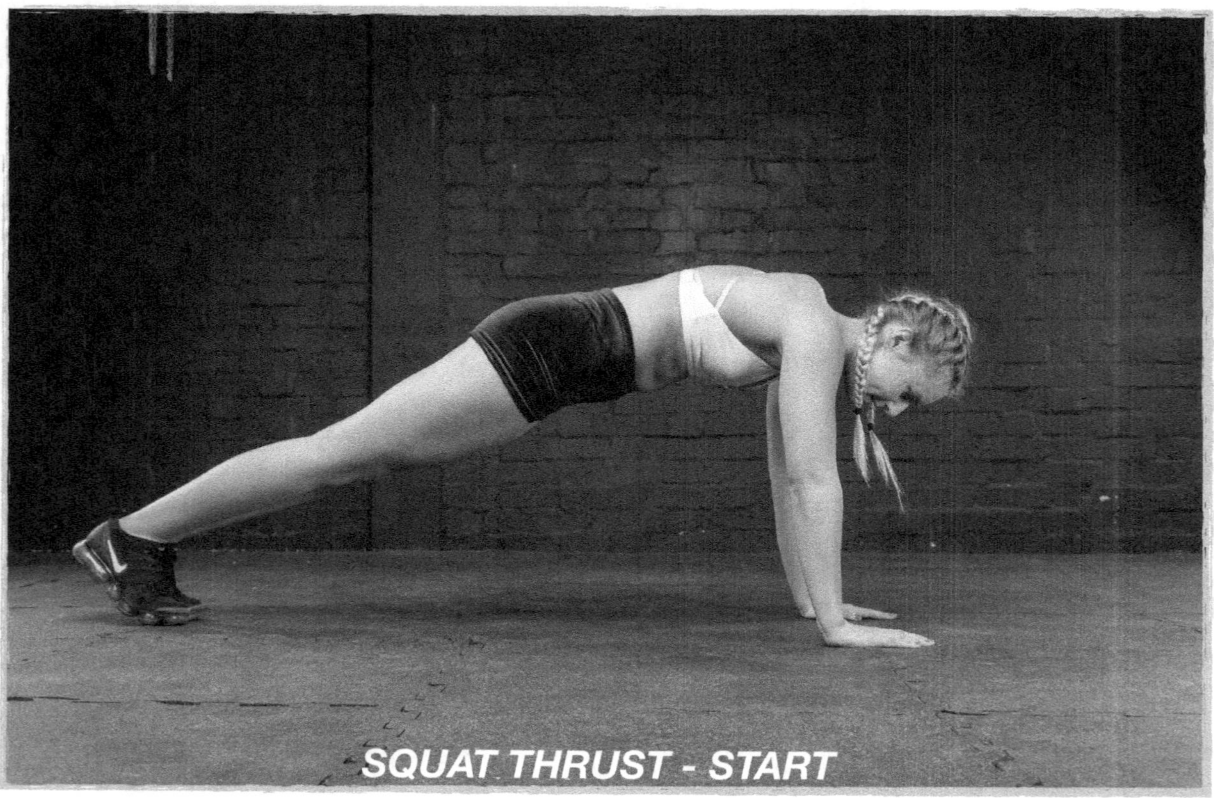

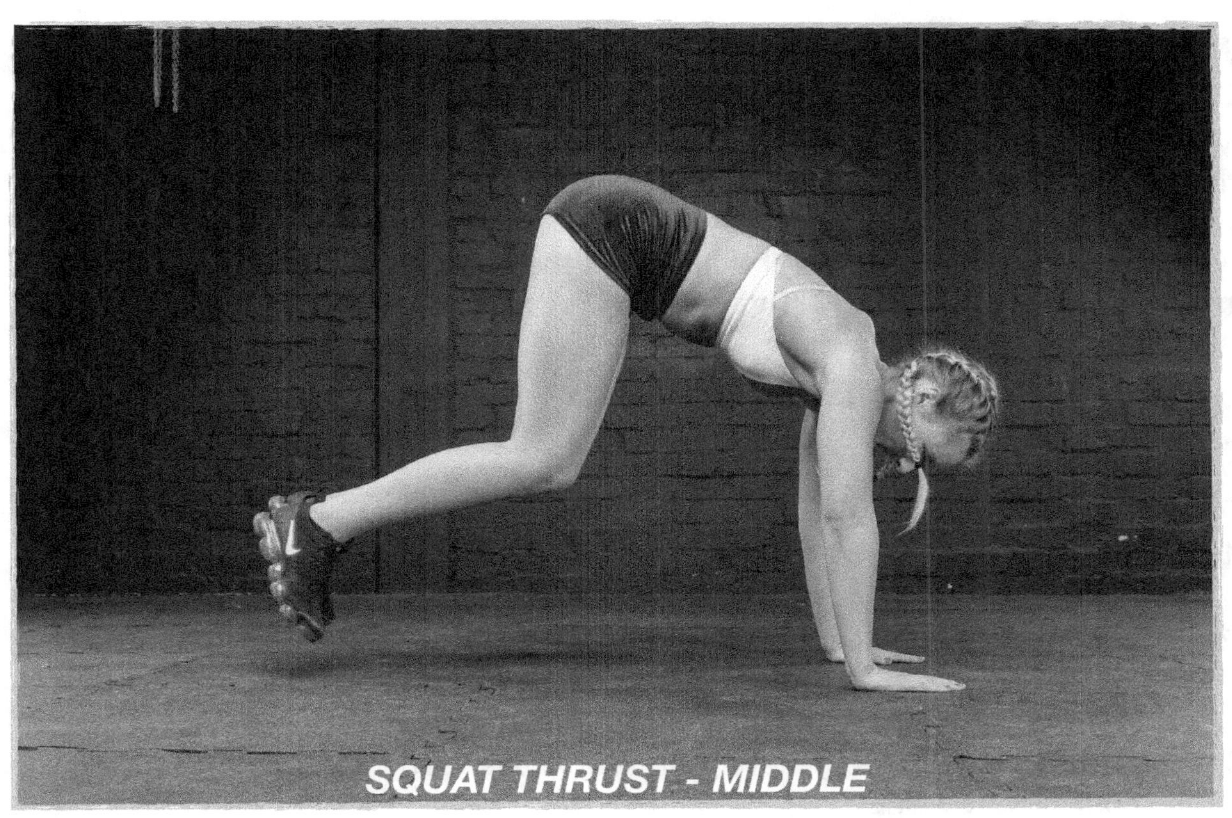

SQUAT THRUST - MIDDLE

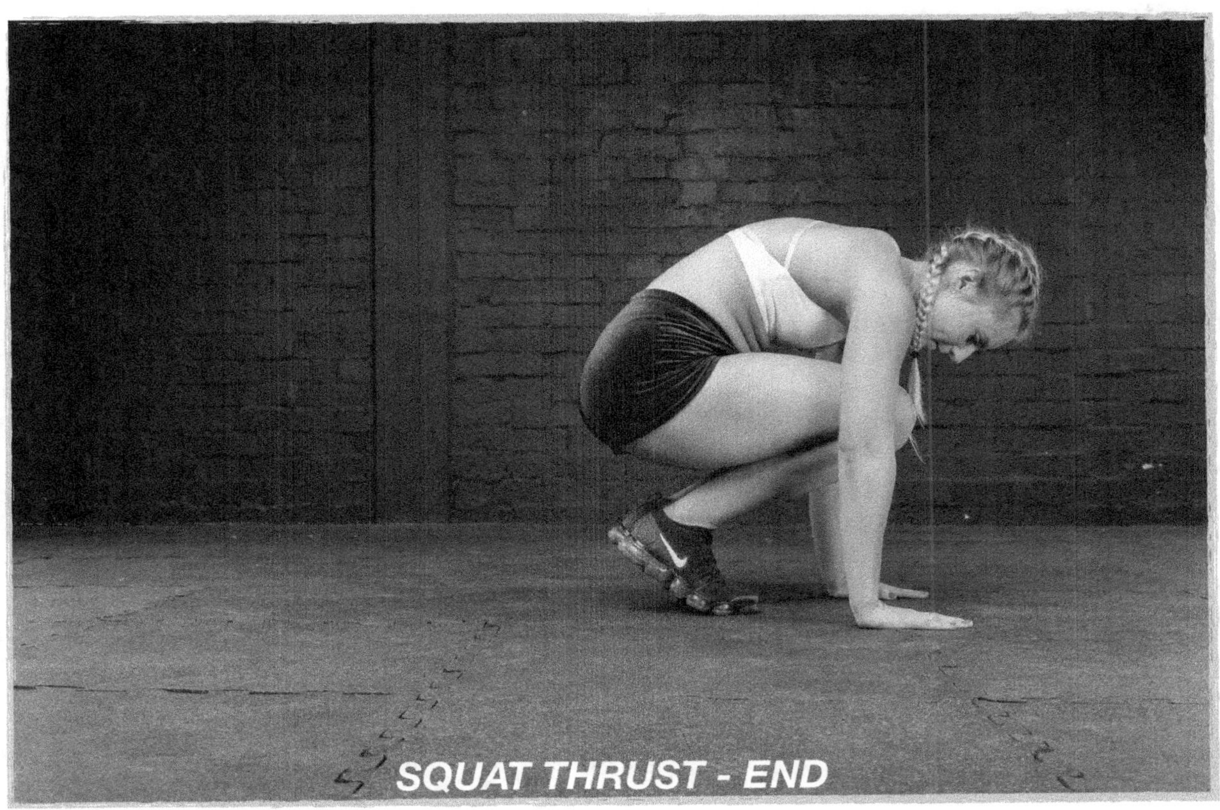

SQUAT THRUST - END

10.5 JUMPING SQUATS

As well as the lunge, the squat can also be made into a fat burning exercise by adding a jump to it. This becomes the jumping squat, and can be made as difficult and challenging as you like. Again, as with other lower body exercises, the muscles worked in the jumping squat are the largest in the body, which means they use tremendous amounts of energy. This makes jumping squats one of the best fat burning exercises.

HOW DO I SET THE EQUIPMENT UP?

You will need some floor space, with no obstacles around you.

HOW DO I DO THEM?

1. To perform jumping squats stand with your feet shoulder width apart and your knees slightly bent.

2. Squat down until your hips are level with your knees, using the same technique as for the normal body weight squat.

3. From this bottom position push up hard with the legs, and jump as high as you can into the air.

4. As you land bend your knees to absorb the shock, and continue with the exercise.

HOW MANY SETS AND REPS?

You can perform jumping squats for a specific number of reps, or for a specific period of time. Try 5 sets of 12 reps, or 5 sets of 20 seconds, with 30 to 60 seconds rest between each set.

HOW DO I ADJUST THE DIFFICULTY?

To make jumping squats easier you can reduce the range of motion, only squatting down half way on each rep. To make them more difficult you can increase the range of motion, dropping lower on each rep. You can also reduce the height of the jump (to make them easier), and increase the height of the jump (to make them harder).

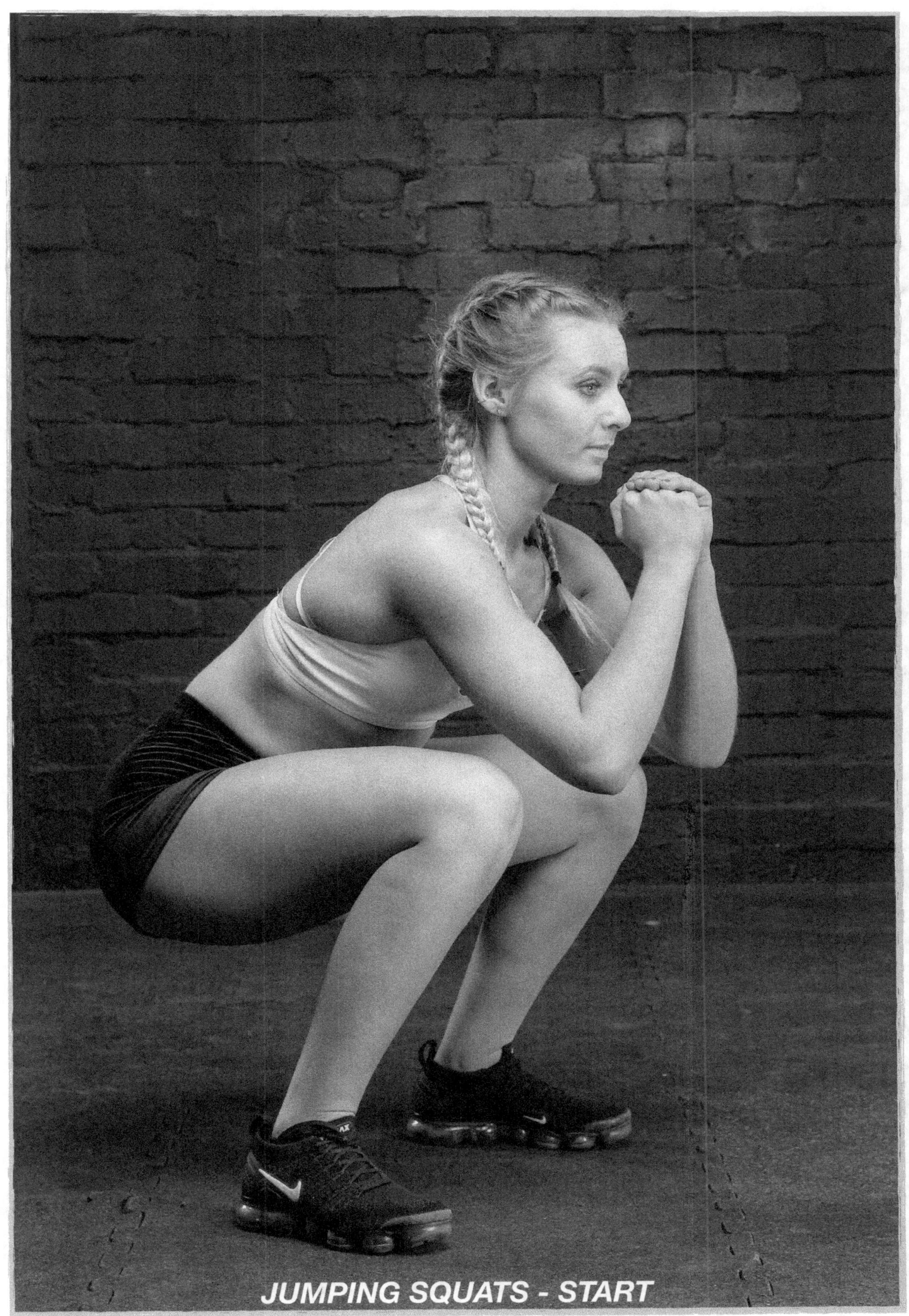

JUMPING SQUATS - START

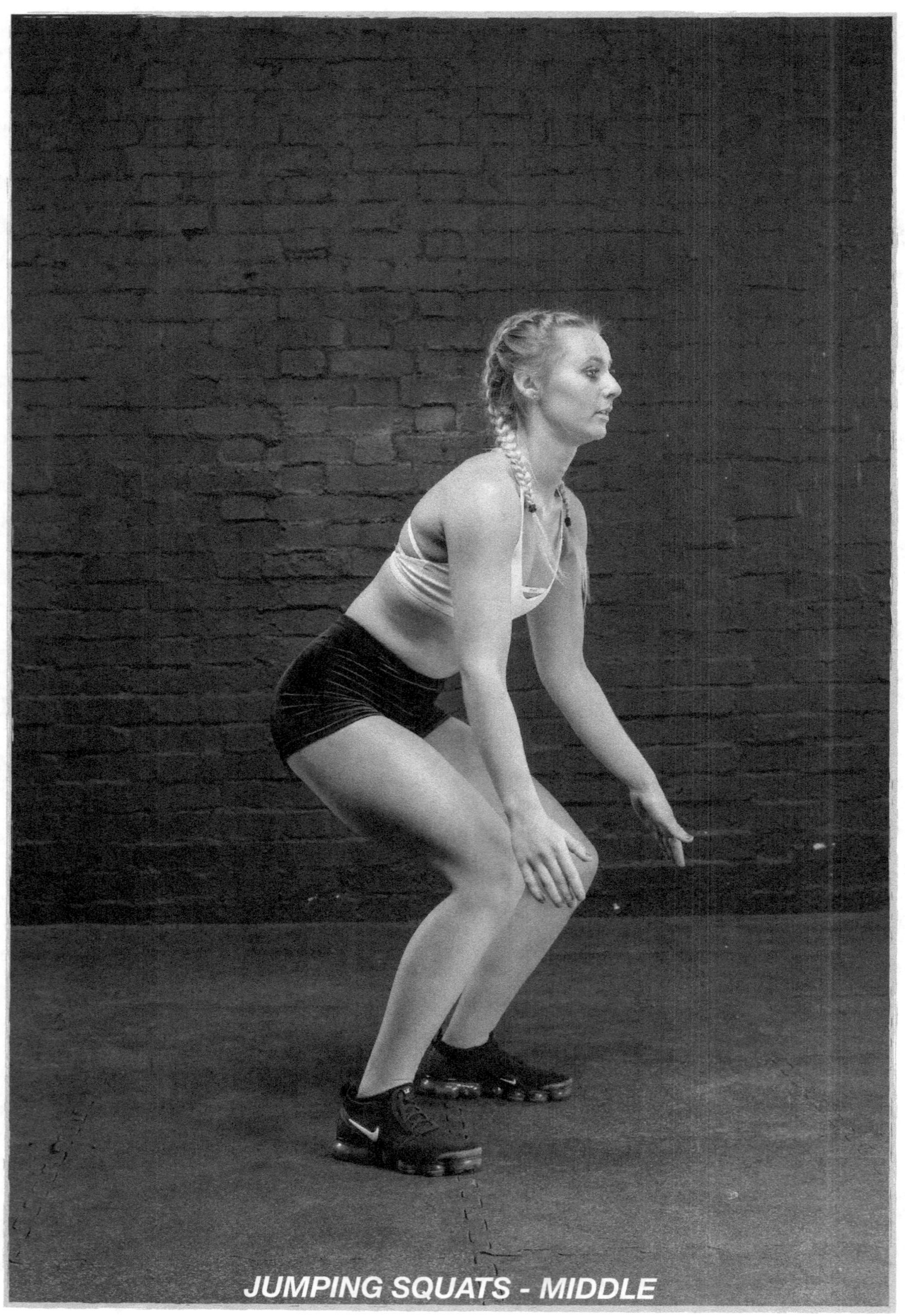

JUMPING SQUATS - MIDDLE

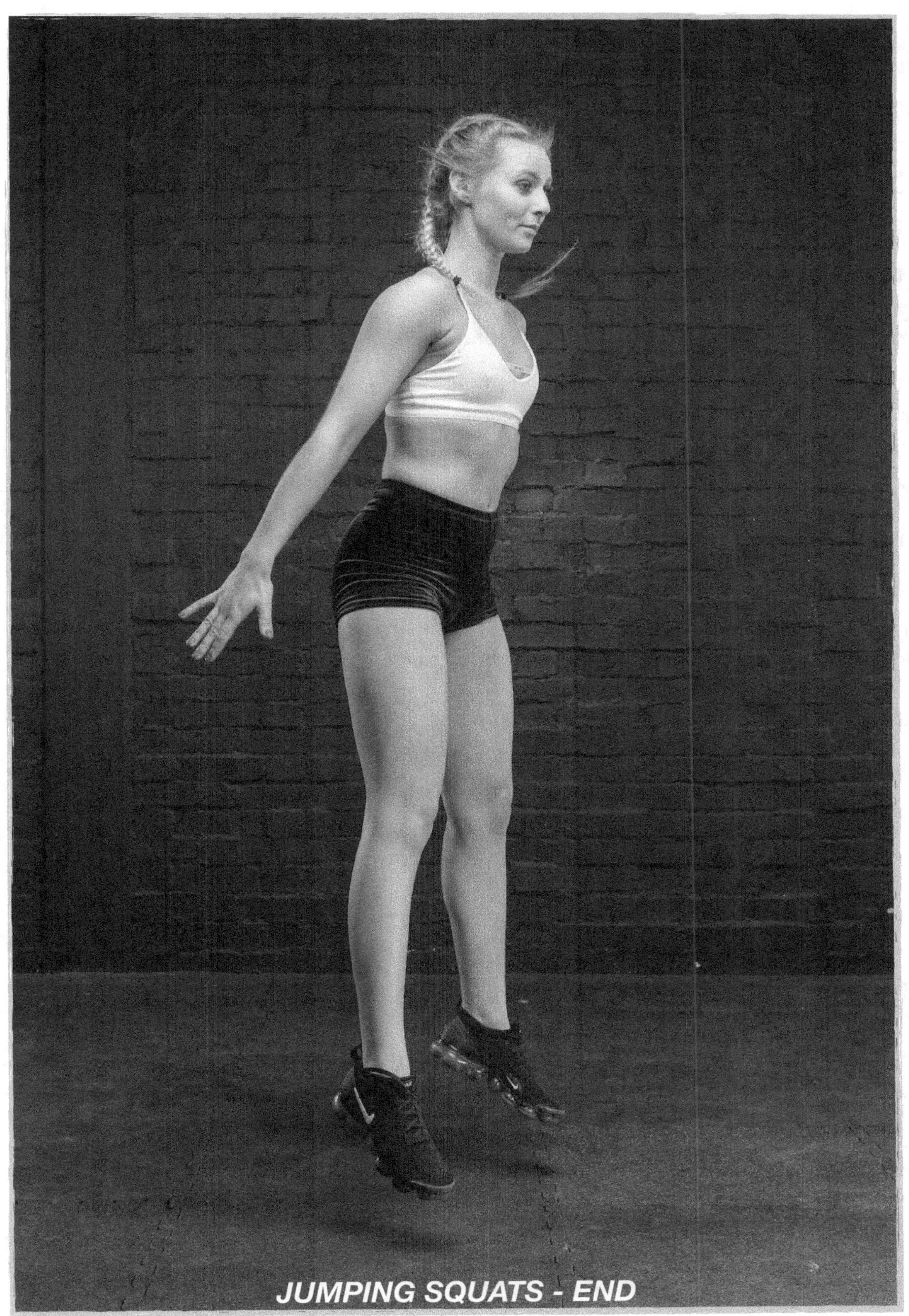

JUMPING SQUATS - END

10.6 KILLERS

Killers are a painful sounding exercise, but really they're just jumping lunges (actually, this still sounds painful!). Like any jumping exercise they use loads of energy, work the largest muscles in the body (the bum and legs), and give a fast and effective cardio workout. It goes without saying that you need to be OK with normal lunges before attempting these!

HOW DO I SET THE EQUIPMENT UP?

For killers you will need some floor space, preferably on a surface that is non-slip.

HOW DO I DO THEM?

1. Stand with your feet shoulder width apart, arms hanging loosely by your sides.

2. Take a large step forward, and sink down into the bottom position of the lunge. Both of your knees should be bent at 90 degrees, torso upright, with your head and neck in a neutral position.

3. From here jump into the air as high as you can. As you do, move your front foot backwards and your rear foot forwards, so that they cross over in the air.

4. Land with your feet in a lunge position and bend your knees immediately.

5. Sink into the lunge position as you land, arriving at the same bottom lunge position that you start in. This counts as one rep.

HOW MANY SETS AND REPS?

For killers you should try and do either 5 sets of 10 reps, or 5 sets of 20 to 30 seconds.

HOW DO I ADJUST THE DIFFICULTY?

To make killers easier you can reduce the height that you jump, reduce the distance between your feet, and reduce the depth of the lunge. To make them harder you can increase the height that you jump, increase the distance between your feet, and perform a deeper lunge on each rep.

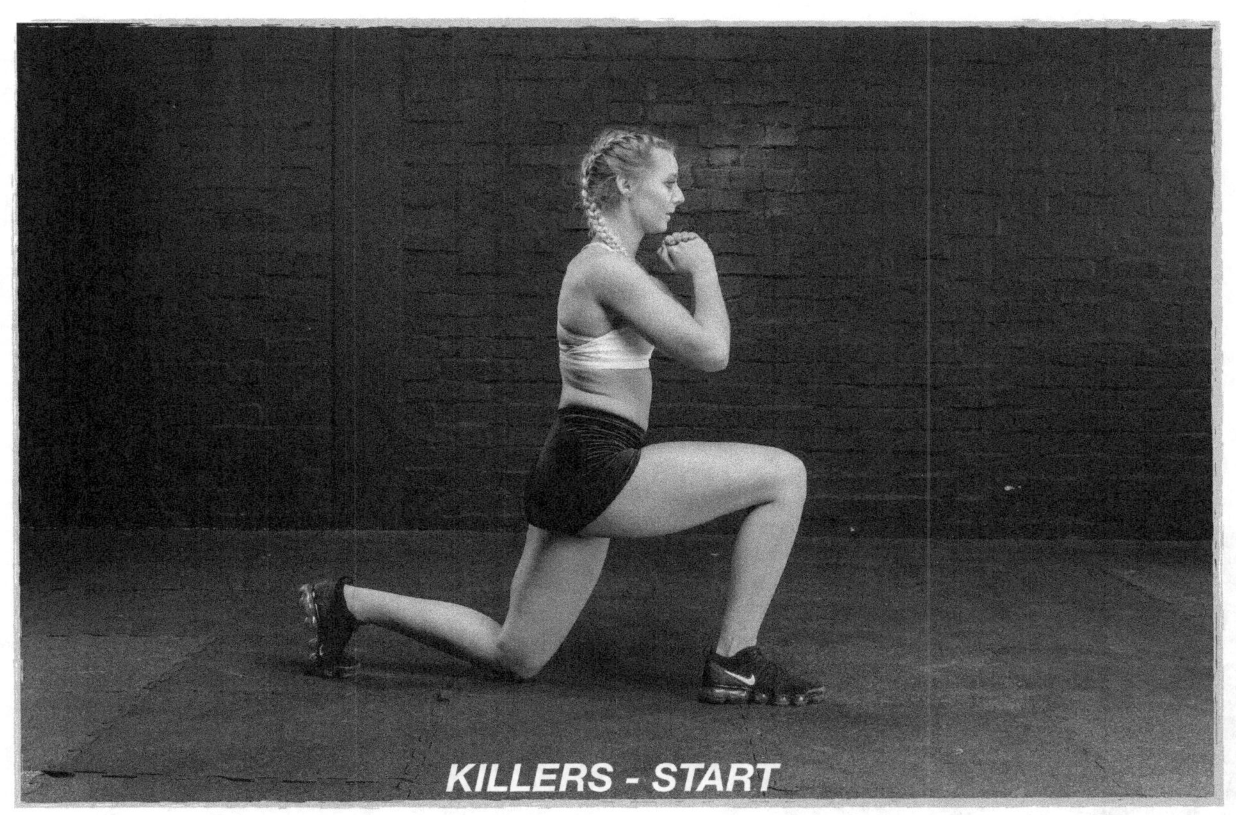

KILLERS - START

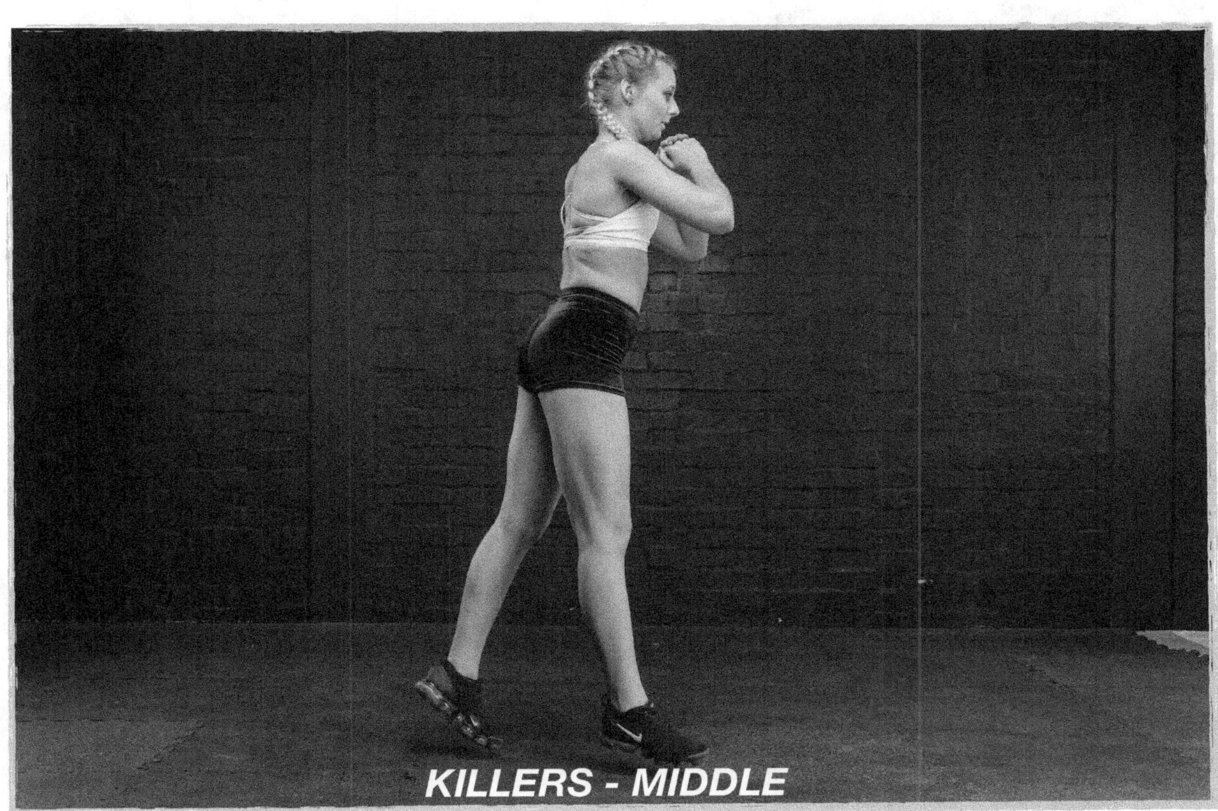

KILLERS - MIDDLE

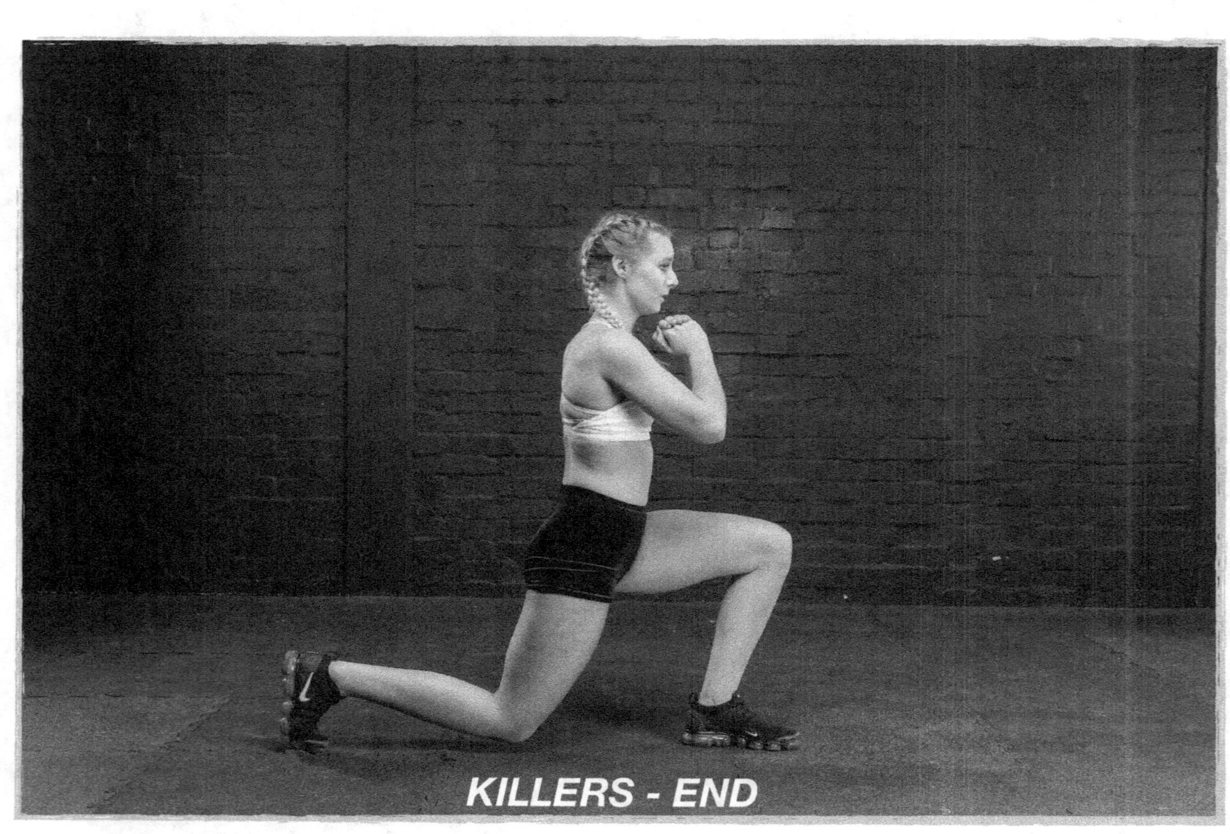
KILLERS - END

10.7 BEAR CRAWLS

Bear crawls sound like they might be a nice, cuddly exercise, but they definitely are not! Walking on the hands and feet whilst keeping the hips low is very tough, and makes for an exceptional cardio exercise. It works the upper body, core, lower body, and the heart and lungs. Yeah, it looks slightly funny running around like a bear, but the benefits are so good it's worth putting up with the funny looks.

HOW DO I SET THE EQUIPMENT UP?

For bear crawls you will need some floor space, preferably with enough room to move for 10 metres or so. If you do perform them outside, make sure that the ground is free of obstacles, or wear gloves for extra safety.

HOW DO I DO THEM?

1. To perform the bear crawl, crouch down on your hands and feet.

2. Now stretch your feet out behind you slightly, so that your knees are bent and your back is horizontal.

3. Now move your right hand and left foot forward together, then your left hand and right foot, and so on, moving forwards in a walking motion.

HOW MANY SETS AND REPS?

Bear crawls can be done for either distance or time. If you are doing distance, perform 5 sets of 10 to 20 metres crawls, with 30 to 60 seconds rest between each set. If you are doing time, perform crawls for 20 seconds, with 30 to 60 seconds between each set.

HOW DO I ADJUST THE DIFFICULTY?

Bear crawls are more difficult if you keep the hips low, so if you need to make them easier then raise the hips up slightly to put less stress on the core. You can also perform them backwards for an added challenge once the normal version becomes too easy (yeah, right!).

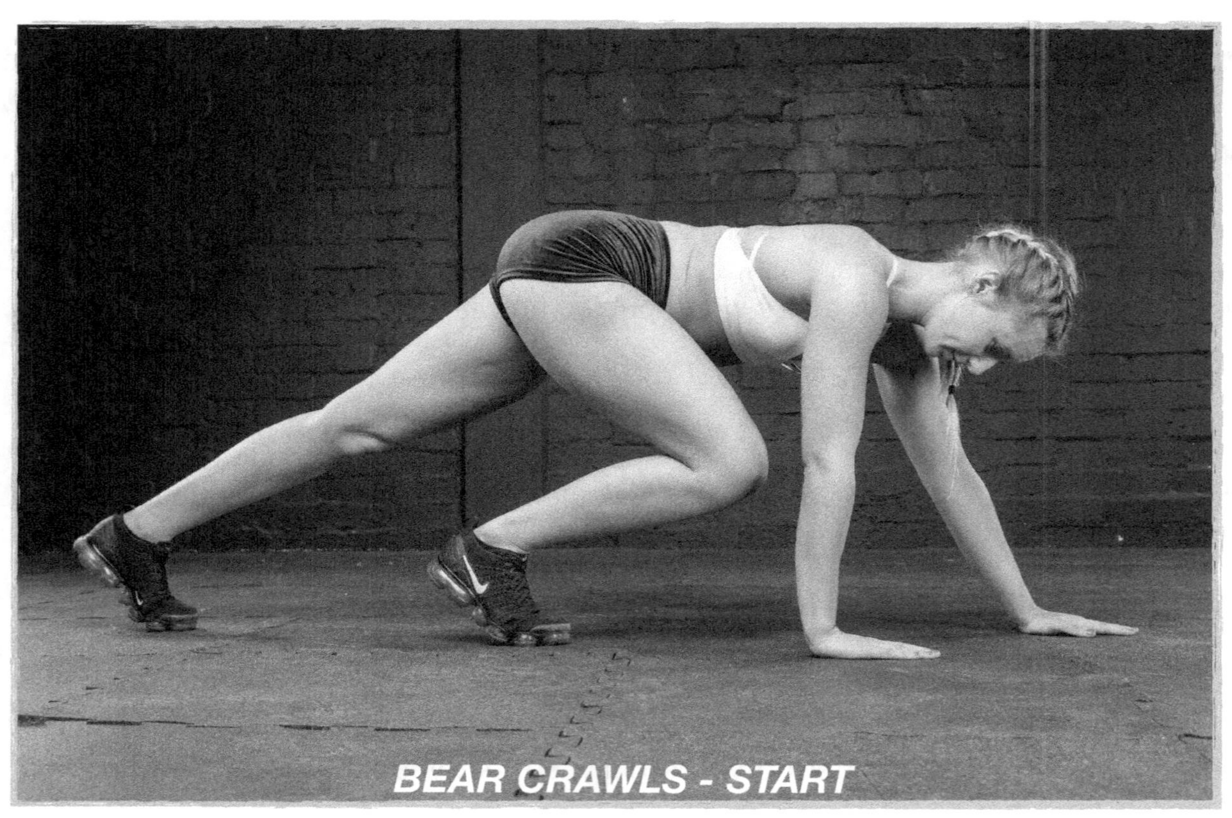

BEAR CRAWLS - START

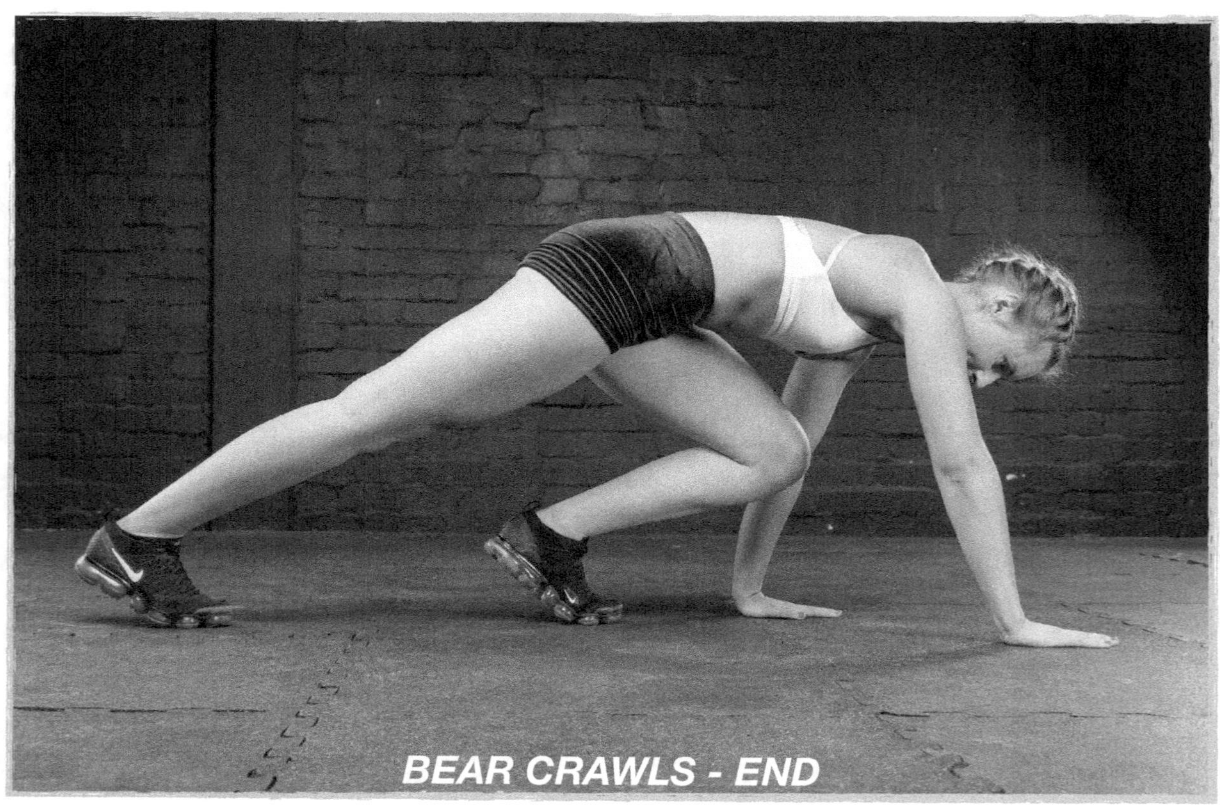

BEAR CRAWLS - END

10.8 BURPEES

We'll end with the greatest fat burning exercise of them all: the burpee! Nothing gets the heart pumping and the lungs busting like burpees, and rightly so. They use most of the muscles in the body, and done at a fast pace are much more physically demanding than any cycling class in the world. If you want to melt fat off your body, do these!

HOW DO I SET THE EQUIPMENT UP?

For burpees you will need some floor space, and possibly an exercise step or platform to make them easier.

HOW DO I DO THEM?

1. Stand up straight with your arms by your sides, feet shoulder width apart.

2. Crouch down, placing your hands flat on the floor, shoulder width apart.

3. Jump your feet into the air and move them backwards, so that you land in a push-up position.

4. Now jump your feet forwards so that you arrive back in the crouch position again.

5. Stand up and jump into the air, landing with bent knees. This counts as one rep.

HOW MANY SETS AND REPS?

For burpees there are a number of approaches when it comes to the sets and reps. The first method is to perform 5 sets of 10 as quickly as possible, with 30 to 60 seconds rest in between each set. Another method is to do 5 sets of 20 seconds, doing as many reps in each 20-second block as you can, taking 30 to 60 seconds rest in between each set.

Read more about how to structure your cardio workouts in the *High Intensity Cardio Programs* section, on page **210.**

HOW DO I ADJUST THE DIFFICULTY?

To make burpees easier you can do a number of things. First, you can slow down the speed that you do them. Second, you can move your feet backwards and forwards one step at a time, instead of jumping them. Third, you can just stand instead of jumping into the air.

To make burpees harder (are they not hard enough already?!) you can do a couple of things. First, you can do them faster, aiming to perform each rep as quickly as possible. Second, you can add a push-up to the crouching part of the movement.

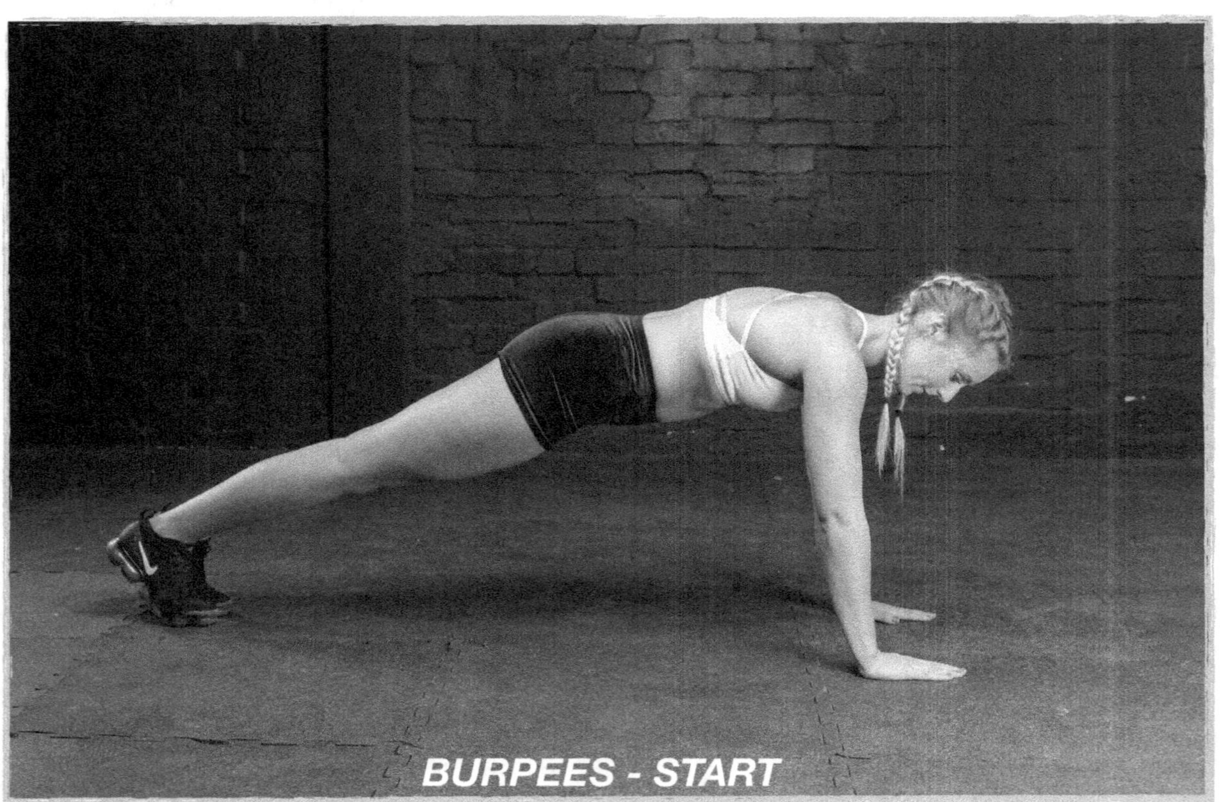

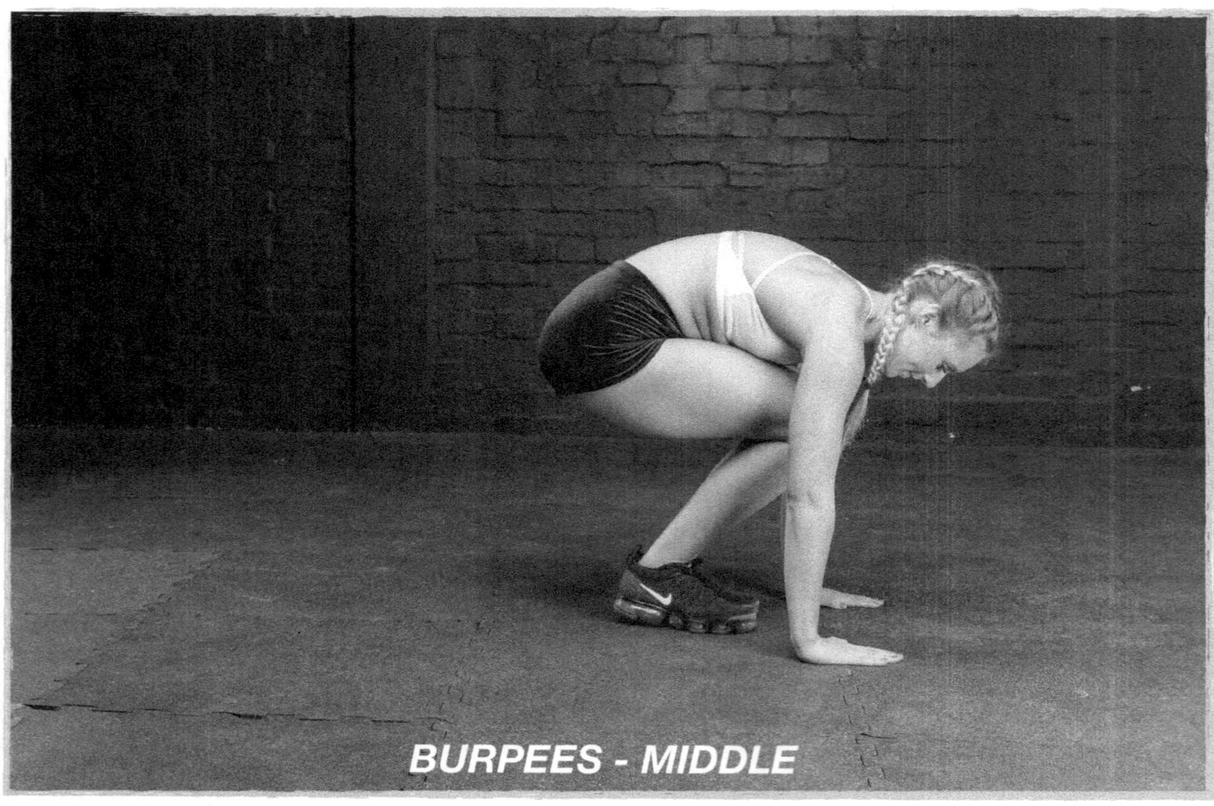

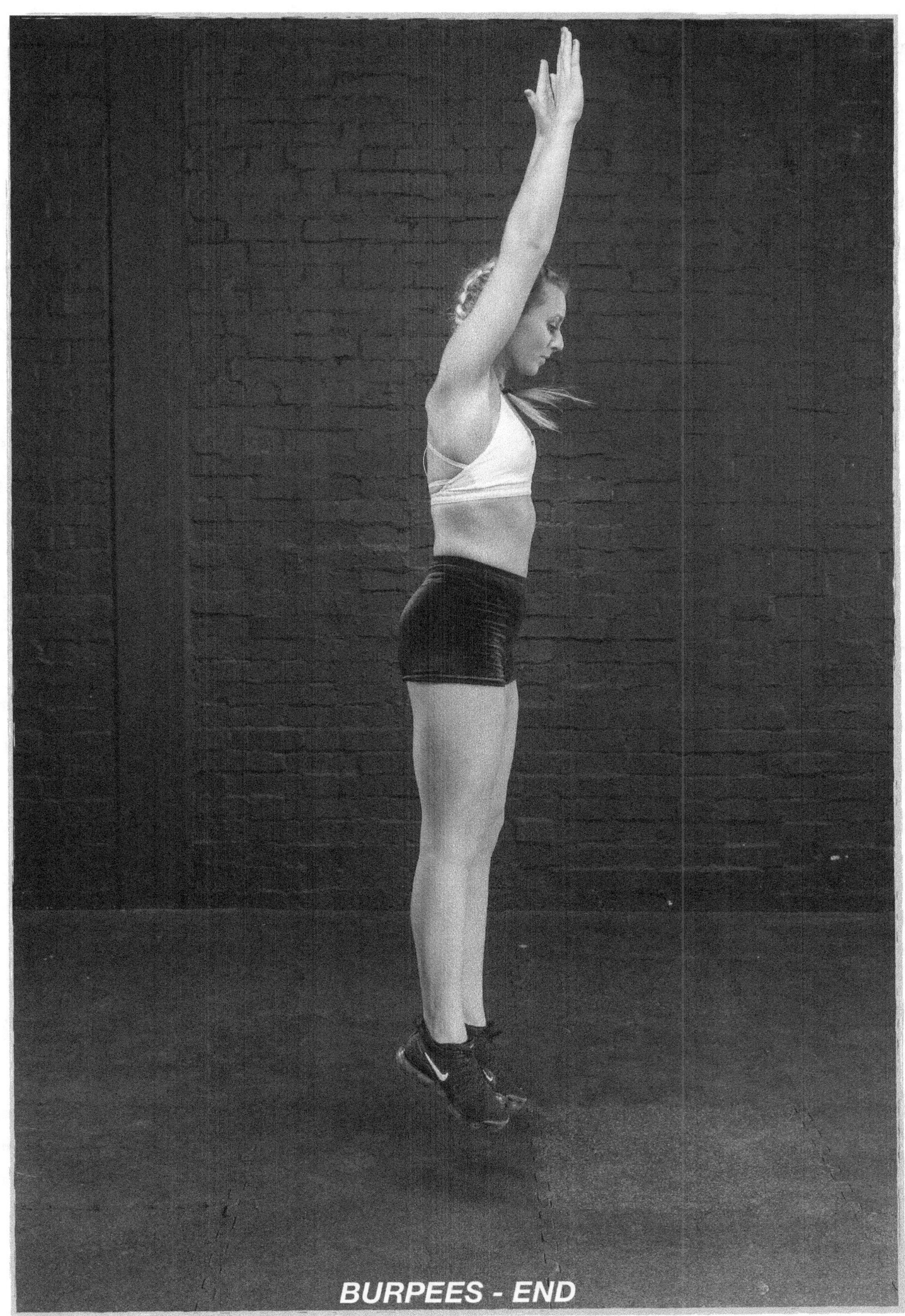

BURPEES - END

11. RESISTANCE EXERCISE PROGRAMS

Knowing how to perform all of the exercises is one thing, but now we have to put them together into some programs. Programs make it so much easier to follow a workout and get results, as they make sure that you always know what you're doing, when you're doing it, and how long you're doing it for.

Obviously, there will be a wide range of abilities amongst our readers, so we have a total of four programs, which should suit the vast majority of people.

It's worth saying that even though we have these different programs there's so much variation between people that some adjustment may be necessary in order for the program to work for you. There are a number of ways that the programs can be adjusted, and we're going to explain those here.

Firstly, if a program is too hard, or a particular exercise is too hard, then make sure to read the sections within the exercise descriptions explaining how to make them easier or more difficult.

Rest time is another factor that can be adjusted, and most likely will need to be adjusted based on your own abilities. The rest time amounts that we give are only a guide, and if you need to add more, or less, then feel free to do so.

11.1 HOW OFTEN SHOULD I BE WORKING OUT?

Good question! Our advice is to start with three times per week, and then go from there. A Monday, Wednesday, Friday routine works very well, as this gives enough rest between workouts, and the entire weekend off. The programs should take around an hour, depending on your ability, so three hours a week is easily achievable for the vast majority of people.

As you progress you may want to do more, either keeping to three sessions a week and doing longer individual workouts, or increasing the number of workouts you do to four or five per week. Be careful here, as it can be easy to over train, and do too much. Your body repairs itself, and gets stronger and fitter when you are resting, and you cannot rest if you are spending all your time in the gym.

11.2 BEGINNER PROGRAM

If you're a beginner then it can be daunting to start an exercise program, but if you want to get the body of your dreams then you're going to have to start one, and our beginner program will help you get where you want to go! Although weighted exercises are great, and allow steady progression, if you are a beginner it is sensible to start with primarily body weight exercises. This program will give you all you need to get started, and help to build a great physique that you can then progress with.

The program is in a table form, which you can see on the next page. Simply follow the program from top to bottom, doing all of the reps and sets (or as many as you can), and taking the correct amount of rest time (remember to adjust this depending on how you feel)!

Below you'll find a table showing each of the exercises in the program, with valuable hints and tips that you should to know before starting.

KNEELING PUSH-UP	Remember to vary the height of the platform if you need to make it easier or harder
LEDGE DIP	You can use bent knees to make them easier, or straight legs to make things more difficult
ROW	Try out both grips (fingers over/fingers under) to find where your weaknesses are
DEAD HANG	See above
BENCH PRESS	Start with just the bar if possible, or if the barbell is too heavy, try a group exercise barbell
BICEPS CURL	Start light and work up in weight. Remember to adjust the angle of the bench for comfort
PLANK	Drop to the knees to make things easier, or stretch out the arms to make things tougher
SIDE PLANK	Make sure your shoulders, hips, and knees are in line
ARCH	Concentrate on keeping your legs straight, and squeeze those shoulder blades together
BODY WEIGHT SQUAT	Really concentrate on form, and make sure that you squat down low enough
BRIDGE	Make sure a straight line forms with your shoulders, hips, and knees
CALF RAISE	Start unweighted to begin with, and then move onto using dumbbells

BEGINNER PROGRAM

WARM UP

ARMS, CHEST, AND SHOULDERS

EXERCISE	REPS	SETS	REST
KNEELING PUSH-UP	8 – 12	3 – 5	30 – 60 SECONDS
LEDGE DIP	8 – 12	3 – 5	30 – 60 SECONDS
ROW	8 – 12	3 – 5	30 – 60 SECONDS
DEAD HANG	1 (LONG AS POSSIBLE)	3 – 5	30 – 60 SECONDS
BENCH PRESS	8 – 12	3 – 5	30 – 60 SECONDS
BICEPS CURL	8 – 12	3 – 5	30 – 60 SECONDS

ABS AND CORE

EXERCISE	REPS	SETS	REST
PLANK	30 SECONDS	3	30 – 60 SECONDS
SIDE PLANK	30 SECONDS	3 (EACH SIDE)	30 – 60 SECONDS
ARCH	30 SECONDS	3	30 – 60 SECONDS

LEGS AND BUM

EXERCISE	REPS	SETS	REST
BODY WEIGHT SQUAT	8 – 12	3 – 5	30 – 60 SECONDS
BRIDGE	8 – 12	3 – 5	30 – 60 SECONDS
CALF RAISE	8 – 12	3 – 5	30 – 60 SECONDS

STRETCHES

EXERCISE	REPS	SETS	REST
SHOULDER STRETCH	30 SECONDS	1	5 – 10 SECONDS
CHEST STRETCH	30 SECONDS	1 (EACH ARM)	5 – 10 SECONDS
BACK STRETCH	30 SECONDS	1	5 – 10 SECONDS
CORE STRETCH	30 SECONDS	1	5 – 10 SECONDS
HAMSTRING STRETCH	30 SECONDS	1 (EACH LEG)	5 – 10 SECONDS
GROIN STRETCH	30 SECONDS	1	5 – 10 SECONDS
GLUTE STRETCH	30 SECONDS	1 (EACH LEG)	5 – 10 SECONDS
CALF STRETCH	30 SECONDS	1	5 – 10 SECONDS
QUAD STRETCH	30 SECONDS	1 (EACH LEG)	5 – 10 SECONDS

FINISH!

11.3 *INTERMEDIATE PROGRAM*

So, once you've got to grips with some of the easier exercises you can move onto the intermediate program. This is a natural progression from the beginner program, and includes some harder movements, and some harder variations of the beginner exercises. You'll still be working all the muscle groups you need to, so don't worry about missing a body area! Like before, simply follow the program from top to bottom, aiming to hit all of the rep and set targets (or as many as you can).

As before, the table below shows each of the exercises found in the program, and any hints and tips that you may need to know before starting.

PLATFORM PUSH-UP	Remember, the height of the platform can be adjusted to make the exercise easier or harder
NEGATIVE DIP	If you struggle here go back to the ledge dip, but with straight legs
ASSISTED CHIN-UP/PULL-UP	Use heavier bands to make things easier, or lighter bands to increase the challenge
TRICEPS EXTENSION	Start light and move up. Make sure the area is clear so you can drop the weight if needed
SHOULDER PRESS	Make sure to start light, and be sure to unpack and rack the weight safely onto the bars
CRUNCH	Remember to keep the head neutral, and curl the shoulders and upper back off the floor
SIT-UP	Pivot from the hips, and don't pull on your head too much
LEG EXTENSIONS	Keep the legs and feet close to the floor, and try and keep the middle of the back from rising
RUSSIAN TWIST	Have a more vertical back to make things easier, and more horizontal for more challenge
LUNGE	Aim to get both knees to 90 degrees, and make sure your torso stays upright
STEP-UPS	Make sure the step is sturdy, and try starting with light weights
BARBELL SQUAT	Pay attention to your technique, and make sure you squat deep enough

INTERMEDIATE PROGRAM

WARM UP

ARMS, CHEST, AND SHOULDERS

EXERCISE	REPS	SETS	REST
PLATFORM PUSH-UP	8 – 12	3 – 5	30 – 60 SECONDS
NEGATIVE DIP	1	3 – 5	30 – 60 SECONDS
ASSISTED CHIN-UP/ PULL-UP	3 – 8	3 – 5	30 – 60 SECONDS
TRICEPS EXTENSION	8 – 12	3 – 5	30 – 60 SECONDS
SHOULDER PRESS	8 – 12	3 – 5	30 – 60 SECONDS

ABS AND CORE

EXERCISE	REPS	SETS	REST
CRUNCH	8 – 12	3 – 5	30 – 60 SECONDS
SIT-UP	8 – 12	3 – 5	30 – 60 SECONDS
LEG EXTENSIONS	8 – 12	3 – 5	30 – 60 SECONDS
RUSSIAN TWIST	8 – 12	3 – 5	30 – 60 SECONDS

LEGS AND BUM

EXERCISE	REPS	SETS	REST
LUNGE	8 – 12	3 – 5	30 – 60 SECONDS
STEP-UPS	8 – 12	3 – 5	30 – 60 SECONDS
BARBELL SQUAT	8 – 12	3 – 5	30 – 60 SECONDS

STRETCHES

EXERCISE	REPS	SETS	REST
SHOULDER STRETCH	30 SECONDS	1	5 – 10 SECONDS
CHEST STRETCH	30 SECONDS	1 (EACH ARM)	5 – 10 SECONDS
BACK STRETCH	30 SECONDS	1	5 – 10 SECONDS
CORE STRETCH	30 SECONDS	1	5 – 10 SECONDS
HAMSTRING STRETCH	30 SECONDS	1 (EACH LEG)	5 – 10 SECONDS
GROIN STRETCH	30 SECONDS	1	5 – 10 SECONDS
GLUTE STRETCH	30 SECONDS	1 (EACH LEG)	5 – 10 SECONDS
CALF STRETCH	30 SECONDS	1	5 – 10 SECONDS
QUAD STRETCH	30 SECONDS	1 (EACH LEG)	5 – 10 SECONDS

FINISH!

11.4 ADVANCED PROGRAM

The advanced program is where you will perform the harder movements, but don't worry! As the exercises get harder they bring more benefits to both your physique and your fitness. In this program there are a mix of body weight and weighted exercises, and there is freedom here to make it as difficult as you want it. Add weight when you can, reduce the weight where you need to, and try and hit all of the rep and set targets.

As before, see the table below for hints and tips on each of the exercises in this program.

Exercise	Tip
PUSH-UP	If you struggle to hit the required number of reps do what you can and you'll get stronger
TRICEPS DIP	Try reducing the range of motion if you struggle here, and make sure your technique is good
CHIN-UP/PULL-UP	Chin-ups are easier, so work on these first. Pull-ups are harder, but work similar muscles
OVERHEAD PRESS	Make sure to un-rack the bar safely, and look forward when pushing overhead
DISH	Make sure to keep your back pressed into the ground as much as you can
ROLLOUT	Start small and build up, and make sure the weight/wall you use is suitable and sturdy
HANGING KNEE RAISE	If you struggle with grip strength spend more time doing dead hangs
LATERAL LUNGE	Make sure you squat deep enough, and move left and right evenly to address imbalances
SINGLE LEG SQUAT	Use as much assistance from the arms as you need, and you will get stronger over time
HIP THRUST	Make sure the bench is secure, and raise your hips up as high as your shoulders
DEADLIFT	Pay attention to proper technique, and only lift within your limits

ADVANCED PROGRAM

START!

WARM UP

ARMS, CHEST, AND SHOULDERS

EXERCISE	REPS	SETS	REST
PUSH-UP	8 – 12	3 – 5	30 – 60 SECONDS
TRICEPS DIP	3 – 8	3 – 5	30 – 60 SECONDS
CHIN-UP/PULL-UP	3 – 8	3 – 5	30 – 60 SECONDS
OVERHEAD PRESS	8 – 12	3 – 5	30 – 60 SECONDS

ABS AND CORE

EXERCISE	REPS	SETS	REST
DISH	30 SECONDS	3 – 5	30 – 60 SECONDS
ROLLOUT	8 – 12	3 – 5	30 – 60 SECONDS
HANGING KNEE RAISE	8 – 12	3 – 5	30 – 60 SECONDS

LEGS AND BUM

EXERCISE	REPS	SETS	REST
LATERAL LUNGE	8 – 12	3 – 5	30 – 60 SECONDS
SINGLE LEG SQUAT	3 – 5 (EACH LEG)	3 – 5	30 – 60 SECONDS
HIP THRUST	8 – 12	3 – 5	30 – 60 SECONDS
DEADLIFT	8 – 12	3 – 5	30 – 60 SECONDS

STRETCHES

EXERCISE	REPS	SETS	REST
SHOULDER STRETCH	30 SECONDS	1	5 – 10 SECONDS
CHEST STRETCH	30 SECONDS	1 (EACH ARM)	5 – 10 SECONDS
BACK STRETCH	30 SECONDS	1	5 – 10 SECONDS
CORE STRETCH	30 SECONDS	1	5 – 10 SECONDS
HAMSTRING STRETCH	30 SECONDS	1 (EACH LEG)	5 – 10 SECONDS
GROING STRETCH	30 SECONDS	1	5 – 10 SECONDS
GLUTE STRETCH	30 SECONDS	1 (EACH LEG)	5 – 10 SECONDS
CALF STRETCH	30 SECONDS	1	5 – 10 SECONDS
QUAD STRETCH	30 SECONDS	1 (EACH LEG)	5 – 10 SECONDS

FINISH!

12. HIGH INTENSITY CARDIO PROGRAMS

As important as resistance and strength training is for muscle building and muscle shaping, fat burning exercises are also important, to make sure that your heart and lungs stay healthy, and to help with losing body fat and getting the body you want! Doing the high intensity cardio exercises by themselves is great, but can get a little boring. Also, doing them in a circuit, or as a workout in their own right, is often a very good way of balancing out your workouts, and making sure that you get the most benefit.

There are a number of ways that you can do the high intensity cardio exercises. You can do a couple of them at the end of every strength workout, or even do a couple of days where you do them exclusively.

In this section we are going to look at a number of different approaches that you can take to make your fat burning days more interesting. Note that you can use any of the eight fat burning cardio exercises for these: just choose your favourite one (or your worst!), and get on it!

12.1 TABATA

The Tabata method of cardio is very popular, and is very simple to perform. Invented by a Japanese exercise physiologist, Tabata consists of a 20 second round of exercise, followed by 10 seconds of rest, repeated 8 times. This equals a total time of four minutes, with 160 seconds of exercise, and 80 seconds of rest. You can use any exercise you like, but we have found that burpees work especially well. There is no rep requirement for each block of 20 seconds; just do as many as you are able to do. We have laid out the structure of the Tabata method below to make it as easy to understand as possible.

START

Round 1
20 seconds of exercise
10 seconds rest

Round 2
20 seconds of exercise
10 seconds rest

Round 3
20 seconds of exercise
10 seconds rest

Round 4
>   20 seconds of exercise
>   10 seconds rest

Round 5
>   20 seconds of exercise
>   10 seconds rest

Round 6
>   20 seconds of exercise
>   10 seconds rest

Round 7
>   20 seconds of exercise
>   10 seconds rest

Round 8
>   20 seconds of exercise
>   10 seconds rest

FINISH

12.2 3oo

The film 300 was made famous for the gruelling training regime that the actors had to go through to get in shape for it. There was also the 300 workout that became a thing of legend in gym circles. Although that particular version used lots of different strength and cardio exercises to get to a total of 300 reps, we are going to do the same but with six of our fat burning exercises. The method is extremely simple; do 50 reps of all six exercises (the rep based ones) to equal 300 reps!

Note that if this is too difficult, you can strip it down and do 10 reps of each, or 20, or any number that suits your physical ability.

START
>   50 Star Jumps
>   50 Burpees
>   50 Mountain Climbers
>   50 Squat Thrusts
>   50 Killers
>   50 Skipping Reps

FINISH

12.3 No EXCUSES

This routine comes from the mind of Ross Enemait, a boxing trainer who specialises in low-tech fitness. It's unbelievably effective, and can be used with easier and more difficult exercises to make it suitable for beginner and elite readers alike.

No Excuses works very simply: you take four exercises of your choice, and then do each exercise for 60 seconds, then each exercise for 45 seconds, then each exercise for 30 seconds, and then each exercise for 15 seconds. This all adds up to exactly ten minutes, and is a real killer! You can set a stopwatch and let it run, and then change over when each section of time passes. It can help to have a friend here to shout out when to change (and also to give encouragement, as you'll need it!).

Look at the diagram below if you are struggling to visualise how it works.

START

Starjumps - 60 seconds
Mountain Climbers - 60 seconds
Burpees - 60 seconds
Skipping - 60 seconds

Starjumps - 45 seconds
Mountain Climbers - 45 seconds
Burpees - 45 seconds
Skipping - 45 seconds

Starjumps - 30 seconds
Mountain Climbers - 30 seconds
Burpees - 30 seconds
Skipping - 30 seconds

Starjumps - 15 seconds
Mountain Climbers - 15 seconds
Burpees - 15 seconds
Skipping - 15 seconds

FINISH

12.4 ONE HUNDRED

This one is easy, but very tough! You simply pick one exercise, and do one hundred reps as fast as possible. The rules are that you can rest whenever you need to, but that you must try and get to one hundred reps as quickly as possible. It works best with exercises that are reps based, obviously, so pick ones like star jumps, burpees, mountain climbers, and so on. Remember to time yourself and try and beat it the next time you do it!

START

Pick an exercise, and then do 100 reps as quickly as possible

FINISH

12.5 ROUNDABOUT

This circuit is great when you don't have much time, or when you wish to get a huge amount of work done with varied exercises and want to blast your body. Roundabout uses five different exercises, and can be scaled for beginners or more advanced readers.

Starting with the first exercise you do one rep, then move on to the second exercise and do one rep, and so on. Once you've done one rep of each exercise you do two reps of each exercise, then three reps of each exercise, and so on, going as high as possible without resting! Once you have to rest, then stop and make a note of how high you got so you can try and beat it next time!

The exercises you should use are listed next. Note that you can swap these for more suitable ones if you wish:

Exercise 1: Star Jumps
Exercise 2: Squat Thrusts
Exercise 3: Mountain Climbers
Exercise 4: Killers
Exercise 5: Burpees

START

Do 1 rep of each exercise
Do 2 reps of each exercise
Do 3 reps of each exercise
Repeat, increasing the number of reps by 1 each round

FINISH

12.6 *Triple hit*

This next circuit is a great one, and can be made more or less difficult very easily. Basically, this one works by increasing the amount of work that is done and decreasing the amount of rest in each round. Start with 15 seconds of work, then rest for 45 seconds, then work for 30 seconds and rest for 30 seconds, and then work for 45 seconds and rest for 15 seconds. This counts as one round. You can then carry on, doing as many rounds as you like, or take a longer rest and do a round every few minutes or so.

We have shown three rounds here, which are repeated as many times as is required, or performed for sets and then repeated as necessary. Choose any exercise for this.

For example:

START

15 on 45 off
30 on 30 off
45 on 15 off

REST

12.7 Cardio crunch

This circuit uses the treadmill, bike, or any other cardiovascular exercise as the main feature, and then injects small bursts of the high intensity exercises to mix things up. You can make this as easy or as hard as you like, so there is plenty of scope for beginners and sadists alike! Try the following to start, and adjust as needed!

START

Round 1

Run/bike/swim/X-trainer for 250 metres
Perform 10 burpees

Round 2

Run Run/bike/swim/X-trainer for 500 metres
Perform 15 burpees

Round 3

Run/bike/swim/X-trainer for 750 metres
Perform 20 burpees

Round 4

Run/bike/swim/X-trainer for 1000 metres
Perform 25 burpees

FINISH

12.8 PARTNERS IN CRIME

For this workout you can pick your other half, a friend, or someone who you like (or dislike, as they'll suffer doing this)! This circuit works with both people facing each other, and doing a set number of reps of an exercise. Once they have finished the other person does the same. The idea is to get your own reps done as quickly as possible, so that the other person doesn't get much rest. Then you can get more rest (hopefully), and so the circuit continues! Keep going for as long as you can, or for a set amount of time. You can use any exercise for this, but try the format below and expand it from there.

START

    Round 1
        Person A - 10 Star Jumps
        Person B - 10 Star Jumps

    Round 2
        Person A - 10 Killers
        Person B - 10 Killers

    Round 3
        Person A - 10 Squat Thrusts
        Person B - 10 Squat Thrusts

    Round 4
        Person A - 10 Jumping Squats
        Person B - 10 Jumping Squats

    Round 5
        Person A - 10 Burpees
        Person B - 10 Burpees

FINISH

13. EXERCISE DIARY

As great as having programs to follow is, an awesome way to make sure that you are progressing is to record what you are doing! Many people use workout logs or exercise diaries to do this, where they record how many sets and reps of an exercise they do, as well as what exercises they perform, as well as other info like rest time, how hard they worked in the session, and so on. To make things as easy as possible, and to make sure that you can record your workouts in the same space as the info about the workout, we have filled the next twenty pages with blank exercise diary pages, where you can fill out as much detail about your workouts as you like. Note that you don't have to record them; but it's very helpful if you do! You can record as much or as little information as you like, and then look back on them to see how far that you've come.

The example table next shows how to fill out the table, and then the following pages contain twenty tables that you can fill out yourself!

DATE: 22 February 2019		**TIME:** 2 pm		**WORKOUT:** Beginner	
EXERCISE	**SET 1**	**SET 2**	**SET 3**	**SET 4**	**SET 5**
1 Kneeling push-up	REPS: 8	REPS: 10	REPS: 10	REPS: 10	REPS: 12
2 Ledge dip (straight legs)	10	10	10	10	10
3 Dead hang	15 seconds	15 seconds	15 seconds	10 seconds	10 seconds
4 Sit-ups	12	12	12	12	12
5 Squat	10	12	12	10	8
6 Hip thrust	8	8	8	8	8

MEAL	**MEAL DESCRIPTION**	**GOOD/ BAD?**
BREAKFAST	2 scrambled eggs with 1 slice toast. Water.	Good!
LUNCH	Tuna salad with olive oil based dressing. Snack bar for desert.	Good!
DINNER	Steak, sweet potato fried, and green vegetables.	Very good!

DATE:		TIME:		WORKOUT:	
EXERCISE	**SET 1**	**SET 2**	**SET 3**	**SET 4**	**SET 5**
1	REPS:	REPS:	REPS:	REPS:	REPS:
2					
3					
4					
5					
6					
7					
8					
9					
10					
11					
12					
13					
14					
15					

MEAL	MEAL DESCRIPTION	GOOD/ BAD?
BREAKFAST		
LUNCH		
DINNER		

DATE:		TIME:		WORKOUT:	
EXERCISE	**SET 1**	**SET 2**	**SET 3**	**SET 4**	**SET 5**
1	*REPS:*	*REPS:*	*REPS:*	*REPS:*	*REPS:*
2					
3					
4					
5					
6					
7					
8					
9					
10					
11					
12					
13					
14					
15					

MEAL	MEAL DESCRIPTION	GOOD/ BAD?
BREAKFAST		
LUNCH		
DINNER		

DATE:		TIME:		WORKOUT:	
EXERCISE	**SET 1**	**SET 2**	**SET 3**	**SET 4**	**SET 5**
1	*REPS:*	*REPS:*	*REPS:*	*REPS:*	*REPS:*
2					
3					
4					
5					
6					
7					
8					
9					
10					
11					
12					
13					
14					
15					

MEAL	MEAL DESCRIPTION	GOOD/ BAD?
BREAKFAST		
LUNCH		
DINNER		

DATE:		TIME:		WORKOUT:	
EXERCISE	**SET 1**	**SET 2**	**SET 3**	**SET 4**	**SET 5**
1	REPS:	REPS:	REPS:	REPS:	REPS:
2					
3					
4					
5					
6					
7					
8					
9					
10					
11					
12					
13					
14					
15					

MEAL	MEAL DESCRIPTION	GOOD/ BAD?
BREAKFAST		
LUNCH		
DINNER		

DATE:		TIME:		WORKOUT:	
EXERCISE	**SET 1**	**SET 2**	**SET 3**	**SET 4**	**SET 5**
1	REPS:	REPS:	REPS:	REPS:	REPS:
2					
3					
4					
5					
6					
7					
8					
9					
10					
11					
12					
13					
14					
15					

MEAL	MEAL DESCRIPTION	GOOD/ BAD?
BREAKFAST		
LUNCH		
DINNER		

DATE:		TIME:		WORKOUT:	
EXERCISE	**SET 1**	**SET 2**	**SET 3**	**SET 4**	**SET 5**
1	REPS:	REPS:	REPS:	REPS:	REPS:
2					
3					
4					
5					
6					
7					
8					
9					
10					
11					
12					
13					
14					
15					

MEAL	MEAL DESCRIPTION	GOOD/ BAD?
BREAKFAST		
LUNCH		
DINNER		

DATE:		TIME:		WORKOUT:	
EXERCISE	**SET 1**	**SET 2**	**SET 3**	**SET 4**	**SET 5**
1	REPS:	REPS:	REPS:	REPS:	REPS:
2					
3					
4					
5					
6					
7					
8					
9					
10					
11					
12					
13					
14					
15					

MEAL	MEAL DESCRIPTION	GOOD/ BAD?
BREAKFAST		
LUNCH		
DINNER		

DATE:		TIME:		WORKOUT:	
EXERCISE	**SET 1**	**SET 2**	**SET 3**	**SET 4**	**SET 5**
1	REPS:	REPS:	REPS:	REPS:	REPS:
2					
3					
4					
5					
6					
7					
8					
9					
10					
11					
12					
13					
14					
15					

MEAL	MEAL DESCRIPTION	GOOD/ BAD?
BREAKFAST		
LUNCH		
DINNER		

DATE:		TIME:		WORKOUT:	
EXERCISE	**SET 1**	**SET 2**	**SET 3**	**SET 4**	**SET 5**
1	REPS:	REPS:	REPS:	REPS:	REPS:
2					
3					
4					
5					
6					
7					
8					
9					
10					
11					
12					
13					
14					
15					

MEAL	MEAL DESCRIPTION	GOOD/ BAD?
BREAKFAST		
LUNCH		
DINNER		

DATE:		TIME:		WORKOUT:	
EXERCISE	**SET 1**	**SET 2**	**SET 3**	**SET 4**	**SET 5**
1	REPS:	REPS:	REPS:	REPS:	REPS:
2					
3					
4					
5					
6					
7					
8					
9					
10					
11					
12					
13					
14					
15					

MEAL	MEAL DESCRIPTION	GOOD/ BAD?
BREAKFAST		
LUNCH		
DINNER		

DATE:		TIME:		WORKOUT:	
EXERCISE	**SET 1**	**SET 2**	**SET 3**	**SET 4**	**SET 5**
1	REPS:	REPS:	REPS:	REPS:	REPS:
2					
3					
4					
5					
6					
7					
8					
9					
10					
11					
12					
13					
14					
15					

MEAL	MEAL DESCRIPTION	GOOD/ BAD?
BREAKFAST		
LUNCH		
DINNER		

DATE:		TIME:		WORKOUT:	
EXERCISE	**SET 1**	**SET 2**	**SET 3**	**SET 4**	**SET 5**
1	*REPS:*	*REPS:*	*REPS:*	*REPS:*	*REPS:*
2					
3					
4					
5					
6					
7					
8					
9					
10					
11					
12					
13					
14					
15					

MEAL	**MEAL DESCRIPTION**	**GOOD/ BAD?**
BREAKFAST		
LUNCH		
DINNER		

DATE:		TIME:		WORKOUT:	
EXERCISE	**SET 1**	**SET 2**	**SET 3**	**SET 4**	**SET 5**
1	REPS:	REPS:	REPS:	REPS:	REPS:
2					
3					
4					
5					
6					
7					
8					
9					
10					
11					
12					
13					
14					
15					

MEAL	MEAL DESCRIPTION	GOOD/ BAD?
BREAKFAST		
LUNCH		
DINNER		

DATE:		TIME:		WORKOUT:	
EXERCISE	**SET 1**	**SET 2**	**SET 3**	**SET 4**	**SET 5**
1	*REPS:*	*REPS:*	*REPS:*	*REPS:*	*REPS:*
2					
3					
4					
5					
6					
7					
8					
9					
10					
11					
12					
13					
14					
15					

MEAL	MEAL DESCRIPTION	GOOD/ BAD?
BREAKFAST		
LUNCH		
DINNER		

DATE:		TIME:		WORKOUT:	
EXERCISE	**SET 1**	**SET 2**	**SET 3**	**SET 4**	**SET 5**
1	*REPS:*	*REPS:*	*REPS:*	*REPS:*	*REPS:*
2					
3					
4					
5					
6					
7					
8					
9					
10					
11					
12					
13					
14					
15					

MEAL	MEAL DESCRIPTION	GOOD/ BAD?
BREAKFAST		
LUNCH		
DINNER		

DATE:		TIME:		WORKOUT:	
EXERCISE	**SET 1**	**SET 2**	**SET 3**	**SET 4**	**SET 5**
1	REPS:	REPS:	REPS:	REPS:	REPS:
2					
3					
4					
5					
6					
7					
8					
9					
10					
11					
12					
13					
14					
15					

MEAL	MEAL DESCRIPTION	GOOD/ BAD?
BREAKFAST		
LUNCH		
DINNER		

DATE:		TIME:		WORKOUT:	
EXERCISE	**SET 1**	**SET 2**	**SET 3**	**SET 4**	**SET 5**
1	REPS:	REPS:	REPS:	REPS:	REPS:
2					
3					
4					
5					
6					
7					
8					
9					
10					
11					
12					
13					
14					
15					

MEAL	MEAL DESCRIPTION	GOOD/ BAD?
BREAKFAST		
LUNCH		
DINNER		

DATE:		TIME:		WORKOUT:	
EXERCISE	**SET 1**	**SET 2**	**SET 3**	**SET 4**	**SET 5**
1	REPS:	REPS:	REPS:	REPS:	REPS:
2					
3					
4					
5					
6					
7					
8					
9					
10					
11					
12					
13					
14					
15					

MEAL	MEAL DESCRIPTION	GOOD/ BAD?
BREAKFAST		
LUNCH		
DINNER		

DATE:		TIME:		WORKOUT:	
EXERCISE	**SET 1**	**SET 2**	**SET 3**	**SET 4**	**SET 5**
1	REPS:	REPS:	REPS:	REPS:	REPS:
2					
3					
4					
5					
6					
7					
8					
9					
10					
11					
12					
13					
14					
15					

MEAL	MEAL DESCRIPTION	GOOD/ BAD?
BREAKFAST		
LUNCH		
DINNER		

DATE:		TIME:		WORKOUT:	
EXERCISE	**SET 1**	**SET 2**	**SET 3**	**SET 4**	**SET 5**
1	REPS:	REPS:	REPS:	REPS:	REPS:
2					
3					
4					
5					
6					
7					
8					
9					
10					
11					
12					
13					
14					
15					

MEAL	MEAL DESCRIPTION	GOOD/ BAD?
BREAKFAST		
LUNCH		
DINNER		

14. CREATING YOUR OWN EXERCISE PROGRAMS

We know what you're thinking: *"I could never write an exercise program!"* But you're wrong! In this section of the book we'll show you how to write your own program, so that you can tailor it to suit your exact needs.

The first thing you need to know in order to write your program is the goal or goals that you are aiming for. Are you trying to lose weight? Are you trying to get stronger? Are you trying to get more flexible? Are you looking to get healthier overall? Or are you just interested in general fitness?

Once you've decided on what goal you're aiming towards, then you'll have to pick the exercises that will help with that goal. Obviously for weight loss you need to build or maintain muscle mass, and decrease the amount of body fat you have. If this is your goal you need to do some resistance exercises and lots of fat burning high intensity cardio.

If your goal is to get stronger, then you need to be doing full body resistance exercises, such as squats, push-ups, pull-ups, deadlifts, and so on. Don't worry too much about the high intensity cardio exercises, unless you want to get fitter as well. If your goal is flexibility, then you will have to spend more time doing stretches, including at the beginning and end of your sessions. If your goal is to get more cardiovascular fitness, then you don't need to do so much of the resistance work. If your goal is to simply lose weight, then you need to do more fat burning exercises and not so many resistance ones (although resistance exercises won't do any harm). You'll also need to make sure your diet is clean as well!

Another variable is the number of sessions that you need to do per week. We think that you can easily get good results doing 3 to 5 sessions per week. There is no real need to do two sessions per day (morning and night), unless you are training for a very competitive sport at a high level. And an hour total time for each session is also completely realistic.

Something else that has to be taken into consideration is the order of the exercises. We recommend doing the whole body exercises first. These are the ones that use lots of muscles groups at the same time, and that require balance, coordination, or muscular control. Do these first so that you can perform them to the best of your ability, and then do the simpler, less difficult movements last.

Over the next few pages are the blank exercise program pages, where you can fill in lots of detail about the program that you are creating. There is room for the type of program that it is, the name that you want to give it, what exercises that are in the program, the number of sets and reps, and the amount of rest time needed.

WORKOUT NAME:

START!

EXERCISE	REPS	SETS	REST

FINISH!

15. FREQUENTLY ASKED QUESTIONS

In this last section we'll answer some common questions that crop up when it comes to the topic of exercise and working out. If you have a question that isn't answered here, feel free to contact us at fisforfitness@mail.com, or visit any of our social media pages and give us a shout! You can also follow us on social media to stay up to date with articles, features, and other things to do with fitness!

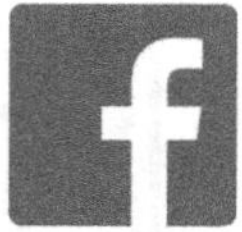 www.facebook.com/FisforFitness

 @fisforfitness1

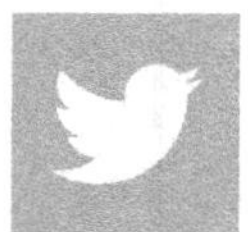 @FisforFitness1

Q. DO I HAVE TO DO THE BODY WEIGHT EXERCISES? CAN'T I JUST GO STRAIGHT TO THE WEIGHTS?

A. You can, but in our opinion this is a mistake. You'll still make progress and change your body shape if you go straight to weighted exercises, but perfecting body weight exercises will give you a very solid base on which to progress. Things like push-ups, pull-ups, squats, lunges, and other body weight exercises are great for teaching your body how to move, teaching your muscles how and when to contract, and learning to move your body through space.

Q. DO I REALLY NEED TO BE A MEMBER OF A GYM?

A. No, this isn't a necessity, but there are some pieces of equipment that are difficult to get for a home gym, that a real gym has both the room and funds for. Things like squat racks are quite large, so unless you have a garage or other indoor space with enough room for one, it is beneficial to have a gym membership. That being said, if you really cannot get to a gym, or hate the idea of joining one, then only using body weight exercises is a perfectly feasible method of achieving the body you want. If you need further proof, just look at gymnasts and those athletes that use only their body weight to train; they are in great shape, and never really set foot in a traditional "gym".

Q. MY PARTNER'S A BIT APPREHENSIVE ABOUT ME DOING RESISTANCE TRAINING. IS THERE ANYTHING I CAN SAY TO ALLEVIATE THESE FEARS?

A. Yes! First, if your partner doesn't exercise or train, then maybe they would like to go to the gym with you? After all, those that train together stay together! Secondly, resistance training is arguably more important for women to do than men to do, as men are naturally stronger than women, and do not suffer from diseases like osteoporosis (weakening of the bones) anywhere near as much as women do.

Q. I'VE HEARD STORIES ABOUT PEOPLE INJURING THEMSELVES DOING RESISTANCE TRAINING. IS THERE ANY RISK TO ME DOING IT?

A. There is risk in many things in life, and resistance training is no different. However, if you follow our instruction the likelihood of you injuring yourself is very low. You have to remember that there are two main reasons why you might injure yourself when doing resistance training. These are:

- *USING WEIGHTS THAT ARE TOO HEAVY*

Using a weight or resistance that is too heavy or high for your level will put too much of a demand on your joints, muscles, bones and other connective tissues, and may increase the risk of injury. *ALWAYS* work with a weight and resistance that is correct for your ability. If you're unsure, use a weight that's too light and work up in small increments, email us, or ask a qualified professional in your gym who can advise further.

- *POOR TECHNIQUE*

Poor technique can cause injury because the correct muscles will not be engaged properly, and there will be too much load on certain parts of the body. For example, deadlifting with a rounded back means that the stress on your back will be uneven, and disc ruptures and other nasty injuries will be more likely. Deadlifting is one of the best exercises for strengthening the back, but doing them with poor technique is one of the best ways to injure it.

If you have to cheat to get the weight up, or complete the exercise, then the weight is too heavy or the exercise is too advanced for your level. Back off a little, and use a lighter weight that allows you to complete the movement with perfect technique. You will progress faster and have a greatly reduced risk of injury if you do this.

Q. DO I NEED TO TAKE SUPPLEMENTS? IT SEEMS LIKE LOTS OF FITNESS PERSONALITIES TAKE THEM AND ADVERTISE THEM, SO MAYBE I'M MISSING OUT?

A. No, you most certainly don't have to take supplements, unless you really are struggling to get all of the correct nutrients into your diet. Supplements do serve a purpose, but for the vast majority of people they will be of little benefit. More effort should be put into perfecting your diet than buying supplements, as if your diet is good then there will be no need for supplements! Obviously, if you are preparing for pregnancy, or have an underlying health condition that requires you to supplement vitamins or other minerals, then this is fine, and you should follow the recommendation of your doctor or health professional.

Q. I'M PREGNANT/TRYING TO GET PREGNANT. CAN I DO THE EXERCISES IN THIS BOOK?

A. Yes, but it's best to seek the advice of your doctor, midwife, or health professional before starting any exercise routine, especially if you're pregnant. The relaxin hormone that accompanies pregnancy can cause problems with ligaments and other connective tissues; especially in exercises that use weights, and deadlifting huge amounts of weight when blood pressure is an issue is a bad idea. Common sense is the best course of action here.

If you're trying for children then it is a very good idea to get in shape. Being in shape will make it easier to get pregnant, and your body will cope more easily with the physical demand of being pregnant.

Q. I HAVE NO IDEA HOW STRONG I AM. HOW MUCH WEIGHT SHOULD I START OUT WITH ON THE WEIGHTED EXERCISES?

A. Obviously it depends on what exercise you are doing, but as a general rule you should start out with the lightest weight you can. There will always be plenty of time to add more, and making sure that your technique is perfect is more important than lifting lots of weight.

Q. IS THERE A SPECIFIC ORDER I SHOULD DO THE EXERCISES?

A. If you are following the programs as written then simply follow the order that they are listed in and you will be fine. If you are doing your own program, or want to do a few exercises in your workout and not follow one of the programs, then do the exercises that use lots of muscle groups first. So, deadlifts before biceps curls, and squats before triceps extensions.

Q. I'M FAIRLY NEW TO EXERCISE, AND VERY NEW TO RESISTANCE EXERCISE. SHOULD I FOCUS ON INDIVIDUAL MUSCLE GROUPS, OR MORE WHOLE BODY EXERCISES?

A. This is an easy question, and the answer is that you should concentrate on whole body movements. There is an old saying that says that you shouldn't major in the minors. All this means is that when exercising, it is much better to do things that use as many muscles as possible at the same time, instead of small muscles on their own. That is part of the reason why the exercises that we have picked are the ones we have picked!